Cancer in context:
a practical guide to supportive care

James Brennan
Consultant Clinical Psychologist
Bristol Haematology and Oncology Centre
and Senior Lecturer in Palliative Medicine
University of Bristol, UK

in collaboration with

Clare Moynihan
Senior Research Fellow and Research Associate
Institute of Cancer Research
and Royal Marsden Hospital Foundation Trust
London, UK

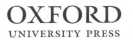
OXFORD
UNIVERSITY PRESS

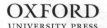
OXFORD
UNIVERSITY PRESS

Great Clarendon Street, Oxford OX2 6DP

Oxford University Press is a department of the University of Oxford.
It furthers the University's objective of excellence in research, scholarship,
and education by publishing worldwide in

Oxford New York

Auckland Bangkok Buenos Aires Cape Town Chennai
Dar es Salaam Delhi Hong Kong Istanbul Karachi Kolkata
Kuala Lumpur Madrid Melbourne Mexico City Mumbai Nairobi
São Paulo Shanghai Taipei Tokyo Toronto

Oxford is a registered trade mark of Oxford University Press
in the UK and in certain other countries

Published in the United States
by Oxford University Press Inc., New York

© Oxford University Press, 2004

A catalogue record for this title is available from the British Library

ISBN 0 19 851525 1 (Pbk)

10 9 8 7 6 5 4 3 2 1

Typeset by Cepha Imaging Pvt Ltd., India
Printed in Great Britain
on acid-free paper by
Ashford Colour Press Ltd., Gosport, Hampshire

Oxford Medical Publications

Cancer in context

For my family

Michael, Sally, Andrew, Ginny,
Penelope, Harriet, Tom,
Kate, and Zoë

Acknowledgements

In the course of many stories I've heard, it has often seemed to me that a good deal of people's distress in having cancer could have been lessened if their care had been handled differently. So this book is an attempt to pull together academic research, people's recorded experiences of the disease, and what people have told me about the effect of cancer on their lives and the healthcare they have received.

My friend and colleague Clare Moynihan and I also wanted to redress what we saw as an imbalance within the relatively new field of psychosocial oncology. In our view, the field has emphasized psychological morbidity, such as depression and anxiety, at the expense of understanding cancer within the wider context of people's lives.

Whenever possible I have tried to provide the evidence base for what I am arguing, though admittedly the way the evidence has been interpreted and joined up is largely my own. In an attempt to make the book easier to read I have used numbered references but, in doing so, have had to obscure the names of countless dedicated clinicians and clinical scientists. Although I have attempted to represent their work fairly, I have also done my best to square my reading of the academic literature with what I have learned from clinical practice. In fact, rather than keep up any affectation of impartiality, I have revealed some of my own assumptions in Chapter One, which also provides a background and map to many of the ideas discussed in other chapters.

What we seem to have ended up with is a textbook of supportive care in oncology, albeit with several omissions. We are very thankful for being able to illustrate parts of the book with poignant snapshots that were recorded in a number of personal diaries kept by people with cancer (*see* Introduction). So, first, thanks to the people who gave us their permission to quote from their diaries or those of their loved ones. To them we apologize for surgically isolating particular moments from their experiences.

I also gratefully acknowledge the many wonderful people who have been my patients. This book is very much an expression of what they have taught me.

A large amount of the research for this book was conducted while I was on sabbatical in Australia. My thanks to Professor Alex Wearing and the Psychology Department of the University of Melbourne, and Dr David Horne for making this possible.

A number of people affected by cancer, professional colleagues, and friends have commented on all these chapters and I am indebted to them for this considerable task. Naturally all mistakes and omissions are entirely mine. In preparing this book I interviewed a number of professional colleagues about their clinical roles, especially about the pressures they face in their daily work. Other people helped with literature searches, hospitality, generosity, wisdom, and kindness.

Thank you all.

Andy and Pam Stuart-Menteth	Nick Ambler
Fiona Caselton	Lucy Davis
Melanie Dias	Chris B.
Haeilli Ford	Lindsay Grice
Sue David	Deborah
Yvonne Hunter	Helen Morgan
Cathy Lacey	Fiona Hamilton
Penny Schofield	Tom Bailward
Annabel Pollard	Diana Harcourt
Elizabeth Ballinger	Joan Clewlow
Sancha Aranda	Tom Wells
Doreen Akkerman	Ailsa Wilson
Thomas Johansen	Jonathan Evans
Elisabeth Whipp	Sarah Ganley
Jenny Altschuler	Richard Leach
Angus Earnshaw	Paul Cornes
Gaye Senior-Smith	Juliet Gilchrist
Tristan Grey	Peter Harvey
Jane Beckinsale	James Johnston
Marion Harris	Lisa Rajan
Rachel Gunary	

Particular thanks to my colleague Suzanne Cowderoy for her level-headed advice, encouragement, and support, and to other dedicated colleagues at the Bristol Haematology and Oncology Centre. I also gratefully acknowledge the help of freelance editor James Loader whose fresh pair of eyes came at just the right time.

Finally, abject gratitude and apologies to my family across all its generations, and unreserved thanks to Harriet, my wife, whose forbearance has been matched only by her love and support during this long process.

Inevitably the following pages are only a very small part of the story. The main story must be rediscovered afresh with each and every patient, family, or friend. Trying to integrate phenomenology, academic research, and clinical practice is perhaps a bit reckless, but I hope this book is useful to you in some way.

J.H.B.

Although I have had a relatively small part to play in the gestation of this book, its content, in part, arrives out of conversations between myself and my staunch friend and ally James Brennan. He has always been the ready recipient of my jobs and my woes and especially of my despairing belief that we as service providers and researchers are making as much of a negative impact on people with cancer as the disease itself. There are too many other people who deserve thanks for their kindness and who have helped me to arrive at the place I am now. I am sorry to have left them out of the list of acknowledgements below but I hope they know who they are.

My children Rose and Leo Moynihan

All the patients who I have had the privilege of speaking with including Sean Hourigan who allowed me to make a magnificent film of an interview wtih him and who taught me so much.

My colleagues in the Academic Department of Radiotherapy especially Professor Alan Horwich
My colleagues in the Department of Psychological Medicine, especially Dr. Maggie Watson
My funders, The Bob Champion Trust and Cancer Research UK
The Tavistock Clinic Cancer Group
The Sociology of Cancer Group
The BACUP Research Committee
Priscilla Alderson
Louise Burchell
Jane Cook
Shron de Mello
Nell Dunn and Dan
Penny Hopwood
Geraldine Leydon
Klim McPherson
Naomi Pheffer
Joseph Sweetman

I do of course take full responsibility for my imput in this book!

C.M.

Contents

Introduction   *xix*

1 Human context   *1*
  Human nature   *3*
    Emotions   *4*
    Language and culture   *6*
    Mental maps   *9*
    Change and development   *14*
  The catastrophe of cancer   *16*
    Shock   *19*
    Denial and avoidance   *20*
    Integration   *21*
    Different adjustments   *21*
    Core human assumptions   *25*
  What helps people with cancer?   *35*
  Quality of life   *38*
  Summary   *40*
  References   *41*

2 Personal context   *47*
  Changed lives   *47*
  Expectations about illness   *49*
  Shock of diagnosis   *51*
  Denial and avoidance   *53*
  Delays to diagnosis   *56*
  'Why me?'—the meaning of cancer   *57*
  Coping with treatment   *60*
  Relationship with the healthcare team   *61*
  Practical concerns   *63*
  Relationships with family and friends   *65*
  Impact on self   *68*
  Hope   *71*
  The body   *73*
  Existential beliefs   *77*
  Ending treatment   *80*
  Living with uncertainty   *82*
  References   *84*

3 Other people *91*

What is social support and why is it important? *92*

What kind of social support do people with cancer need? *93*

What is emotional support? *94*

The social context of social support. *95*

Helpful and unhelpful reactions to cancer *96*

Family context *98*

Family turmoil *99*

Family roles, relationships, and communication *100*

Families and the healthcare team *102*

Supporting families *103*

What and when to tell children *106*

People on their own *110*

Older people *111*

Partner relationships *113*

Partner relationships and communication *114*

Gender differences in partner support *120*

Gay and lesbian couples *124*

Communication advice for couples *126*

Sexual problems *127*

Caring *134*

The stress of caring *135*

Assessing distress among carers *137*

Supporting carers *137*

References *139*

4 Social context *147*

Background and introduction *148*

Social class *152*

Introduction *152*

Social class, language, and health beliefs *153*

Social class and unemployment *155*

Social class and practicalities *156*

Social class, service providers, and support *156*

Summary *157*

Gender *158*

Introduction *158*

Gender and pain *159*

Gender and emotions *160*

Gender and support *161*

Yonger men *161*

Older men *162*

Gender and cancer information   *164*

Gender and sexuality   *165*

Gender and infertility   *167*

Gender and body image, disability, impairment, and stigma   *169*

Summary   *172*

Homeless people   *172*

Introduction   *172*

Defining 'homelessness'   *173*

Homelessness and health   *173*

Homelessness and cancer   *174*

Homelessness: psychosocial factors   *175*

Homelessness and support   *176*

Summary   *177*

Ethnicity   *178*

Introduction   *178*

Defining 'race', 'culture', and 'ethnicity'   *178*

Race   *178*

Culture   *179*

Ethnicity   *179*

Ethnicity and essentialism   *179*

Ethnicity and social class   *180*

Ethnicity: West versus East   *180*

Ethnicity, religion, and death   *182*

Ethnicity and diet   *184*

Racism and ethnicity   *185*

Ethnicity and giving support: communication, advocacy, and interpreters   *189*

An interpreter   *190*

An advocate   *191*

Summary   *193*

Refugees and asylum seekers   *194*

Introduction   *193*

Defining 'refugees' and 'asylum seekers'   *194*

Asylum seekers, refugees, and health   *194*

Asylum seekers, refugees, and mental health   *195*

Asylum seekers and refugees: registration and information   *196*

Asylum seekers, refugees, and discrimination   *197*

Asylum seekers and support   *197*

Treatment for psychological problems   *197*

Summary   *198*

Conclusion   *198*

References   *199*

5 Clinical context *207*

General practice *208*

Diagnosis *211*

Speed of diagnosis *211*

Eliciting key concerns *212*

Concerns associated with early phases of treatment *213*

Surgery *214*

Hospital admission *215*

Preparation for surgery *216*

Continuity of care *217*

Psychiatric durgs *217*

Radiotherapy *226*

Preparation for radiotherapy *227*

Main areas of radiotherapy information *228*

Side-effects of radiotherapy *229*

The role of radiographers *229*

Chemotherapy and hormone therapy *231*

Preparation for chemotherapy *232*

Side-effects of chemotherapy and hormone therapy *234*

Common treatment difficulties *242*

Fatigue *242*

Nausea and vomiting *245*

Pain *247*

Depression *253*

Intense fear *255*

Worry *258*

Insomnia *260*

Rehabilitation *262*

Mobility *263*

Activities of daily living *264*

Psychosocial rehabilitation *264*

Rehabilitation teams *265*

Recurrence *266*

Palliative care *267*

Psychosocial issues for people who are dying *268*

Bereavement care *277*

References *282*

6 Communication *295*

Communication and ethics *298*

Disclosure of diagnostic information *298*

Consent, collaboration, and choice *299*

Information *302*
 Information supply and demand *302*
 Written information *305*
 Video *307*
 Audiotapes *307*
 Internet and computer-based information *308*
 Information and support centres *308*
Staff–patient relationships *309*
 What do healthcare professionals want in their patients? *309*
 What is appropriate professional distance? *311*
 What are patients looking for in the professionals who care for them? *313*
Patient-centred communication *315*
 Cultural assumptions and differences *316*
 Working through interpreters *318*
 Language *319*
Eliciting concerns *320*
 Assessing the whole person *321*
 Conducting a patient-centred clinical interview *323*
 Problem-solving *328*
 Clarifying and challenging assumptions *329*
Specific communication issues *330*
 Giving bad news *330*
 Discussing resuscitation *335*
 Identifying vulnerability *336*
 Working with people with special needs *338*
 Working with someone clinically depressed or suicidal *342*
 Working with denial and avoidance *346*
 Anxiety, worry, and uncertainty *348*
 Working with someone acutely confused or cognitively impaired *350*
 Angry, difficult, or disliked patients *351*
Professional issues in communication *353*
 Communication between professionals *353*
 Healthcare teams and patient confidentiality *354*
 Communication training *355*
References *355*

7 Professional context *363*
 Part 1 *365*
 Stress and burnout in healthcare professionals *365*
  Sources of stress *365*
  Effects of stress *366*
  Burnout *367*

Cancer professionals   368
Doctors   369
Nurses   375
Radiographers   377
Other healthcare professionals   379
Medical secretaries, receptionists, and porters   379
Preventing burnout and reducing stress   380
Management strategies to prevent burnout   380
Strategies to reduce stress in healthcare   381
Team functioning   384
Part 2   386
User-involvement   386
Voluntary support   387
Complementary therapy and alternative medicine   389
Informed consent   391
Guilt and responsibility   392
Spiritual abuse   392
Colluding with denial   393
References   393

Appendices

1 Common self-report questionnnaires   399
Psychological and social distress   400
Hospital Anxiety and Depression Scale   400
General Health Questionnaire   400
Brief Symptom Inventory   400
State-Trait Anxiety Inventory   401
Profile of Mood States   401
Social Problems Inventory   401
Quality of life   401
Functional Assessment of Chronic Illness Therapy   401
European Organisation for Research on Treatment for Cancer   401
World Health Organization Quality of Life assessment instrument   402
Schedule for the Evaluation of Individual Quality of Life   402
Short Form 36   402
Life Evaluation Questionnaire   402
Symptoms   402
Memorial Symptom Assessment Scale   402
Edmonton Symptom Assessment Scale   403
Cancer Rehabilitation Evaluation System   403
Functional Assessment of Cancer Therapy—Fatigue   403
Brief Fatigue Inventory   403

Brief Pain Inventory   *403*

McGill Pain Questionnaire   *403*

Maslach Burnout Inventory   *404*

References   *404*

2 Managing the stress of cancer: a psychosocial guide for people with cancer   *407*

Information   *408*

Shock   *408*

What can you do?   *409*

Out of control   *409*

What can you do?   *409*

Who am I now?   *410*

What can you do?   *411*

Feeling overwhelmed   *412*

Making sense   *412*

Taking control   *413*

Worrying   *413*

Useless (unproductive) worrying   *414*

Productive worrying   *414*

Getting on with living   *415*

Other people   *415*

Changing relationships   *415*

Advice for couples facing cancer   *416*

Index   *419*

Introduction

Extraordinary medical advances in the treatment of cancer have been made over the past few decades. The acceleration of cancer research across the world over the past fifty years has enabled scientists and clinicians to prolong, if not save the lives of unprecedented numbers of people—especially children. The emergence of molecular biology and genetics has yielded much and promises more, and there has been significant progress in disentangling the causes and risks of cancer and what can be done to prevent it and detect it early.[1] On a 'human scale', this progress has meant fresh hope for people facing a disease that historically has caused so much suffering; in the richer parts of the world clinicians are increasingly regarding some forms of cancer as long-term or chronic illnesses.

Yet for all this promise, cancer continues to represent a death sentence for a vast number of people across the world. The truth is hard to grasp. More than 7.8 million people are estimated to have died from cancer in the year 2000, and currently one in seven people worldwide will die of the disease.[2] In the industrialized West, where health services are considerably better funded than most other nations, as many as one in four people will die from cancer. In the UK, 154 460 people died from cancer during 2001,[3] while in the United States an estimated 1 220 100 people were diagnosed with cancer in 2000, and over half a million people were expected to die from it.[4] In 2003 this corresponds to about 1500 Americans dying from cancer every day.

Cancer is not a new disease. It is improved life expectancy, and to a lesser extent the lifestyle of the West, that is largely responsible for the fact that, globally, the incidence of cancer is rising.[5] In 1990, 8 million people were diagnosed with cancer worldwide. By 2000, the number of new cases of cancer had risen to an estimated 10 million. The World Health Organization (WHO) predicts that by 2020 there will be more than 15 million new cases of cancer every year, of which over two-thirds will arise in developing countries, where the disease is often diagnosed at a late stage and where health resources tend to be meagre.[6] The lifestyle factor mainly contributing to this increase, and 'dwarfing all others', is smoking.[7] Multinational tobacco corporations continue to market their addictive product in the poorer countries of the world, whose governments are more than grateful for the foreign advertising and tax revenues, while turning a blind eye to the inevitable future pressures on their health services, let alone the personal suffering of those who will die, and the family and friends who survive them.

In the developed West, 50% of people with the disease can now be cured, yet cancer continues to be seen as a sentence of inevitable and often imminent death. In fact, even among people who can be cured, this unwelcome confrontation with their mortality can ignite a personal catastrophe that can fundamentally change their lives.

The normal assumptions of everyday 'reality' often shift in a way that is psychologically and socially traumatic. The experience violates the most deep-seated assumptions by which many people have lived their lives. And it is against this backdrop of personal turmoil that healthcare professionals offer some of the most notoriously difficult and demanding treatments in medicine, treatments that have their own consequences and emotional outcomes.

This book is about the impact of cancer on people's lives and the vital role that healthcare professionals play in shaping this experience and minimizing the distress involved. It is a guide for healthcare staff who support patients and their families through the many changes and challenges that cancer entails.

> Supportive care for cancer patients is the multi-professional attention to the individual's overall physical, psychosocial, spiritual and cultural needs, and should be available at all stages of the illness, for patients of all ages, and regardless of the current intention of any anti-cancer treatment.[8]

> (Ahmedzai 2001)

The quality of healthcare that people with cancer receive has a demonstrable effect on their level of distress. But of course that is not the only factor. Each patient's day-to-day needs reflect the unique 'context' of their lives: their partner, family and friends, their age, gender, and cultural background, their prior beliefs about cancer and illness generally, the social conditions of their lives, other stresses they may already be facing, and so on.

Faced with the shocking crisis of cancer, people not only turn to healthcare 'experts' and figures of authority for guidance and answers, but as Susan Sontag pointed out in 1978, they draw on the prevailing cultural assumptions of the time to make sense of their experiences.[9] The dominance of a military language of fighting, winning, and surviving battles with cancer that Sontag reported 35 years ago, continues to this day, though these days the terms often mingle with sporting metaphors.[10] She argued that a person's recovery from illness, depicted as their private 'battle' with cancer, is frequently portrayed as their personal responsibility, a reflection of their character rather than as mostly a matter of biology. If cancer is represented as a punishment, then the victim can be blamed for the onset and course of their illness.

Trends over the past few decades seem to have vindicated Sontag's argument regarding personal responsibility.[11] The growing public awareness in the West that 'smoking kills' parallels the increasing emphasis on individuals being accountable for their health through diet and exercise (even if the advice seems to change). Public health campaigns which encourage self-examination of the breasts and testicles, and which urge people to attend screening appointments (cervical smears, mammograms) add to this sense of personal responsibility. Within cancer care itself patients are increasingly given responsibility for choosing aspects of their medical treatment, and even psychological research has targeted the individual's response ('fighting' spirit, optimism, active coping, etc.) as being critical to their emotional outcome.

With this emphasis on personal responsibility, where should people with cancer turn for support and guidance? Who are the experts? In the West, at least, it seems that patients look to healthcare professionals to understand their predicament and help them with it. Yet, paradoxically, there seems to be growing public disillusionment with the way scientific medicine applies its knowledge to individual patients, despite its scientific progress and accomplishments. Modern healthcare has been criticized for being 'spiritually deprived',[12] focusing almost exclusively on the biological concerns of the patient (the tumour), at the expense of other needs: emotional, social, and spiritual. The complexity of modern cancer treatments may have obscured its importance but the supportive care that a trusted clinician can give their patient has been one of medicine's most powerful tools since its beginnings.

This is not merely a point of nostalgia. Ironically, the very success of scientific medicine has led to the astonishing costs, time-pressures, diminishing resources, and all the other familiar arguments for why the *quality* of healthcare may in some ways have deteriorated in recent years. Quantity of throughput is certainly a poor measure of quality of care, and a 'cure *or* care' mindset is ethically untenable. Modern medicine requires modern skills of communication and supportive care because the consumer public is learning to communicate in increasingly informed ways, and expects more than it has been getting.

For most of the eighteenth century and beyond, the use of leeches and blood-letting was still common medical practice after hundreds of years of use. In fact, it had become so popular that the governors of St George's Hospital in London required frequent updates as to the market price of leeches.[13] Ironically, while medicine has increasingly become more scientific, the public has become 'regressively more magico-religious in its outlook' towards medicine.[14] (Stein 1985, p. 26) It is surely no coincidence that over the past quarter century the West has witnessed the mushrooming popularity of complementary therapies and alternative medicine. Do these many non-scientific forms of 'folk intervention' offer something genuinely helpful to people with cancer, or do they merely provide instant religion, a mystical form of hope to people facing a crisis of uncertainty? Or does the popularity of complementary therapies perhaps represent a reaction to the way scientific medicine is practised, a disillusionment with medicine's apparent preoccupation with the physical? Is modern healthcare simply out of step with public expectations; has it brushed aside the very human need for hope in its pursuit of scientific honesty?

Complementary therapies, of course, include a diverse range of approaches, some of which have ethical and communication problems of their own, not least of which can be burdening the patient, once again, with personal responsibility for their own recovery and survival.[15] However, for those who can afford them, complementary therapies typically offer a refreshing blend of sufficient time, open communication, having one's problems seen within the broader context of one's life, ample information, addressing questions of spiritual meaning, being encouraged to be an active participant in one's treatment, having a model of how the treatment works, and so on. In fact, understanding their popularity is not difficult when complementary therapies seem to offer many of the qualities that are deficient or lacking in modern scientific healthcare. Whether they contain 'active ingredients' beyond these powerful non-specific elements is an important but different question.

At roughly the same time that complementary therapies have flourished, psycho-oncology has emerged as an 'ally' to cancer medicine, with the similar aim of improving the quality of life of cancer patients and their families. This small but growing field has been dominated by psychologists and psychiatrists, bringing assumptions and ideas from the field of mental health. Clinicians and researchers have categorized and investigated the many ways that patients respond to their diagnosis, treatment, and survival, and the most effective ways of alleviating their distress. A large number of studies have documented high levels of distress among people with cancer and their families, albeit mostly using the language of mental illness.

But the methodological tools that people use always influences their research findings by limiting the agenda of what it is possible to 'discover'[16] and there has been a tendency in psycho-oncology to examine emotional distress in isolation, rather than binding it to the social context within which it occurs. People exist within complicated changing lives, so research that relies on purely categorical data and cross-sectional 'snapshot' designs often fails to capture the most important information. Responses are plucked from individuals and then interpreted out of the context in which they arose.

For example, a great deal of empirical research, mostly on women with breast cancer (who have become the exemplar of the cancer journey), has been conducted with respect to particular psychological states of mind, but rarely with much reference to people's social context, or how the research findings fit into a broader theoretical picture. Anxiety and depression are frequently treated as unitary 'things' that can be measured by a simple questionnaire, with little reference to their many possible causes or how they might change over time. Yet emotions are never fixed and static. Similarly, ethnicity, age, and sex are often 'controlled for' when assessing the numbers of people who suffer from clinical anxiety, or the number of people who delay in presenting symptoms to their doctors, but too rarely are these variables the subject of enquiry in their own right. Moreover, the 'lay beliefs' of patients have their own logic and rationality and deserve as much respect and understanding as the expertise of healthcare professionals.

High levels of emotional distress are common in cancer, but should distress be regarded as an illness? Certainly, high levels of distress among people with cancer and their families have been well documented,[17] but the preoccupation with quantifying psychiatric morbidity in cancer has overshadowed the need to understand people's distress in context and find ways of preventing as much of it as possible. Much of the distress in cancer is understandable and to be expected given what is occurring, but healthcare staff can do a great deal to shape the experience of their patients and lessen their suffering.

Psychosocial experts on their own have very little effect on the distress of cancer; it is the caring hands and listening ears of doctors, nurses, and radiographers that will always have the greatest impact on how people regard their illness.

The distress of cancer is significant and should be addressed, but simply finding shorthand labels like depression and anxiety to describe emotional suffering offers limited help to people affected by cancer, or the professional staff trying to care for them. Diagnostic labels when applied to emotional states are crude at best, and run the risk that people's needs and concerns become seen, by both professionals and patients alike, as a form of pathology or illness rather than being understood within the unique and complicated context of people's lives. And once distress is defined as an illness, it is in danger of being seen as the preserve of mental health specialists rather than the concern of every healthcare professional. Psychosocial care cannot be a bolted-on extra; it must be integral to cancer care.[18]

We believe it is possible to recognize profound human distress without having to define it as a form of mental illness. In the context of cancer, understanding people's state of mind is more important than knowing their 'mental state', but to understand this we need to consider what is happening at several levels: the biological, personal, inter-personal, socio-cultural, and spiritual. Strong emotions such as despair, fear, and even anger are *natural* emotions that can often be helpful and adaptive. When understood *in context*, (i.e. from the unique perspective of the person experiencing it), 'psychosocial distress' can be seen as an expression of important '*concerns*' within the person or their family. One thing is clear: the way that healthcare staff respond to these concerns has a critical bearing on how patients perceive their situation and, consequently, their level of emotional distress.

Throughout this book we advocate a form of 'patient-centred' care, which shares the same aspirations as palliative care. David Jeffrey[19] has described these as emphasizing:

1. Quality of life, including good symptom control. Quality of life means different things to different people. It also changes with the patient's situation so must be reviewed continually.

2. Understanding the person in the context of their past life experiences and current situation. This is holistic, patient-centred care.

3. Care that includes other people who are important to the patient (e.g. family, partners, etc).

4. Respect for patients' autonomy and choice whenever they wish to exercise it.

5. Open and sensitive communication that addresses the physical, psychological, social, and spiritual needs of patients and their families.

The book has been mainly written for health professionals who directly care for people with cancer. It touches on specialist psychosocial interventions but maintains a primary focus on how general oncology staff can provide optimal supportive care to their patients. No attempt has been made to cover all the main sites of cancer and the particular psychosocial issues associated with them. There are also a number of other areas we have not attempted to include: cancer prevention and screening, childhood cancers, psychoneuroimmunology, cancer genetics, prophylactic surgery, and euthanasia. Nevertheless the underlying principles of this book will hopefully have some applications in these and other areas.

Cancer diaries

Many of the issues we consider are illustrated with short quotations drawn from over 20 personal diaries of people with cancer. We have chosen not to include lengthier clinical examples in favour of presenting these snapshots from people's lives. These diaries were written at the time that cancer and its treatment were occurring and they depict events as they were happening. They are predominantly written by women and were not originally intended for healthcare professionals to read, but were for the diarists themselves or sometimes as a personal message for their partners or children.

The extracts are short, selective, and out of context, but they are the authentic voice of people living through 'the cancer journey', and we believe they speak not only for those who experienced it but for many other people with cancer too. We are enormously grateful for permission to quote from these diaries. [1]

> I found that keeping a diary helped me to organise my thoughts and feelings and to see things more objectively. I also found it useful to look back to remind myself how I had felt at similar stages (e.g. chemo sessions). I found it a useful discipline to confront my feelings on a daily basis – it helps me to remain positive.

(From a letter accompanying one of the diaries)

Structure of the book

The book is divided into seven chapters, each taking a different perspective on the supportive care of people with cancer. Naturally, these perspectives have many points of overlap so we have tried to cross-reference pertinent sections of the text.

Chapter 1 – Human Context   provides a background to some of the core themes and key assumptions used throughout this book. People with cancer face wide-ranging challenges that stretch from the biological to the spiritual. Yet despite the diversity of their concerns there are general processes that underlie how most people respond and adjust to cancer. The distinctive way that human beings make sense of catastrophic change in their lives is

---

[1] These personal testimonies were acquired through an ongoing qualitative research study (the Cancer Diaries Project), conducted by the authors in conjunction with Suzanne Cowderoy, in which people who have had cancer themselves were invited to submit their personal diaries for scrutiny. The project was advertised through UK national daily newspapers and through Cancer BACUP News, the newsletter of the pre-eminent UK cancer information service.

central to understanding how people with cancer manage the unbridled changes and challenges that follow their diagnosis. Using this general framework we can gain a clearer understanding of how distress can be minimized and quality of life maximized.

Chapter 2 – Personal Context   considers the unfolding experience of cancer from the point of view of the patient. It highlights many of the concerns and challenges faced by individual men and women, how these concerns so often lead to high levels of distress, and what healthcare professionals can do to minimize them and prevent unnecessary suffering.

Chapter 3 – Other People   looks at the vital importance of other people in our lives, particularly when we are faced with a major crisis like cancer. Why is 'social support' so important and how does it work? Often the anguish of people closest to the patient is comparable to the distress felt by patients themselves, and although other people can be a valuable source of emotional support to people with cancer, they can also be an additional source of stress. We consider how partner and family relationships are affected over time, and how carers are able to sustain their frequently exhausting role. Finally this chapter also looks at the needs of particular groups within society who face additional challenges due to their age or lifestyle.

Chapter 4 – Social Context   looks at the wider social parameters of people's lives in the context of cancer. Most importantly, it accentuates the part that healthcare professionals play as members of the institution of medicine. This has wide repercussions for the way people experience their cancer. From this wider perspective we hone in on particular issues such as social class, gender, homelessness, ethnicity, refugees, and asylum seekers.

Chapter 5 – Clinical Context   looks in more detail at common cancer treatments and their effects on the people having them. Although many of these treatments are notoriously challenging, healthcare staff can do much to lessen their patients' distress. The chapter follows a trajectory that roughly tracks that of many patients, considers common treatment difficulties, and ends with a brief look at cancer rehabilitation and palliative care. A focus on particular disease sites has been used to illustrate particular psychosocial issues in treatment, but we make no attempt to cover all the main types of cancer.

Chapter 6 – Communication   focuses on the many communication challenges in cancer care, retaining the traditional, if arbitrary, distinction between information and communication. The second half of the chapter looks at communication issues that are sometimes more challenging, such as working with people with special needs, or those experiencing intense emotional distress.

Chapter 7 – Professional Context   looks at the context of the people who work in cancer care. This is not confined to healthcare professionals but acknowledges that there are other important actors on the cancer stage. Cancer care is emotionally draining work and the level of stress and burnout among staff working in cancer is unacceptably high. How can professionals sustain genuinely supportive care without becoming burned out? This chapter asks more questions than it answers, but perhaps some of the questions need to be asked.

References

1. Editorial (2001). Cancer toll in the USA. *Lancet* **357**:1897.
2. World Bank (2003). http://devdata.worldbank.org/hnpstats/DEAselection.asp
3. Cancer Research UK. Statistics. http://www.cancerresearchuk.org
4. Greenlee RT, Murray T, Bolden S, and Wingo PA. (2000). Cancer statistics, 2000. *CA: A Cancer Journal for Clinicians* **50**:7–33.
5. Greaves M. (2000). *Cancer: The evolutionary legacy.* Oxford: Oxford University Press.
6. World Health Organization (1996). *Cancer pain relief with a guide to opioid availability*, 2nd edn. Geneva: WHO.
7. Ferlay J, Bray F, Pisani P, and Parkin DM. (2001). *GLOBOCAN 2000: Cancer incidence, mortality and prevalence worldwide.* Lyon: IARCPress.
8. Ahmedzai SH, Lubbe A, and van den Eynden B. (2001). *Towards a European standard for supportive care of cancer patients. A co-ordinated activity funded by DGV, final report for EC on behalf of the EORTC Pain and Symptom Control Task Force.* 1–25. Cited in N Ahmed, S Ahmedzai, V Vora, S Hillam, S Paz. (2003). Supportive care for patients with gastrointestinal cancer (protocol for a Cochrane Review). In: *The Cochrane Library* (Issue 1), Oxford: Update Software.
9. Sontag S. (1991). *Illness as metaphor.* London: Penguin. (First published in 1978).
10. Seale C. (2001). Sporting cancer: struggle language in news reports of people with cancer. *Sociology of Health and Illness* **23**:308–29.
11. Wilkinson S and Kitzinger C. (2000). Thinking differently about thinking positive: a discursive approach to cancer patients' talk. *Social Science and Medicine* **50**:797–811.
12. Sheard T. (1994). Complementary therapies, existential turmoil, spiritual abuse ... and spiritual deprivation. *Newsletter of the British Psychosocial Oncology Group.* September issue.
13. Williams G. (1986). *The age of agony: the art of healing c1700–1800.* Chicago: Academy Chicago Publishers.
14. Stein HF. (1985). Whatever happened to countertransference? the subjective in medicine. In: HF Stein and M Apprey (ed.), *Context and dynamics in clinical knowledge*, Charlottesville: University of Virginia Press.
15. Coward R. (1989). *The whole truth: the myth of alternative health.* London: Faber.
16. Payne S and Ellis-Hill C. (2001). Being a carer. In: S Payne and C Ellis-Hill (ed.), *Chronic and terminal illness: new perspectives on caring and carers,* Oxford: Oxford University Press.
17. Holland JC. (ed.) *Psychooncology.* Oxford: Oxford University Press.
18. Brennan J and Sheard T. (1994). Psychosocial support and therapy in cancer care. *European Journal of Palliative Care* **1**:136–9.
19. Jeffrey D. (2003). What do we mean by psychosocial care in palliative care? In: M Lloyd-Williams (ed.), *Psychosocial issues in palliative care*, Oxford: Oxford University Press.

Chapter 1

Human context

Human nature 3
    Emotions 4
    Language and culture 6
    Mental maps 9
    Change and development 14
The catastrophe of cancer 16
    Shock 19
    Denial and avoidance 20
    Integration 21
    Different adjustments. 21
    Core human assumptions 25
What helps people with cancer?. 35
Quality of life 38
Summary 40
References 41

It felt like a bad dream. One minute life was chuntering on. The next – well, someone switched the reels, the road forked and I didn't notice. Somewhere, in some parallel universe, life was continuing to chunter on; here, in this one – or was it in the other one? – where I was unaccountably stuck after some through-the-looking-glass moment … mammograms, ultrasound, core biopsies, sitting in a square at Bart's weeping, apologising, on my partner's shoulder in the soft rain, the world suddenly upside down, guilty, I or my body had let us down – him, the kids, me …

In some parts of the West, 50% of patients with cancer can now be cured of their disease[1] and cancer specialists increasingly view at least some forms of cancer as being long-term or 'chronic' illnesses. Over the past few decades, the depiction of cancer as an incurable, painful, and wasting disease has had to be redrawn in the light of huge strides that have been made in the medical treatment of this disease. There may never be a single magic bullet, but clinical science is finding more and more ammunition. Clinicians are increasingly confident about the future of cancer treatments, and the scientific and medical community probably deserves more recognition than it gets for this real progress.

But for most people cancer remains a very frightening disease, one that is still equated with death. There is also nothing pleasant about modern cancer treatments, and everyone knows it. Patients must quickly enter the foreign, often surreal world of high-tech medicine and the immediate start of notoriously aggressive medical treatments. The depiction of cancer treatments as 'cutting, burning, and poisoning' is uncomfortably near to the truth when one looks at the effects of surgery, radiotherapy, and chemotherapy. In fact, the public's perception of cancer is often far more grim than the essentially bleak fact that 50% of patients *cannot* be cured of their disease. Even the word 'cancer' is still associated in the minds of many people with truly worst-case scenarios:[2] the patient riddled with the agonising and disabling effects of widespread metastatic disease.

In reality, however, it is the psychosocial suffering associated with cancer that bears a much closer resemblance to these common images of the disease as wasting and painful. While there may be no room for complacency, the physical suffering of cancer has never been better controlled, thanks to the emergence of the hospice and palliative care movement. But the trauma of a cancer diagnosis heralds turbulent and far-reaching changes to the patient's world, many of which can slowly eat into the fabric of their personal and family life.

It is not only that people must cope with tough treatments and an uncertain future, cancer reminds us of the limited nature of our lives, and this involves a re-examination of our most basic needs and what we ultimately value in life. It impacts on many core aspects of our human nature, and often violates the underlying premises by which people have lived their lives. So to write that the diagnosis of cancer can be psychologically and socially devastating is coarsely to understate its impact. And the same could be said of any other seriously life-threatening illness.

The first part of this chapter is therefore about human nature and the distinctive way that people in general make sense of sudden and dramatic changes in their lives. Issues of life and death inevitably demand that we step back and take a more spacious or consilient[3] view of human beings, adopting as much a scientific wide-angle view as a philosophical one. By drawing together scientific insights made over the past 30 years and more, we can see more clearly how people manage and adjust to frightening changes such as serious illness. Using this as a background, the second half of the chapter describes some of the elemental challenges that people with cancer face, the factors that shape their experiences, and the resources they draw upon.

Being able to contemplate one's mortality is sometimes considered a defining feature of what it is to be human. So *how do* human beings respond when they are faced with the grave threat of their own demise? And how do people 'move on' from this arresting realization? Rather than dwell on how many people develop anxiety or depression, we will try to get behind the labels and consider how cancer inflicts distress on patients' lives, and those of their families and friends, and how this distress can often be prevented and alleviated.

But there is a further question worth considering, an intriguing paradox that cancer shares with other life-threatening illnesses. Along with all the personal distress and social disruption caused by cancer, some people seem to value what having the disease has taught them. They describe their illness as a time of personal transformation in the way they look at their lives, a transition that they are somehow grateful for. These 'personal transitions' are no longer a matter of clinical anecdote—they can be found both in those who survive the disease and amongst those who die from it.

There is certainly no need for mysticism; the positive flipside to cancer is clearly linked to the more obvious distress that the disease causes. It simply appears that when people contemplate their death they are often compelled to look at their lives, and those of the people they care most about. Confronting their mortality often helps people see their lives more clearly, although this is rarely achieved without fracturing some of their most deep-seated assumptions about their lives (a few of which may turn out to have been illusory).[4]

People with cancer do not merely cope with their treatment and return to their unaltered lives. Frequently both they and the contours of their lives change irrevocably. These profound changes seem to have some positive consequences for some people but, as we shall see, they can also cause significant distress to many. Understanding some of these changes can help healthcare professionals provide care that is more in tune with their patients' needs. But before looking at the specific case of cancer, we first consider how people in general react to massive change in their lives, and start by reflecting on what the mind was 'designed' to do. It will, we hope, become apparent why an understanding of this aspect of our *human* nature helps us to prevent and mitigate the distress of cancer.

Human nature

Over the past two centuries it has become clear that the mind is not a formless abstract idea, but has structure, the same way an organism or a healthcare department has. And this structure evolved.[5] The human mind is ultimately shaped and constrained by what the brain was 'designed' through evolution to do. Over many years biologists, archaeologists, ethologists, and psychologists and other disciplines have been considering how our evolutionary origins may still be influencing how we think, feel, and behave. They have been studying the 'primitive beast' within us, our primate origins, our deepest human history. Social scientists meanwhile have studied the complexity of the social world to which people, individually and collectively, are subject but also create.

For most of us the complexity of modern daily life seems so unmistakably different from that of other living creatures that it is easy to neglect the fact that we are 'just another' animal, albeit with some rather special qualities. The centre of gravity and influence over our nature may have gradually shifted from genetic evolution to cultural evolution over the past hundred millennia,[5] but our more primitive human nature nonetheless remains a potent force in modern daily life. All human beings are, first and foremost, biological creatures and are provided with essentially the same mental equipment the world over.

It is a basic premise of evolution that all species adapt to the ecosystems that they inhabit, or they become extinct. Like every other animal people have special adaptations, biological drives and built-in tendencies to behave in one way rather than another.

There is a selfish evolutionary 'purpose' of all adaptations and that is to ensure that genes are successfully passed on from one generation to subsequent generations.[6] In this way the mental equipment that any animal is born with helps it make optimal sense of the world around it (its ecosystem) so that it has the best chance of surviving within it, and thereby passing on its genes to subsequent generations. Thus the basic machinery of the human brain enables people to learn about the world around them: for example, to know how to do things, to know where things are, to work out what other people are like, to know how things work, etc. As we will see, such learning continues throughout life and enables people to adjust to changes in their circumstances. In fact, the capacity to respond effectively and flexibly to complex change turns out to be a particularly human adaptation, and one that people draw on heavily when faced with the challenge of cancer.

All animals ultimately depend on their instincts to help them survive, and to a large extent these instincts are expressed through their emotions. Emotions become aroused when basic needs require satisfying or are threatened.[7] People too depend upon their emotions to survive so, it is little wonder that a life-threatening illness like cancer triggers such high levels of emotional distress in view of the threat it poses. But first let us briefly consider the nature of emotion, and why strong emotions are a natural reaction to change, and to cancer.

Emotions

When people describe an act as 'emotional' they are usually implying a temporary loss of control ('uncontrollable' rage, 'passionate' love), a primitive impulse that has somehow not been tempered by reason or thought. Without a doubt, the emotions *are* more primitive in the sense that they evolved much earlier than modern 'conscious thinking'. Emotions are there to guide the behaviour of animals to ensure their survival; they are innate instinctive programs of biological activity. The powerful 'instinctive' feelings of love and protection that a parent feels towards their children is a potent and tangible example of these 'primitive' impulses. In people, these raw emotions are mixed with the complexity of thought to produce the rich emotional texture of life.

> Early this morning, I was woken up by the cheerful song of a bird greeting the new day. My first thought was: 'How many more Springs will I be privileged to enjoy?' Don't tell me I shouldn't allow these negative thoughts to creep into my mind! Why shouldn't I? Anyway, there is nothing much I can do, but just accept that feeling depressed from time to time is part of the healing process. There are also still moments when I feel very, very angry that I have cancer. I feel very betrayed, having led a healthy life.

Emotions and drives subtly animate and focus mental activity,[3] so people generally become aware of their emotions the more intense they are. Hunger, sexual excitement, delight, fear, loss, anger, and other emotions or drives provide continuous emotional colour to an otherwise monochrome experience of life. Like Darwin, modern scientists argue that people have a few basic emotions from which all others are derived; these include fear, sadness, anger, disgust, and happiness.[8] Although there are slight social variations, the facial expression of these emotions appears to be universal among people, regardless of their culture, age, race, or gender.[9] Humans share most of these basic emotions with other animals, but we have a far larger repertoire which includes more complicated and varied social emotions such as love, jealousy, contempt, envy, pride, and so on. These secondary emotions invariably also involve associated thoughts and occur in particular social situations.

Fear and sadness are the most common emotions in response to catastrophic events, such as having cancer, so we briefly consider them.

Fear

Fear and anger are closely related emotions and aptly illustrate our evolved nature. It has long been noted, for example, that modern humans continue to be far more likely to fear spiders and snakes and other potential threats to the species, than cars and firearms which these days pose a far greater danger. Fear and anger prepare the body to take evasive action in the face of danger; being essential survival tools, they are entirely appropriate responses in the face of threat.

Confronted by a sabre-toothed tiger, for example, our ancestors had two simple choices: either to run away and hide or, if necessary (because one is trapped) fight it out with the beast. Both fighting and running away (the *fight-or-flight response*) require similar reactions from the body, all of which make up the emotions known as fear and anger: the muscles tense up, we breathe more quickly to take in more oxygen, the heart beats faster to pump the oxygen to other parts of the body, enabling it to keep running or fighting; the blood vessels in the muscles dilate, while those of other organs constrict. With so much exertion, we perspire more to keep the body cool. The mind becomes highly focused and alert for threat. The pupils dilate enabling more light to enter the eyes. Digestion stops and appetite is suppressed. All these automated reflexes are designed to ensure that the body quickly becomes an efficient athletic machine, rather than one that continues with temporarily unnecessary functions like eating and digesting.

Sadness

One might reasonably ask what the biological function of sadness could be. How could sadness be biologically adaptive to the species? It turns out that cultures vary in their attitudes towards sadness. 'Western' cultures that emphasize individual self-reliance tend to view sadness wholly negatively, but other cultures place more value on its salutary effects.[8]

Sadness occurs in response to loss, and loss frequently represents an increased level of threat or uncertainty. Withdrawal and inactivity, which often accompany loss, offer the potential for people to remodel their assumptions about the world in light of the loss, before re-entering the world (i.e. 'licking one's wounds'). This has obvious adaptive value. Sadness induces a period of personal reflection and rumination in which the individual can review the priorities they have given to important goals and roles in the light of a loss or the possibility of a loss.[8] Equally, sadness may have functioned to elicit the emotional and practical support of other people.[8] Of course, a period of self-repair and withdrawal carries the risk of depression; avoiding the changed world for too long can lead one to lose touch with changing conditions and one's confidence to deal with them.

Human beings evolved emotions first, their thoughts later, though it is our thoughts and ideas that make people unique within the animal kingdom. Language has allowed us to articulate what we *feel and think* about other people, what we *feel* and *think* about a work of art, an idea, the taste of something, and so on. People have feelings about the things they think, and thoughts about the way they feel (in the case of panic attacks, these abilities mutually escalate out of control). Some 'feelings' are deeply buried in places inaccessible to words but intuitively known, while other feelings can be identified, expressed, and discussed.

As we consider later in this chapter, our particular combination of thought and emotion has proved a fertile partnership. However, where there is a lingering uncertain threat (and cancer poses many such uncertainties), people are likely to be especially vigilant and to worry. Because people are able to think, imagine, and reason about the past, present, and future, they can also experience the physical emotions associated with the imagined situation in the 'here-and-now'.

To summarize, emotions guide our attention and prompt us to act whenever our personal concerns and goals are at stake.[7] Although our emotions may be gently steering us one way or another, providing a sort of biological commentary on what we think and perceive, the culture around us nonetheless shapes our behaviour through the beliefs and assumptions we develop throughout our lives. It is to the importance of the social world that we now turn our attention.

Language and culture

Human beings and other animals may share emotions, but our most special adaptation, and the most important departure from all other species, is our unique capacity for language and imagination. Nearly all species communicate with members of their own kind, some of them using channels of communication not used by humans (e.g. chemical and electrical signals), but no other creature has anywhere near the human aptitude for language or the kind of creative imagination language gave birth to[1].

---

[1]"Survival machines which can simulate [i.e. imagine] the future are one jump ahead of survival machines who can only learn by trial and error. The trouble with overt trial is that it takes time and energy. The trouble with overt error is that it is often fatal. Simulation is both safer and faster. The evolution of the capacity to simulate seems to have culminated in subjective consciousness". (Dawkins 1976, p. 63)

Dawkins R. (1976). The selfish gene. Oxford: Oxford University Press.

Beyond anything else, it is language that defines the way human beings think. It is through words and abstract ideas that we ponder and make sense of the world around us. Language is the main currency of social contact through which people construct the world. It has enabled the human species to thrive.

In language, humans evolved the ability to articulate a wide range of sounds that could be combined in an infinite number of ways to represent symbolically the world around them. Over time we have learned to communicate with one another in sophisticated new ways. What may have started as a grunt to indicate pleasure and perhaps a groan to signify displeasure has, over the 200 000 years since modern humans emerged (i.e. *homo sapiens)*, spawned the thousands of complex languages there are today. It may have been people imitating the sounds of nature, or perhaps adding emphasis to gesture and sign language, that gave birth to early language systems, but words have become symbols for objects and ideas in the world at large.

Language is therefore the author of culture. Language allows information and ideas to be passed from one person to another and for knowledge to be stored from one generation to the next. Language allows both technological knowledge (the creation and use of tools) as well as social knowledge (customs, rituals, contracts, and oral histories, etc.) to accumulate within cultures. The earliest records of truly modern minds are only about 50 000 years old—cave paintings, jewellery, elaborate weapons, and burials,[10] a mere blink in evolutionary time.

It is only very recently, in evolutionary time, that there has been such an acceleration of technologies for storing and distributing the accumulated knowledge of human culture. After tools, drawings, paintings, ceramics, and oral histories, there came writing (only 5000 to 6000 years ago)[9] and eventually libraries that for a long time were confined to a small élite. Finally, the printing press (only 550 years ago) enabled identical copies to be made in vast numbers at a relatively affordable price, and even more recently digital storage systems, telecommunications, and the Internet enable people across the world to share information with one another at the speed of light. Nevertheless even language has its limits; you can share a song but it is much harder to communicate the feeling it evokes.

Each word has some vague nuance of meaning that almost always distinguishes it from similar words. For example, we may never have considered the slight difference between the words *direct* and *straight* but we use them in different contexts to convey subtly different meanings. But the most amazing 'aspect' of language is not that it 'contains' words which 'name' objects (i.e. nouns: tree, rock, man, etc.), words which 'describe' (i.e. adjectives: green, hard, young, etc.) and words which denote actions and the relationship 'between' objects and events (verbs, conjunctions, and prepositions: goes, because, from, to, etc.). What is more amazing is that it also involves the 'use' of *abstract ideas* like love, trust, courage, and beauty. Imagine!

Metaphors enable abstract ideas to be expressed *as if* they were objects or living things (examine the middle sentence in the previous paragraph—the words in inverted commas underline the abstract metaphorical nature of language).[11] Being able to juggle abstract ideas and play imaginatively with symbols (conceptual thought) defines the way human beings think, compared with animals or computers.[12] The fact that our brains can carry, even within their billions of connections, the abstract idea of 'sincerity' is a mind-brain feat to be reckoned with. Using analogy and metaphor, people are able to manipulate abstract images and ideas—the very currency of ethics and morality, and the raw material of imagination and creativity in both the sciences and the arts.

Developing minds

From the moment we are born we learn what to expect in the world around us; we begin to develop our own 'mental maps' of the physical world. Our brains have evolved to be this way. Babies crawl about their worlds exploring, prodding, and tasting what they find; they are not taught to do this. If we could not learn that space underneath an object causes it to fall, or that fire that is too close to us causes pain, we would soon be in trouble. As it is, by the time babies are between 6 and 12 months they have learned not to crawl over the edge of a cliff.[13] (Psychologists have studied this with more care than this may suggest.)

The human brain is also particularly attuned to the social world around it, because we are an intensely interdependent or social species. No one can afford to be an island. Childhood is spent not only learning about how physical objects in the world fit together but how other people work too. Each child's developing mind is shaped and enlarged by their unique experience of other people, especially their relationship with their earliest caregiver (usually the mother). For example if the caregiver is loving, reliable, and responsive to their needs, the child is likely to develop loving, caring, and trusting relationships later in life.[14] Likewise, children who feel safe and secure are happier, take more risks, are more likely to explore the world around them; they also tend to be more social, creative and better at problem-solving than children who feel threatened.[15]

As they grow up, children increasingly think of themselves in relation to other people.[16] They use other people as yardsticks by which to compare themselves and alter their behaviour. It is through the relationships we form with one another that we learn to trust, fear, love, hate, despise, tolerate, and care for one another. The systems of social bonds and contracts formed between people are the building blocks of society.

From a very young age and with little effort or awareness, people collect and communicate ideas from the social world around them: talking with friends, watching television, fetching water, shopping, eating with the family, working, reading—in other words, mundane experiences which draw from and create the culture that makes up everyone's distinctive everyday reality. Accordingly, because each person grows up and develops within a unique social background, they develop different abstract ideas or 'assumptions' about the world.

In short, people develop their own 'mental maps' of the social and physical world. For example, when people encounter cancer, they bring with them all the assumptions and expectations that they have picked up throughout their lives: how dangerous cancer is, its causes, what treatments exist, how to handle it, what to expect from others, and so on. These assumptions and expectations, and the social conditions of people's lives, are critical to how cancer is then experienced. Chapter 4 explores in more depth how the social context of people's lives often defines their experience of cancer and the healthcare they receive.

For the most part, we are unaware of the assumptions we have developed and carry around with us because much of the knowledge people possess has been implicitly or intuitively acquired, literally 'constructed' from the social context or culture in which they have lived their lives. People soak up cultural assumptions, or memes,[6] from the world around them, 'learning by osmosis'.[17] Knowledge is fluently picked up through contact with other people: we learn about their experiences and they react to ours. Contact with other people provides everyone with important social reference points, support, advice, information, and so on. Again, the main medium for social communication is language, mostly spoken language. Our mental maps of the social world enable us to negotiate it and find our place within it.

From a young age, therefore, children begin to form abstract ideas, or assumptions, about people and their relationships to one another, and by the age of four or five they have worked out that other people have minds much like their own, but with their own different perspectives. The development of this 'theory of mind' is hugely significant in a person's life.[2] It is from this unique human insight (that other people have their own consciousness, feelings, intentions, perspective, etc.) that people subsequently develop varying degrees of 'emotional literacy': being able to 'read' other people's motivations, to recognize deception, to trust and co-operate, to empathize with another's feelings, as well as recognize and contain their own feelings. This growing awareness of other people, in turn, leads children to develop a vague collection of implicit assumptions about themselves.[18] This is the beginning of a 'self-concept'.

Mental maps

A deep depression strikes me from time to time making me sob my heart out. I need time to assimilate, to tame the word MALIGNANT which has disrupted my life so suddenly. Cancer burst into my life, threw it into confusion. I have great difficulty getting my act together and thinking straight. I am going through each day like a somnambulist. Nothing seems real. The intruder MALIGNANT derailed my life. Until this "black Wednesday", I used to walk on a wide, bright road. The world was mine, I was in control of my life … I realise that there will be a lot of mountains to climb before the familiar wide road will come in sight. Do I really want to return to it? I am not sure.

---

[2] These days many psychologists consider this 'theory of mind' mechanism to be, like language, an evolved, specialised, and innate structure (Leslie 1987; Plotkin 1997) though not everyone agrees (Gopnik and Wellman 1994).

Leslie AM. (1987). Pretense and representation: the origins of "theory of mind". *Psychological Review* **94**:412–26.

Plotkin H. (1997). *Evolution in mind – an introduction to evolutionary psychology.* London: Penguin.

Gopnik A, Wellman HM. (1994). The theory theory. In: LA Hirschfield and SA Gelman (ed.) *Mapping the mind – specificity in cognition and culture,* Cambridge: Cambridge University Press.

Only human consciousness includes the abstract idea of time. There is as yet no evidence that other animals can form abstract ideas, let alone communicate about the past or the future. Each of us has a memory of our past ('*life narrative*') and a sense of our future ('*life trajectory*'). People are uniquely able to reflect upon the past and use this knowledge to anticipate and imagine a future. This is particularly pertinent to cancer because time often takes on a completely new meaning in the face of an illness that threatens one's sheer existence. As mentioned already, one unfortunate legacy of this capacity to anticipate possible future threats is the exclusively human misery of worry, a common experience among people with cancer.

The ability to draw general conclusions (assumptions) from previous experience so as to be able to predict the future makes humans far more flexible and imaginative than any other animal in solving and overcoming the challenges they face. Our ability to anticipate the future arms us to control it.[3] The unrivalled and insatiable creativity of people is evident in the human-made world around us, however imperfect. All technology and art are the products of this unique skill at modelling real and imagined worlds.[6] By learning and remembering which caves housed sabre-tooth tigers and which were safe to inhabit, by learning who would be a reliable, trustworthy hunting companion or child-carer, and by learning the skills of hunting with stealth and mutual co-operation and above all by using their imagination, our ancestors were able to predict, control and eventually dominate the world around them. However, this feature of the human mind is so commonplace, so basic to our nature that we are hardly aware of it.

> The ability to distil out of our everyday experience useful maps and models of the world around us is very down-to-earth; so mundane that it is, in many ways, the unsung hero of the cognitive repertoire[17].

> (Claxton 1998, p. 21)

[3]Human beings are considered to occupy the 'cognitive niche' within the ecosystem (Tooby and DeVore 1987), being especially skilled at reasoning and analysing the world using intuitive theories or mental maps that they have developed over their lifetime. Our special quality is the combination of 'animal craftiness and emotion' (Wilson 1998), our ability to devise and apply our exquisitely complex mental maps of the world which are infused by the raw emotions which also biologically drive us. In other words, the human mind-brain is built to learn from the past, understand the present, and anticipate the future:

> Humans achieve their goals by complex chains of behavior, assembled on the spot and tailored to the situation. They plan the behavior using cognitive models of the causal structure of the world. They learn these models in their lifetimes and communicate them through language, which allows the knowledge to accumulate within a group and over generations (Pinker 1997, p.186).

Pinker S. (1997). *How the mind works*. New York: W.W. Norton.

Tooby J and DeVore, I. (1987). *The reconstruction of human behavior: primate models*. Albany: NY, SUNY Press. Cited in Pinker S. (1997). *How the mind works*. New York: W.W. Norton.

Wilson EO. (1998). *Consilience – the unity of knowledge*. London: Little Brown and Co.

In summary, human beings are extraordinarily agile and adaptable, capable of flexibly adjusting their behaviour in response to the situation they find themselves in. We are able to do this because, from the moment we are born and throughout our lives, we continue to refine our *mental maps* of how the world works. These mental maps involve *assumptions* about the world; they enable people to understand the unfolding moment-to-moment events of their lives, and to recombine the knowledge they have acquired to predict the future. Imagining a future enables us to anticipate and solve problems and to develop new plans and goals.[4]

Unlike real maps, however, mental maps are flexible and dynamic; they are continually being refined and adjusted; indeed, many are very abstract and poorly understood, even by ourselves. Intuitive feelings are examples of such implicit knowledge. In the same way that real maps can depict a particular place in terms of its physical features, political boundaries, rainfall patterns, etc., mental maps are similarly varied and only those that are relevant to the context are active in any given moment.[19] And a person's mental maps arc uniquely their own; every sound, image, person, fact, word, object, and so on, has a particular nuance of meaning that has been built up over the lifetime of the individual.

Coherence

Throughout childhood and beyond, people continue to refine their assumptions of the physical and social world, creating evermore complex 'representations' of the social

---

[4] This basic idea that people set goals, plan activities and order their behaviour on the basis of assumptions or personal theories of the world is an idea shared by many authors, though expressed using different terms. Bowlby (1969), for example, wrote of 'internal working models', and Parkes (1971) wrote of the 'assumptive world'. Other authors who share this so-called social-cognitive view include Janoff-Bulman (1992), Figley (1985), and Horowitz (1986). Cognitive theorists use the term 'schema' to refer to cognitive structures that 'guide the screening, encoding, organizing, storing, and retrieving of information' (Beck and Clark 1988, p. 24). Like Champion and Power (1995) we prefer to use the terms mental models or mental maps because they imply a more flexible and dynamic quality.

Beck AT and Clark DA. (1988). Anxiety and depression: an information processing perspective. *Anxiety Research* **1**:23–36.

Bowlby J. (1969). Attachment and loss: Vol 1. *Attachment,* London: Hogarth Press.

Champion LA and Power MJ. (1995). Social and cognitive approaches to depression: towards a new synthesis. *British Journal of Clinical Psychology* **34**:485–503.

Figley CR. (1985). Trauma and its wake: the study and treatment of post-traumatic stress disorder. New York: Bruner/Mazel Horowitz MJ. (1986). *Stress response syndromes,* 2nd edn. New York: Jason Aronson.

Janoff-Bulman R. (1992). *Shattered assumptions: towards a new psychology of trauma.* New York: The Free Press.

Parkes CM. (1971). Psycho-social transitions: a field for study. *Social Science and Medicine* **5**:101–15.

and physical world around them. We learn to predict with reasonable accuracy what to expect from one day to the next, and from one moment to the next: night follows day, the bathroom door is always across the hall from my bedroom, Mummy loves me, rain gets you wet, that is the sound of my cat in the next room, etc. The physical and social world is experienced as *coherent*, fitting together, making sense, largely predictable. Having coherent mental maps of the world enables people to predict and interpret events as they unfold and thus feel safe. From a biological point of view the unpredictable is a far greater threat than what is predictable and there is little doubt that people with cancer face great threats that undermine their ability to predict their future, or sometimes even make sense of the present.

> I can't take in what he's saying. My head is swirling with waves of shock as I try to absorb a piece of fact for which there is no appropriate slot in my mind. It's like putting a coin into a dispensing machine that keeps getting rejected and clattering out into the metal tray at the bottom … It'll take a long time to create a slot in my mind that will accept this new and unwelcome statement my body is making about itself.

When experiences defy our expectations, and we are unable to make sense of the changes we are confronting, there ensues a period of turmoil in which the world feels uncertain and less safe. That is, until more coherent mental maps have been re-established and one has adjusted to the new situation. If something unexpected happens, say your friend John lets you down, your mental maps of the world are subtly changed (your assumption that John is a trustworthy friend is perhaps weaker than it was before). If something *very* unexpected happens, such as receiving a cancer diagnosis, a more fundamental reorganization of one's mental maps will be required. By contrast, when something predictable happens (it grows dark towards the end of the day; a dropped plate crashes to the floor), it reinforces or strengthens that part of the mental map that gave rise to the expectation (the assumption that night always follows day; that unsupported objects fall!) This kind of adaptive learning, or adjustment, is occurring all the time. It is depicted in Fig 1.1.

New information enters through our five senses but it can only be *understood* on the basis of what we already know; something completely new has no meaning (though our brains will try to construct one). Similarly, if our expectations were not guiding our attention, moment-to-moment reality would seem like a chaotic and incoherent babble of input from the senses. People are constantly 'constructing' the meaning of everything they experience on the basis of what they already know about the world and expect to find within it. For example, people's prior knowledge and assumptions about cancer profoundly colour their experience of it.

> A. was introduced to me as a breast-care specialist and Macmillan nurse, the latter giving me the shakes a bit. I immediately envisioned emaciated bodies being wheeled around in beds in hospices …

We try to fit what we see, hear, taste, smell, and feel into the categories and scenarios we have learned and which appear to be relevant to the current context. Expectations are

The Social-Cognitive Model of Adjustment[20]

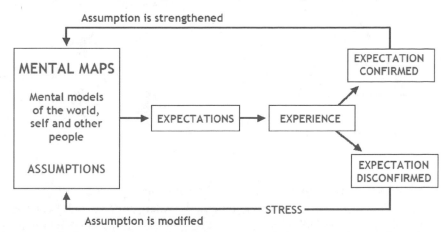

Fig. 1.1 From the moment we are born, we are constantly drawing conclusions about the world around us so as to be able better make sense of it. All experiences lead people to refine their mental maps of the world, a continuous process of self-regulation or adjustment.

derived from prior knowledge of the world fashioned by the present context. When our expectations are not met, we feel temporarily disoriented. The disconcerting sensation of walking up a stationary escalator, or the 'strange taste' of coffee when you thought it was going to be tea, are trivial examples of expectations which have been 'disconfirmed' by experience (see Fig. 1.1). Information that is incompatible with a person's assumptions can either be ignored or reinterpreted,[8] or the assumption itself must be modified.

Cognitive scientists have long been aware that a person's mental maps are vulnerable to many sources of misinterpretation and error. The assumptions we hold are powerful in shaping our experience. People 'see' the world according to their expectations (known as 'top-down processing'). We perceive and comprehend the world through eyes that have been coloured by our experience of the world. For example, people who hold strong beliefs are generally convinced that their assumptions have been repeatedly confirmed by their experiences; studies have shown that, despite being presented with contrary evidence, people maintain stereotypes because their expectations influence what they think they 'see' and therefore remember (a phenomenon known as 'illusory correlation').[21]

The assumptions people hold about the world constantly cause them to *add* or *subtract* from their perception of what is 'out there', shaping the input from their senses to 'fit' with what they have learned to expect. This can be demonstrated with two classic illusions in which the assumptions we hold 're-shape' the information from our senses (see Fig. 1.2). In the first, many people read the sentence in the triangle as "Paris in the spring" because that is what their brains assume is there; having read the words as a whole (or *gestalt*), the brain disposes of what it does not expect to see.

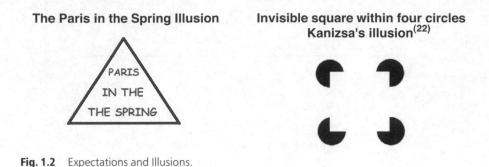

Fig. 1.2 Expectations and Illusions.

In the second, our prior experience of objects hiding one another leads the brain to 'see' the familiar objects of a square and four circles where none exist on the page. In this example, our brains add the 'missing' elements. One of the reasons we find magic and illusion such fun is that, like comedy, they gently violate all sorts of assumptions our mind-brains have previously developed about the world.

Change and development

How do people react to change? Developmental psychologists have studied how young children create categories to describe the world around them (e.g. animals, houses, vehicles, etc.). Not surprisingly, they start off with simple, literal, and often over-inclusive ideas about the world (e.g. using 'Daddy' as a label for all men), but quickly develop more general concepts ('fathers'). Using these categories, children also begin to develop, refine, and rework more general theory and reasoning abilities, developing abstract ideas which reflect the child's unique social context as well as their developing brains.[23] In other words, young children rapidly begin to develop their own assumptions and belief systems.[24]

By the time they reach adulthood, people have developed extraordinarily rich mental maps, full of ideas, know-how[17] and assumptions about how the world, other people, and they themselves generally work. By this point, assumptions include spiritual and moral beliefs, ideas that are perhaps the most abstract of all. Furthermore, each individual's unique personal history is represented to themselves as a kind of story, or *life narrative* (i.e. their memory of their lives). A life narrative provides people with a sense of continuity, a private story *that accounts for* one's passage through life. The projection of this story into the future has been termed one's 'life trajectory'.[20] Importantly, a person's life narrative is their personal story that to them feels coherent and 'makes sense'. As we will see, it can be difficult sometimes to integrate very frightening events, such as cancer, into one's existing life narrative.

However, what becomes more obvious in adulthood (though it is certainly evident in childhood as well) is a form of a resistance to change. The 'grooves of thought' become so worn[17] that new ideas are unable to bypass existing assumptions and there is a resistance to the new information. Although the human mind is designed to be curious, creative, and draw conclusions from experience, cognitive scientists agree that it also has a built-in tendency to be conservative, particularly when deeply held assumptions and beliefs are at stake.[25] If one of the key functions of the mind is to be able to predict what is likely to happen next, then the more deeply held the assumption the more important it is to the overall 'architecture', or coherence of the person's models of the world. We therefore have a strong investment in maintaining our most fundamental beliefs. To alter them requires huge amounts of mental and emotional processing,[26] what Freud referred to as 'working through'.[27] Guy Claxton uses the following metaphor:

> Wholesale reorganisation of the mental household is not to be undertaken lightly. If someone suggests that we rearrange the furniture, so to speak, we might be willing to try it; but if they propose that the house would look better if we were to move the foundations a few metres to the right, they are inclined to meet rather stronger resistance. Just so with fundamental changes to the structure of our knowledge.
>
> (Claxton 1998, p. 79)

People tend to be resistant to significant change because, as everyone knows, change is always stressful, whether it involves organizational restructuring, starting a new job, unemployment, marriage, having children, divorce, mid-life crisis, retirement, or indeed major illness. This should not be overstated however – only events that are appraised by the person as being *negative* cause significant distress.[5] Change can sometimes require the reassessment of large tracts of our mental maps and, while this transition is going on, the world feels less coherent, safe, and predictable. Not surprisingly, people prefer to avoid this kind of stressful situation if they can and we discuss some of the ways people do so below. Of course, most of us invite change into our lives and enjoy a sense of exploration and discovery although, depending upon our sense of control and safety, we are inclined to call it 'exciting', 'interesting', or 'stimulating' rather than 'stressful'.[6] Nonetheless, similar processes of learning and mental adjustment are taking place.

---

[5] It is important to emphasize that change *per se* is not the most potent ingredient here. Change to a less desirable state is considerably more stressful than change to a more desirable one (Mirowsky and Ross 1989), despite the widely held and mistaken belief that positive events are significant contributors to emotional distress. Positive experiences may be stressful and engender turmoil for the individual, for the reasons we have stated, but it is only their negative elements that are experienced as distressing. In this sense, one can think of distress as being the polar opposite of good quality of life. Neither are pure constructs but both describe the relationship between what is expected and what is experienced.

Mirowsky J and Ross CE. (1989). *Social causes of psychological distress.* New York: Aldine de Gruyter.

[6] It seems that people particularly enjoy the challenge of confronting new situations, thereby extending their mental maps, provided they are able to exercise some control over the situation, or at least limit its uncertainty (Csikszentmihalyi and Csikszentmihalyi 1988).

Csikszentmihalyi M and Csikszentmihalyi IS. (1988) *Optimal experience: psychological studies of flow in consciousness.* Cambridge: Cambridge University Press.

In time, what may have been frightening can feel more familiar, and even normal.

> In some ways I feel more positive now. My first reaction was to book my place in a hospice in June/July. Subsequently, I was very conscious that my life was limited, but felt impelled to be positive. As time goes on, and with the chemo affecting my daily life less than I expected it has become easier to feel that things are normal.

Thankfully, given time, most organizations settle down again, new jobs begin to feel familiar and parents learn to do their best. People negotiate the changes they face and eventually make a truce, or 'come to terms', with the change and its implications. Throughout the period of adjustment, people's mental maps gradually incorporate the changes that have taken place, until the mental household feels recognizable and predictable again. Moreover, change is not always negative. It can often stimulate positive, unforeseen outcomes, fresh opportunities, and new goals.

So far, we have looked at how people generally deal with change in their lives. We now consider the specific threats involved in cancer. What happens when people are *forced* to move the 'foundations of the mental household' in response to cancer? What are the core, deep-seated assumptions that underpin a person's mental maps of the world? What do people bring to their encounter with cancer and what conclusions do they draw about their lives? What happens when these changes occur among several people at the same time, such as the members of a family facing cancer? And how can healthcare professionals best minimize this distress?

The catastrophe of cancer

The psychiatric label that most closely describes the psychological experiences following a cancer diagnosis is Post Traumatic Stress Disorder (PTSD). Here, the individual is required to cope with a surreally terrifying and horrific event beyond their control, and that occurs entirely without warning (a terrorist attack, plane crash, war, rape, kidnapping, etc.). In the early stages there is an unreal, dreamlike quality to unfolding events—television pictures of New York City on September 11, 2001 had this quality for viewers in distant parts of the world, days or even weeks after the event, let alone for those who were directly affected. What follows for those who develop PTSD is a period of denial or avoidance of the enormity of what has happened, together with symptoms such as intrusive flashbacks and nightmares about the traumatic events, and a state of heightened autonomic arousal (i.e. generalized anxiety or vigilance).

There is thus a tension within the person between trying to keep the traumatic memories at bay through *avoidance* (including denial and even amnesia), and the *intrusion* of thoughts and images of the event (the flashbacks and nightmares) which work to integrate the memories into the individual's mental maps of the world.[28, 29] The latter process has been termed the 'completion tendency'[30]—the need to integrate catastrophic events into one's life narrative. In fact, this tension between the need to absorb dangerous new information and the need to keep it at

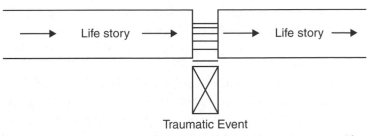

Fig. 1.3 Traumatic experiences must be integrated with the individual's ongoing life story

bay also underlies other difficult transitions such as bereavement.[31] *Avoidance* is merely seen as a mechanism for slowing down and filtering the absorption of traumatic information, while *denial* acts as a more extreme form of avoidance, sometimes permitting no absorption.[7]

In short, traumatic experiences leave people grappling with a new and unfamiliar world. The person must somehow integrate the new events into their ongoing life story. But because traumatic events require a massive reassessment of people's most deep-seated assumptions, the person's only alternative is to keep the full implications of the events at bay (*see* Fig. 1.3) until they can be safely examined and integrated.

In 1994, for the first time the American Psychiatric Association in their diagnostic manual, DSM-IV,[32] permitted the diagnosis of post-traumatic stress disorder when the traumatic event is a medical crisis such as life-threatening illness. However, in no sense are we proposing that cancer necessarily qualifies patients for a diagnosis of PTSD. Rather, like others, we are merely suggesting that there are similar processes at work, which provide useful ideas for reducing some of the psychological ill effects of cancer.[20, 33, 34]

In fact, the similarities of PTSD and cancer are obvious: a sudden, unexpected, life-threatening event over which there is little personal control, together with high levels of distress and anxiety. Admittedly, the experience of cancer is far from a single event, and denial is rarely prolonged. But there usually follows a protracted period of adjustment during which the individual fluctuates between trying to absorb the reality of what has happened to their lives and retreating to a form of mental sanctuary in which the full reality is avoided or kept at a distance. Even among long-term survivors of cancer, the presence of PTSD-like symptoms is associated with higher levels of distress.[35]

Before considering how people with cancer react to the many changes in their lives, recall that any understanding of how people 'come to terms with', or *adjust* to a

---

[7] In much of this text we use the word 'denial' to denote various degrees of *avoidance*, because the term 'denial' is probably more familiar to healthcare staff.

catastrophic event such as cancer, must also be able to explain the paradox mentioned earlier: the fact that some people emerge from these events having learned something valuable about their lives and their relationships. How is this possible in the context of such high levels of distress?

People who experience traumatic events, just like people with cancer, frequently report changing fundamental views about their lives, themselves, and their relationships with others.[36] Perhaps it takes a catastrophic event, like cancer, to make us aware of the deep-seated, most basic assumptions by which we have lived our lives. Many people with cancer actively appear to turn their lives around and take unprecedented strides in personal growth and development. They often describe it as a personal wake-up call. They may become clearer about the priorities of their lives and set about reordering their plans for the future. Or they may simply realize that they have been living for some promised reward in the future at the expense of appreciating the small pleasures of everyday life. Loved ones may also experience their own positive personal transitions which can, in turn, impact on their relationship with the patient. The positive effects of cancer on people's lives is no longer a matter of clinical anecdote, many studies testify to this intriguing flipside of serious diseases.[8] American researchers have naturally even coined a term for it: post-traumatic growth.[36]

Here's how the French writer Hervé Guibert poignantly described his sense of discovery during his struggle with AIDS:

> An illness in stages, a very long flight of steps that led assuredly to death, but whose every step represented a unique apprenticeship. It was a disease that gave death time to live and its victims time to die, time to discover time, and in the end to discover life.[37]
>
> Hervé Guibert (1955–1991)

---

[8] A comprehensive review of these studies is currently unavailable. A few studies are mentioned here merely to demonstrate the point. Nearly 80% of long-term bone marrow transplant survivors reported positive changes in existential beliefs (such as what is important in life), over 50% reported positive changes to future plans and activities, and over 80% reported positive changes to relationships. Furthermore, positive changes appeared to protect people from some of the negative effects of what they had been through (Curbow *et al.* 1993). In a similar vein, long-term follow-up of patients with advanced cancer who achieved remission found they had a greater appreciation of life, time, other people and their relationships. They became less concerned about the 'nonessentials' of life (Kennedy *et al.* 1976). Among Hogkins disease survivors, increased enjoyment of the small pleasures in life was 'almost universal' (Cella and Tross 1986). Among 34 men with testicular cancer and their wives interviewed four years after their treatment had ended, about 90% of the couples reported that their relationship had been strengthened by having endured cancer together with positive effects on intimacy, communication, and sensitivity to feelings (Gritz *et al.* 1990). Following a radical mastectomy, 73% of women reported at least one positive consequence such as a more positive outlook on life, closer family ties, a better understanding of how they feel (Zemore *et al.* 1989). Finally, a study which examined patients with cancer being evaluated for possible BMT described frequent reports of positive psychological gains: improved outlook on life, enhanced relationships especially with partners, and greater satisfaction with religious concerns (Andrykowski *et al.* 1993).

Shock

> How can this possibly be? It's a nightmare. A terrible, terrible nightmare. I plead to wake up from it. I do, but it is still there. I try to bargain. No-one is listening. Nothing changes. The tears flow. Cancer. Everyone's worst fear. A statistic. A reject. I am still in shock. Everyone is shocked. I can't eat. This lump of fear in my throat prevents me swallowing. I hide the news. I don't want everyone knowing. This can't be real. It's a dreadful mistake. What am I supposed to do?

When someone is diagnosed with cancer, the most common response is shock (*see* Chapter 2). In view of cancer's reputation, the person's worst nightmare has often come to pass and many people find it difficult to absorb the enormity of what they have been told. There often follows a period characterized by a dissociated, dreamlike numbness that can last from hours to days. The person's mental maps of the world fail to offer an effective guide to what is happening. The 'shocking' implications of the diagnosis have yet to sink in. There is such lack of coherence and continuity with what has gone before that it is difficult to make sense of unfolding events (the dreamlike quality of the experience). However, the bad dream does not finish and the patient and their family are forced to grapple with their changed world. In other words, the initial shock reaction yields to a more prolonged period of adjustment; the terror and disorientation of diagnosis give way to a gradual realization that life will never be the same again.

> A few people have said, not in so many words but to the effect that now my treatment is over, that's it, and I can go back to work, to life again. But there is no going back, only forward I suppose. Things will never be the same again.

Whenever possible, people use what they know to interpret and respond to unfolding events in their lives. In other words, people cope with new events using the assumptions they have learned from past experiences and, not surprisingly, people come to cancer with widely varying expectations. As events unfold patients learn from the people around them (family, friends, other patients, healthcare staff) how they should best respond.

Andrykowski MA, Brady MJ and Hunt JW. (1993). Positive psychological adjustment in potential bone marrow transplant recipients: cancer as a psychosocial transition. *Psycho-Oncology*, 2:261–76.

Cella D and Tross S. (1986). Psychological adjustment to survival from Hodkin's disease. *Journal of Consulting and Clinical Psychology* 54:616–22.

Curbow B, Somerfield MR, Baker F, Wingard JR, and Legro MW. (1993). Personal changes, dispositional optimism, and psychological adjustment to bone marrow transplantation. *Journal of Behavioral Medicine* 16:423–43.

Gritz ER, Wellisch DK, Siau J, and Wang H-J. (1990). Long-term effects of testicular cancer on marital relationships. *Psychosomatics* 31:301–12.

Kennedy BJ, Tellegen A, Kennedy S, and Havernick N. (1976). Psychological response of patients cured of advanced cancer. *Cancer* 38:2184–91.

Zemore R, Rinholm J, Shepel LF, and Richards M. (1989). Some social and emotional consequences of breast cancer and mastectomy: a content analysis of 87 interviews. *Journal of Psychosocial Oncology* 7:33–45.

Preparation

The more that people are prepared for something and the more their expectations are in line with what they subsequently experience, the less the shock and difficulty they will have in absorbing the new experience or information. For those facing a diagnosis of recurrent cancer, for example, psychological distress is related to the extent to which patients are surprised by the recurrence. In one study, those who 'knew it could happen' appeared to do better psychologically than those who were confident it would not.[38] The importance of being prepared is one of the reasons why most authors agree that providing patients with some form of warning of bad news can slightly cushion its impact (*see* Chapter 6).

Psychological and educational preparation by healthcare staff is therefore essential for patients about to undergo unfamiliar treatments and, for most people, this means all cancer treatments (*see* Chapter 5—Clinical Context). Patients can only make sense of information about their illness by fitting it into their existing knowledge and assumptions,[39] so information must always be tailored to fit with the patient's existing knowledge base (*see* Chapter 6—Communication).

Denial and avoidance

> I guess I'm not letting myself think about it too deeply – shove it to the back of my mind … You know it's happening, you know it's real, but you don't think about it too deeply because you couldn't cope with it if you did.

In cancer, as in post-traumatic stress disorder, many people find it hard to integrate the distressing changes they face. The implications are often too enormous to be easily and quickly absorbed; they are simply too incompatible with existing assumptions. Cancer frequently violates a number of long-standing and deeply held assumptions about one's life, the world, and other people (*see* Core Human Assumptions). The more that the individual's mental map of the world requires wholesale reorganization, the higher the level of stress and resistance to the information (*see* Fig. 1.4). People sometimes therefore deploy a 'defence mechanism', to slow down the rate at which they absorb the new information and its implications.

Psychological defences, such as denial or avoidance, are often useful and adaptive because they help to filter the absorption of new information. In fact, denial and avoidance are not the only sanctuaries in such situations; rationalization and intellectualization are also used (i.e. plausible explanations which turn the threat into a logical, almost normal state of affairs). For others, avoidance is achieved by becoming immersed in busy activity that provides distraction from the threat of cancer and a semblance of normality to people's lives. It is important to reiterate that a temporary or occasional retreat into some form of avoidance is not pathological but can be helpful and adaptive. Avoidance and denial only become serious problems when they block open communication (*see* Chapter 2—Denial and Avoidance, and Chapter 6—Working with Someone in Denial).

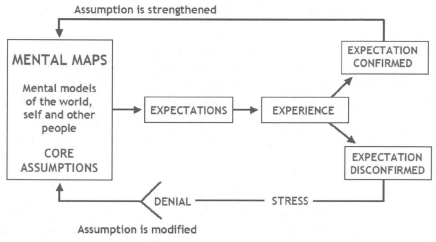

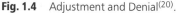

Fig. 1.4 Adjustment and Denial[20].

Integration

> Most of my energy is spent putting up with the side-effects of my chemotherapy. There is frankly little left to convince myself that everything is, or will be, okay again. It won't! Nothing will ever be as it was before the 6th September 1995. Never ever. After all, I have lost a breast, haven't I? Since my life has been disrupted, I do everything in a robot-like way: I carry out my everyday tasks automatically and conscientiously, but my thoughts are miles away. It's a very big job to restructure one's life after a traumatic experience.

Adjustment is never a single or linear process. The implications of cancer are not immediately obvious and may take many months to reveal themselves—one's long-term prognosis, other people's reactions, the extent of permanent disability, the future of a particular relationship, long-term plans, etc. At the same time, people with cancer are coping with other stressful experiences: their cancer treatment, childcare demands, lack of income, etc. Over the coming months or years, cancer survivors may be required to modify some of their most cherished assumptions about their life, other people, and themselves (i.e. the lower loop in Fig. 1.4).

The ultimate task of adjustment is for people to confront and manage the implications of their illness and treatment, to overcome obstacles that are surmountable, and to integrate these events and changes into their mental maps and 'life narratives', so that they can re-engage productively with the rest of their lives. This is ideally accomplished by obtaining the support of other people, notably family, friends, and healthcare professionals. As we will see, the use of words and emotional disclosure is a potent way in which people integrate change in their lives.

Different adjustments

Before discussing the deeply held assumptions that are often violated when someone has a life-threatening illness, we consider the huge range of individual differences in the way people respond to catastrophic events in their lives. These differences reflect three primary factors:

(a) Different social contexts through which events are experienced (*see* Chapter 4). The social class, cultural background, age, and gender of the individual will all influence the way illness is perceived and handled by the individual, their family, and their community. Pre-existing stresses, such as poverty or homelessness, may mean that the individual has an already weakened sense of control over their life. The different ways healthcare is delivered also shape the individual's reaction to serious illness (Chapters 5 and 6). For example, healthcare services which inadvertently diminish patients' sense of control over their lives can contribute to patients' feelings of helplessness and dependence.

(b) Different mental maps of the self, world, and other people. As described above, people acquire from their social environment the varying assumptions about the world, themselves, and other people that make each person unique. These mental models of the world include assumptions about illness generally and, more specifically, the meaning of a cancer diagnosis and how to respond to it. These personal reactions to cancer are explored in Chapter 2 while the impact of cancer on those closest to the patient is considered in Chapter 3. The meaning ascribed to cancer is central to the way it is experienced.

(c) The diversity of people's characteristic styles of responding to information that is incompatible with their assumptions.[9] People react to cancer with different levels of optimism, stoicism, helplessness, or denial because of what they have learned from previous experiences, and in response to the way others handle their illness. Some people react to change in their lives with enthusiasm and optimism; other people feel overwhelmed by their sense of loss. Some people remain open to learning from new experiences; others withdraw in dread and fear. It seems that some people confront the challenge of their illness with less recourse to avoidant strategies than others. Some patients actively seek out new information as a way of feeling in control, while others prefer to know relatively little, sometimes preferring to place their trust entirely in the hands of their doctors.

Most people's mental maps are reasonably flexible and permeable structures that gradually permit the integration of new information. Some people, however, hold more rigid or overvalued models (e.g. the world is completely safe), or have a history of repressing or avoiding incompatible information (e.g. due to childhood trauma or neglect).[8] Like any brittle object, such rigid assumptions are more likely to shatter when assaulted by something as far reaching as cancer. These individuals may be more vulnerable to prolonged 'post-traumatic symptoms' (regardless of whether they constitute a diagnosis of PTSD) because they are unable to integrate the catastrophic information into their mental models. Indeed, cancer patients with a previous history of trauma tend to report more post-traumatic symptoms.[40]

When people are anxious they become less creative in their thinking, and are more inclined to resort to well-tried coping strategies or problem-solving assumptions drawn from past experience. Thus people 'cope' by using their existing knowledge of the world to interpret and respond to stressful events as best as they can. Technically coping refers to the way people manage internal and external demands that are felt by the individual to be taxing or exceeding their resources.[41]

Research has shown, for example, that people who are generally optimistic in out-look,[42] or who are able to adopt a coping style of 'fighting spirit'[43] and become actively involved in their treatment (e.g. obtain information), suffer less psychological distress. These people are more likely to confront the reality of their illness head-on and thus engage in the processes of adjustment. People with this sort of personality are more robust and proactive in the face of adversity and this protects them from excessive psychological distress. Others are apparently more passive, avoidant, or helpless. Probably all of us are a combination of these qualities and many more, but we react differently depending on the situation we are faced with and the type of person we are. This poses a major problem for coping research that has tried to identify universally effective coping strategies.[9]

To summarize, while people with cancer are doing their best to cope with the day-to-day challenges of their treatment, the uncertainty of the future, the reactions of their loved ones, and the reorganization of their normal domestic and work routines, they are also engaged in the stressful process of integrating these new experiences into their mental maps of the world. It is frequently this need to attend to many simultaneous concerns that leads people with cancer to feel overwhelmed and distressed. Studies have shown that those who are having to deal with a number of concerns at the same time are more likely to become overwhelmed and feel helpless in response to their can-cer, regardless of what kind of 'coping strategy' they deploy. Helplessness is a known precursor to depression and, not surprisingly, those with multiple concerns suffer more psychological distress.[44]

---

[9] A great deal of research in cancer continues to be concerned with identifying 'coping strategies' that people use in the face of cancer, despite the fact that this approach has yielded limited practical ben-efits to either patients or clinicians (Somerfield 1997) and many of its results are 'trivial or mislead-ing' (Coyne 1997). One problem is that cancer involves many different changes and threats; a person's response depends on the nature of the challenge they are facing, the stage of the disease and its treatment, and the personality of the individual. It is unlikely that one type of coping strategy is helpful in all contexts, anymore than one way of communicating is useful in all situations. Some of the models of coping that have been proposed involve taxonomies of unwieldy complexity that are of little practical use to clinicians (Brennan 2001).

Despite the idiomatic appeal of the term 'coping', what has emerged has been a rather static view of how people respond to cancer, and has 'failed to adequately take into account the existential reality of individuals in life-threatening situations' (Spiegel 1997, p. 170). The search for general purpose coping strategies that work for every individual in any situation seems ultimately futile and it is arguable how useful coping theory is in preventing psychological distress in cancer. People do con-siderably more than cope with cancer.

Emotional reactions such as fear, anger, and sadness are entirely appropriate responses when catastrophic events threaten the most basic assumptions of life (*see* Emotions above). Indeed, emotional distress appears to drive the process of reconstructing meaning.[45] Heightened anxiety, another key feature of post-traumatic stress, is also common among people with cancer.[46, 47] Anxiety is simply the physical and psychological response to danger. Generalized anxiety, moreover, represents a state of increased vigilance towards potential threat, and the main psychological manifestation of vigilance is worry. Worry is an attempt by the mind to anticipate and prepare for future threat, something that other animals, by contrast, are relatively unable to do. (Worry is explored in more detail in Chapter 5.)

Finally, we consider how cancer can lead to both psychological distress as well as positive development by considering the deep-seated assumptions that commonly underlie people's mental maps of the world. Adjustment sometimes leads people to draw unhelpful conclusions that can result in prolonged psychological distress and personal difficulties but, as we have already indicated, the catastrophe of cancer can also lead

---

This is not to say that patients cannot be helped to alter a *generally* passive or helpless stance to one that is more active and engaged. Some forms of psychological therapy help people to get involved with the processes of adjustment we outline in this chapter, enabling them to confront and respond to the implications of cancer. For example, Adjuvant Psychological Therapy (APT) has shown value; this is a cognitive-behavioural intervention designed for people with cancer in which maladaptive or unhelpful assumptions are challenged (*see* Moorey and Greer 2002).

In fact, all *psychological* treatments in cancer tend to focus on how people perceive their illness, its implications and its meaning, and what 'the patient' thinks, feels and does in response to it. By changing people's interpretation of the threat, or sometimes merely their assessment of their own resources to deal with it, people's distress can be reduced. Individual or group treatments involve the opportunity for patients to review the wider implications of their illness and its impact on their assumptions about the world, themselves, and other people. But in as far as people's distress is often to do with the socio-economic conditions of their lives, psychosocial interventions must always consider the social context of serious illness.

Brennan J. (2001). Adjustment to cancer – coping or psychosocial transition? *Psycho-Oncology* **10**: 1–18.

Coyne JC. (1997). Improving coping research: raze the slum before any more building! *Journal of Health Psychology* **2**:153–72.

Greer S, Moorey S, Baruch JD, Watson M, Robertson BM, Mason A, *et al.* (1992). Adjuvant psychological therapy for patients with cancer: a prospective randomised trial. *British Medical Journal* **304**:675–80.

Moorey S and Greer S. (2002). *Cognitive behaviour therapy for people with cancer*. Oxford: Oxford University Press.

Somerfield MR. (1997). The utility of systems models of stress and coping for applied research. *Journal of Health Psychology* **2**:133–51.

Spiegel D. (1997). Understanding risk assessment by cancer patients. *Journal of Health Psychology* **2**:170–71.

people to reassess their lives in ways that result in healthy personal growth and development.

Core human assumptions

For most people cancer is a catastrophic life experience which, like other traumatic events, requires a period of psychosocial adjustment. The illness violates the most basic assumptions by which people have lived their lives. These basic assumptions, both primitive and existential, must alter so that the illness and its implications can be integrated with the individual's mental maps of the world. This enables the person to 'move on' and re-engage with their changed life. Fear, sadness, and other powerful emotions are natural responses in such catastrophic circumstances and health-care staff therefore have a role in helping people orientate to their new situation or condition.

But, of course, people are also embedded in a complicated network of other people (family, partners, friends, colleagues, etc.). Each one of these people will also need to adjust *their* assumptions, so as to accommodate the patient's illness. The many ways that the patient's relationships are affected by cancer is the subject of Chapter 3.

So what are the deep-seated assumptions that are violated when someone develops cancer? (what we have dryly termed 'disconfirmed expectations' in Fig. 1.4). There have been several attempts to answer this. [10] We offer five overlapping themes which, drawn from this literature and from clinical practice, summarize the main areas of concern for people with cancer. Indeed, they map onto the clinical themes that follow throughout the rest of this book.

An important point to grasp is that adjusting 'the mental foundations' of one's life is fraught with danger, and lying within the following assumptions are the seeds of more severe and prolonged distress. Adjustment certainly carries the risk that people become lost, stuck, or despairing, drawing conclusions which turn out to be counter-productive or just plain wrong (e.g. *'There's no point in going on because having cancer means I'm going to die'*), or merely exhausted by the attrition caused by sustained stress. These factors lie behind many of the psychological difficulties faced by people with cancer.

---

[10]A number of authors have attempted to describe the task of adjustment to illness in terms of the resolution of threats or incongruences with existing assumptions about the world. There is a degree of consensus among their conclusions. Cohn and Lazarus (1979) have postulated that illness entails threats to (a) life; (b) bodily integrity and comfort; (c) self-concept and future plans; (d) emotional equilibrium as a result of the other threats; (e) social roles and activities; and (f) threats involving the need to adjust to new social or physical environments. Very similar constructs are described by Moos and Schaefer (1984).

Moorey and Greer (1989) conceptualised the stress of cancer along two dimensions: threat to survival ('our sense of immortality is shattered') and threat to the self-image (mental and physical abilities, personal and social roles, and physical appearance). Janoff-Bulman (1992) takes a similar view

But first, two caveats must be made. The first is that the core assumptions described below cannot reflect all the concerns or priorities of people from every culture. There is a suggestion, for example, that people in India place a higher value on family ties and spiritual concerns compared with people in 'the West'.[48] Different cultures will have different points of emphasis, but we venture that the underlying mental processes are the same and the limited evidence to date suggests that people from different cultures have similar worries and concerns.[49] The second caveat is that, by describing the very broadest, underlying assumptions that are fractured by cancer, we necessarily adopt an imprecise language. Despite many attempts to carve it up into neat categories, human experience is variable, fluid, continuous, and rarely distinct. Bear in mind that much of what people learn about the world is implicit: people are not necessarily aware of what they know, feel, or believe until, for some reason, it is brought into clearer focus.

stating that, at the core of the assumptive world, are abstract beliefs about self, the external world, and the relationship between the two. 'Extreme life events' (such as having cancer), shatter the assumptions that (a) the world is benevolent; (b) the world is meaningful; and (c) the self is worthy.

In 1983, Taylor proposed an influential theory of cognitive adaptation which is essentially similar to the models of adjustment mentioned above. However, Taylor's theory proposes certain strategies which function to restore schema (i.e. similar to assumptions) which, she postulates, are illusions that are characteristic of positive mental health. She maintains that normal human thought involves overly positive self-evaluations, exaggerated perceptions of control or mastery, and unrealistic optimism (Taylor and Brown 1988) though the evidence for this part of her theory has been questioned (Colvin and Block 1994). The theory of adaptation was derived on the basis of extensive interviews with 78 breast cancer patients who appeared to (a) search for a meaning for their predicament (finding a causal explanation for their cancer and restructuring the priorities of their lives as a result of their cancer); (b) gain a sense of mastery (believing that they could exert control over the course of their cancer; for example, believing that they had changed from the way they lived their lives before their diagnosis); and (c) enhance the self (through construing personal benefit from the illness or comparing themselves with others worse off).

Cohn F and Lazarus RS. (1979). Coping with the stress of illness. In: G Stone, F Cohn, N Adler *et al.* (ed.) *Health psychology: a handbook.* Washington: Jossey-Bass.

Colvin CD and Block J. (1994). Do positive illusions foster mental health? An examination of the Taylor and Brown formulation. *Psychological Bulletin* **116**:3–20.

Janoff-Bulman R. (1992). *Shattered assumptions: towards a new psychology of trauma.* New York: The Free Press.

Moos RH and Schaefer JA. (1984). The crisis of physical illness: an overview and conceptual approach. In: R Moos (ed.), *Coping with physical illness: new perspectives,* Vol. 2, New York: Plenum Press.

Moorey S and Greer S. (1989). *Psychological therapy for patients with cancer: a new approach.* Oxford: Heinemann Medical Books.

Taylor SE. (1983). Adjustment to threatening events: a theory of cognitive adaptation. *American Psychololgist* **38**:1161–73.

Taylor SE and Brown JD. (1988). Illusion and well-being: a social psychological perspective on mental health. *Psychological Bulletin* **103**:193–210.

The following core assumptions reflect the main concerns of people with cancer, the key areas of people's lives that are commonly affected by cancer and which require adjustment. They are not presented in any particular order because this varies from person to person.

Life trajectory

Each of us has our own unique story, a personal history stretching back into our childhood. It is vital to our sense of who we are. We experience this as a kind of life narrative that includes what has happened in our lives and what we expect to happen in the future. Consciousness is its ever-breaking wave. We locate ourselves within this unfolding story and project ourselves into the future by having plans and goals, though not every culture may be as future-oriented as those of the West.[50, 51] We look forward and strive towards moments in the future, and we implicitly make assumptions about where we are in our unknown lifespan. Thus, the idea of *life trajectory* is simply to do with the fact that people's lives are structured around these often implicit and unspoken plans, goals, and assumptions about the future.[52, 53]

Goals often vary with age (i.e. the person's stage in life—child, young, middle age, older) but certainly not always. And goals can range from being short-term and clear-cut (e.g. looking forward to seeing friends later in the day, finishing a book) to being long-term and more abstract (having grandchildren, wanting a happy retirement).[20]

It is not difficult to see how people with serious illnesses like cancer lose their normal levels of hope and motivation. Implicit life hopes are often crushed by news of the diagnosis. For most people *survival* becomes the overriding concern, because the threat of death has a compellingly biological tug on our attention. Survival, a concern for others, and managing the cancer treatment which soon becomes the central focus of patients' lives. In this sense, the healthcare that patients receive inevitably shapes the unfolding story of their cancer.

We have written that 'for most people' survival becomes the overriding concern. For most it is, but for some people cancer can be seen as 'the last straw.' This may be the case, for example, among patients and families facing social deprivation (poverty) and dislocation (e.g. homelessness, refugees), people coping with an existing disability or serious illness (multiple sclerosis), or people are already adjusting to stresses that remain unresolved (bereavement, unemployment, etc.). In the context of chronic psychological and social stress, serious illness can quickly overwhelm the remaining vestiges of resistance. Following a diagnosis of cancer, the future can seem bleak indeed, leaving people feeling defeated, hopeless, and often severely depressed.

Cancer treatments are also notoriously tough. They make people feel sore, tired, weak, and sick. Most people understandably focus on the life-saving treatment they are undergoing and put the rest of their lives on hold. The problem here is that many people disengage from the roles and goals that previously sustained them, and they fail to make new plans. Some authors have made a distinction between people whose lives are entirely dominated by their disease, and those who are able to 'encapsulate' it and see it as merely as something very important they must deal with, whilst trying in every other way to function normally.[54]

For the majority of people, life-threatening illness represents a sudden 'amputation of the future'[55]—the underlying assumptions about one's future life trajectory are fractured, if not permanently shattered. Long-standing implicit life goals may become clear and distinct yet their eventual attainment now seems unrealistic or less relevant. As these goals are re-examined, new priorities are often formed. There is little doubt that this can be a *positive* experience for a number of people but, as already described, any kind of change can also be highly stressful. For example, the person who concludes that 'life is too short' to continue with their physically or emotionally draining career, to which they had previously committed their lives, may feel liberated by this insight but 'lost' as to their future direction and purpose.

By the end of treatment many people have often lost touch with their former lives and, in doing so, have lost confidence in themselves. There is an understandable anxiety about having to pick up the pieces of a life whose fabric has largely fallen apart.[56] People with cancer also describe being unable to make plans because of a fear of 'tempting fate'— '*If I make a plan for next year, something is bound to go wrong*'. Other people develop a morbid fear of being shocked and disappointed again (e.g. by a recurrence) and spend their lives anxiously (sometimes obsessively) vigilant, or by living one-day-at-a-time, without any longer-term purpose or hope.

> I still get hit when people talk about the future, and don't like to think about what my chances are, but it is getting easier to enjoy the moment and concentrate on getting through the next six months. That doesn't feel as if I am tempting fate as much as future planning would be, nor does it raise expectations about my future health that may be dashed; that will be hard to accept. But to maximise the moment.

Depression has long been associated with a loss of things to look forward to ('pleasure') and things to achieve ('mastery').[57] Having a 'wished for' future is also thought to be a major component of hope,[58] and working towards a goal provides energy and momentum and may even be fundamental to people's optimal experience.[59] Without enough to motivate them, anyone is at a risk of depression;[57] the high incidence of depression among the long-term unemployed is a case in point.[60] And, in the context of cancer, people's mood is therefore often dependent on the type of goals they set for themselves.[61] The simple fact is: if you stop having things to look forward to, or goals to achieve, you are more likely to feel hopeless and depressed.

A further unfortunate side effect of having little to do with one's time is that it provides fertile ground for the development of worry. When asked what advice they would give to other cancer patients, 60% of post-mastectomy patients in one interview survey advocated 'keeping busy' and 'carrying on with life'.[62]

The implications for prevention are that healthcare staff should enable people to stay engaged with the things that motivate them and, within the obvious constraints of their prognosis, they should encourage patients to continue to develop meaningful plans and realistic goals, to have events to look forward to and things to achieve. Palliative care professionals are generally very familiar with this idea.

Other people

Humans are instinctively social beings. We live our lives in and out of dependent and interdependent relationships. Family relationships are often particularly enduring but other relationships can be intensely important too. When an illness threatens a person's life, everyone around the patient becomes suddenly more aware of who depends on whom for their needs to be met. Again, we do not often consciously examine these assumptions, but the web of our varied personal relationships is essential to our emotional well-being.

On the positive side, other people can be a vitally important resource in helping individuals adjust to cancer and the many changes it brings. Certainly those who lack this resource are more prone to physical[63] and psychological[64, 65] health problems. But on the negative side, these relationships can sometimes be the source of additional stress for the patient (see Chapter 3).

The effect of cancer is to draw people's attention to their implicit assumptions about their most important relationships. This can frequently be very reassuring and lead to a strengthening or affirmation of existing relationships[66, 67]—again, a positive experience for some people. But cancer can also lead to a crisis within relationships when these implicit assumptions are found to be inaccurate or wanting. For example, women are sometimes deeply disappointed by the response (or lack of it) of their male partners, and this is particularly distressing when the woman feels she has spent many years within the relationship supporting her husband. One study found that almost 40% of breast cancer patients changed their view of who they regarded as their most important source of support, mostly changing it from their male partner to another woman.[68]

As we describe more fully in Chapter 3, the entire system of family relationships has to adjust to the presence of illness in one of its members. Each family member's adjustment to cancer, however, occurs in the context of the other members' adjustment. This carries the risk that the needs of certain family members become eclipsed by those of others, and that the normal developmental requirements of the family become neglected.

Parents' (biologically-driven) assumptions that they will be there to respond to the needs of their children throughout their childhood must sometimes yield to a different expectation of the future. It is distressing even to question this assumption, but cancer inevitably forces parents to do just that. Single people face the challenge of making new friends and dating, such as when to talk about their cancer and its treatment, how much to tell, how to convey one's infertility; and, of course, bearing rejection if it does occur.

The implications for prevention are that healthcare professionals need to ascertain how much support their patients have access to and to ensure that this is adequate to meet their needs. Families are usually deeply concerned and hungry for information though it is up to the patient to determine the flow of information. Healthcare staff must also be sensitive to the high levels of distress among family members who are themselves having to adjust to the implications of the illness and the often massive disruption to family and other relationships.

Self-worth and personal control

Earlier in this chapter we described how children from a young age begin to form views about themselves, based on their experiences and contact with other people. From the moment they grasp that other people have *their own* experience of the world, children also begin to learn the hard lesson that, while they are unique, they are also fundamentally the same as all other human beings. Throughout life a person's sense of themselves, their self-concept, alters according to the social role they are performing: a sexual partner in one context, parent in another, employee, friend, … etc.[69]

People's views of themselves are notoriously resistant to change, but they can be easily undermined as a consequence of life-altering experiences like cancer. Among the many assumptions of the self that people acquire are beliefs about their personal safety and control in the world, as well as their value in the eyes of others. These are particularly salient to the experience of cancer.

Of all the social causes of psychological distress, *lack of control* stands out as central.[70] To feel safe, a person must feel in control of their situation or, failing that, they must believe that someone they *trust* is in control. When people feel trapped in a situation that is neither predictable nor controllable, fear and trauma are likely to ensue. At the very least, psychological and physical health are likely to suffer.[71] This is as true for adults as it is for children. Again, it is not difficult to see why people with cancer feel a loss of control when they suddenly find themselves dependent on other people, predominantly doctors, to control a disease that they fear may be *out* of control. Patients also very quickly have to cope with a bewilderingly complex and often intimidating medical environment[72] over which they may feel little control (*see* Chapter 2).

People are especially receptive to outside influences at times of change and uncertainty[73, 74] so they naturally look to the healthcare team for guidance and reassurance. In the context of cancer, the doctor and the extended healthcare team can provide a large measure of safety by (a) demonstrating that they always have something to offer, (b) showing that they are sincerely concerned about the overall welfare of the individual and their family, and (c) providing whatever level of information and control the patient wants. Taking charge, adopting a 'fighting spirit' or 'active coping' all appear to help people retain their sense of control. The clinical lesson is that healthcare staff should encourage people with cancer, indeed any serious illness, to retain and regain as much control over the events of their lives as they feel ready to handle. By acting upon the world and feeling a sense of 'agency', people not only feel safer, they gain a sense of purpose and hope (*see* Chapter 2—Hope).

Some people seem to respond to the challenge of cancer with particular vigour and optimism. Over 95% of patients in one study were able to offer an explanation for why they in particular had developed cancer, and two thirds believed they could exercise some control over the course of their treatment, and over the recurrence of their cancer—for example, many people believed they had removed a potentially carcinogenic aspect of their lifestyle, such as their diet.[4] In the context of so much uncertainty, perhaps there is an overwhelming need in almost everyone to regain a sense of control by reconstructing a *safer* mental map of the world. Certainly, as the outlook for people with cancer in the West improves, people increasingly want to become fully informed and actively involved with their own treatment.

But not everyone wants to be active collaborators in their treatment, nor receive detailed information about their condition. Indeed, some people prefer to entrust their safety entirely in the hands of the medical team treating them, although this is often a temporary position that relaxes with time, especially if the individual feels well supported by their family and the healthcare team. However, this wide variation in the need for information and control is the source of a well-known communication challenge for healthcare professionals (*see* Chapter 6).

For some people, it may be difficult to assert control when healthcare staff appear to be better educated, have a higher social status, speak in a bafflingly technical language (which, worryingly, they expect one to understand), speak with a different accent, are from a different ethnic background, appear to be only interested in the tumour, and are seemingly too busy and important to delay with questions. To be assertive in such a situation takes an assertive person. Once a sense of powerlessness and lack of control become the prevailing expectation (and it may pre-date the cancer), the person will be *more* passive, *more* resigned to their helplessness and *less* able to retain any expectation of solving problems that do come up, let alone communicate effectively with healthcare staff.

Feeling a sense of control has an intimate relationship with a person's sense of worth or self-esteem.[75] The sheer length and physical burden of cancer treatments leads many people with cancer to withdraw from social roles (work, interests, and social activities) which previously let them know about their potency, competence, and value in the world, information that may have been vital to their sense of self-worth. Patients in treatment often report experiencing days on end when they feel they have achieved nothing useful and have become a chronic burden on others. Social discrimination from a number of sources (e.g. employment, insurance, etc.) is likely to reinforce this perception that the person has little value to others. People with cancer may even express shame about their own level of distress which they regard as patent evidence of their 'poor coping'. Furthermore, a deterioration in their physical condition can lead people to feel not only unattractive but helpless and of less value to others (*see* The Body).

The independent, self-sufficient maverick businessperson who is unable to work owing to illness or the demands of treatment, may find themselves deprived of an important source of feedback about their value in the world. Instead, perhaps for the first time, they are forced to depend upon others and must tolerate being substituted at work. Likewise, the 'all-caring, nurturing super-mother' finds herself physically and emotionally too exhausted to maintain the primary role from which she may have derived much of her self-worth.

In summary, serious illness, like retirement or unemployment, can lead to sudden and deep changes both in a person's roles and spheres of influence, and in the responses of other people. Without this regular social feedback, people can quickly lose confidence in themselves and seriously doubt their value to others. Such self-doubt and loss of self-esteem are obvious precursors to depression[76] and are common experiences among people with cancer. Finally, people with high self-esteem are likely to receive greater social support than those who are low in self-esteem[69] leading to something of a self-fulfilling prophecy. Furthermore, if patients feel that healthcare staff define them by their illness (i.e. professional interest is limited to the tumour) people with cancer may come to do this themselves (*see* Chapter 2—Impact on Self). The effect of this on patients' self-worth can be rapid and severe.

The body

We spend our entire lives in our bodies. Our bodies are so central to our identity or self-concept that we rarely consider the assumptions we have developed about them. It is through the sensory apparatus and functions of the body that we interact with the world and one another. On a moment-to-moment basis we are unaware of any mind–body split; our corporal and sentient selves are inextricably bound to one another. We are as much our bodies as ourselves.

As we age, however, we become aware of subtle changes in the capabilities, appearance, and sensation of our bodies. These changes occur slowly enough for most of us to adjust to them without associated psychological difficulty (e.g. wrinkles, balding, going grey); indeed, it is often the experience of a sudden change in one of these facets of the body (capability, appearance, or sensation) that prompts us to seek medical help.

Life-threatening illnesses, by definition, involve a threat to the integrity of the body. It is hard enough to absorb the fact that a growing cancer in the body threatens to end one's life. On top of this we must adjust to the fact that the treatment, if not the illness itself, may lead to massive changes in our physical capabilities, appearance and sensation, all of which have implications for how we interact with and are seen by the social world. With diagnosis comes the sudden realization that our bodies are not the reliable organs we once thought they were, they have let us down. The assumption that the body is simply an obedient servant to the cognitive master is forever laid to rest. Indeed, for a high proportion of patients there remains more than a residual suspicion, more of a morbid fear, that one day the body will once again provide shelter for the enemy. For a smaller number of patients this manifests itself in intrusive ruminations or compulsive urges to check the body for signs that the disease has returned.[76]

The most common and obvious example is that of a sudden change to a person's physical appearance. Any form of disfiguring disease or mutilating surgery can lead to body image problems if the person is unable to adjust their self-image to accommodate their changed appearance. Even where an individual's identity is not highly bound up with their physical appearance they may be at risk of a loss of self-esteem and thus depression. Disfigurement is both a personal and social experience. Adjustment to any form of visible change to the body usually requires adjustments in other people, since our physical appearance is also part of the social world in which we live. In addition to learning to deal with the reactions of others in the broader social world, people with cancer often have to face relationship and sexual difficulties as both the patient and their loved ones attempt to adjust to the new reality (*see* Chapters 2 and 3). Long-term physical disabilities (amputations, loss of speech or ability to eat, etc.) and sensory discomfort (pain, dyspnoea, etc.) involve similarly protracted periods of psychosocial adjustment.

Existential–spiritual

The spiritual side of a person is that which expresses their deepest convictions about the nature of existence. Questions of existential meaning usually involve notions of fundamental causation and purpose, the preciousness of being alive, of being in existence. These questions are naturally important to people because, as we have seen, human beings are always implicitly struggling to understand the world they inhabit. It is in our nature to do so.

Across much of the world beliefs about the nature of existence involves some version of the conviction that people exist in relation to a power greater than human beings and the known natural world. This very common cultural belief is expressed both in private and in larger social movements associated with religions. Being part of a religion provides people with several social advantages. First, they offer a framework in which to find meaning and continuity. Religious beliefs provide the reassurance that, amidst the danger and uncertainty, there is a higher purpose or design, though unfortunately this carries the risk that patients with cancer feel they are being punished for some moral transgression, a form of divine retribution.[11] Religions also frequently provide tools for contemplation and mental adjustment—the frequency of personal prayer, for example, has been shown to relate to higher levels of psychological well-being.[77] Finally, religions often help to embed people in a valuable community of social support (*see* Chapter 3 for a description of social support).

Varied spiritual expectations shape the experience of cancer. Many of these experiences involve the challenge to and/or confirmation of existing assumptions about the moral or rational nature of existence (e.g. 'Why me?'). For example, the Christian axiom, 'the meek shall inherit the earth', whatever its intended spiritual meaning, encourages a popular belief in a world in which good things happen to good people. The law of karma in Hinduism similarly asserts that people deserve the consequences of their actions. Moreover, modern scientific and technological wonders amply demonstrate the power of a Newtonian view of the physical world, all effects having physical causes. These powerful cultural assumptions provide people with solid reference points with which to view the world, but they do little to prepare us for the catastrophe of a life-threatening diagnosis that is experienced as both unfair and inexplicable. The ubiquitous question 'Why me?' can be targeted at one or both of these assumptions in the individual's search for meaning. And if these fundamental constructs about the world are found lacking, what others should be questioned?

People who have lived by a doctrine of religious principles may feel a sense of injustice and spiritual doubt (e.g. that they live in a fair and just world), but perhaps no more so than those with atheistic beliefs. The latter too may feel an abrupt need to re-examine previously held assumptions about the nature of existence, and this may lead them to question their implicit and explicit beliefs (e.g. in a rational universe). In either case, loss of spiritual meaning can result. These experiences are also sometimes connected with those of 'existential loneliness' in which people become acutely aware of the ultimate isolation of their existence as they pass through life to death, an isolation that cannot be transcended through any form of communication.

Such existential–spiritual questions can leave people highly distressed, lost in a sea without reference points. It is painful to adjust one's internal picture of the world if one has to conclude that life is apparently unfair and meaningless, though clearly this is a particularly unhelpful conclusion. Happily, however, many people find their faith being reaffirmed through their illness, but the wish to attribute blame to something or

[11]Of course, religious beliefs not only advantage the individual. The origin of most cultures has involved 'god-given' laws and customs which have served to restrain the impulses of the individual in favour of the community at large, even if rulers have often borrowed this authority for their own ends (Wilson 1998). Even in modern times, to profess no religion at all can set oneself apart in a minority deviant position where one can face rejection and prejudice. In America, where religious belief is the norm, those who claim no religion may even be thought to be 'un-American' (Mirowsky and Ross 1989).

Mirowsky J and Ross CE. (1989). *Social causes of psychological distress.* New York: Aldine de Gruyter.

Wilson EO. (1998). *Consilience: the unity of knowledge.* London: Abacus.

someone is as understandable as it is common. The deity may become an obvious target for blame though the need for accountability can become displaced onto other people (doctors, employers, the government, etc.) or to individuals blaming themselves ('I should have quit smoking'). Even if they discern no way of having caused their cancer, some people grapple with the moral tally of their lives so as to somehow account for their predicament.

What helps people with cancer?

It would certainly be satisfying to be able to end this chapter with some novel conclusions about how best to help people with cancer adjust to their illness and enjoy the highest quality of life whatever their prognosis. Understanding the main concerns and feelings that cancer patients experience can enable doctors, nurses, and radiographers to provide healthcare that minimizes the physical and emotional side-effects of treatment. The truth is that one only has to talk to a few people with cancer to know what helps them manage and adjust to the ordeal they face. Our conclusions should therefore not be surprising, but their implications permeate the text throughout the remainder of this book.

For anyone facing a life-threatening illness, there are two overarching psychosocial concerns that have implications for healthcare professionals.

Safety

Like anyone facing an unforeseen and chilling crisis, people with cancer quickly need to feel as safe as possible. There are a number of ways that healthcare professionals can enable their patients to feel they are in safe, caring, and trustworthy hands. They can:

- make it clear that the healthcare system will never abandon the patient;
- offer patients clear clinical goals to aim for;
- provide every patient with a 'treatment road map' to follow;
- prepare patients for experiences they are not expecting;
- encourage patients to assume as much control over what is happening as can be provided; in other words, enable patients to be active contributors to their treatment if they wish;
- show sensitivity to the unique personal, social, and cultural context which each person brings to their illness and which so fundamentally shapes their experience of cancer;
- normalize patients' reactions and feelings;
- encourage people to retain as many of their (a) normal social roles (parent, sibling, friend, colleague, wage-earner, etc.) and (b) goals (things to look forward to, things to achieve) as possible;
- ensure that patients have easy access to information and emotional support whenever they require it;
- wherever possible, ensure the treatment schedule fits the patient's schedule.

Support and integration

The second, highly related principle of care rests on the fact that people are sustained by the support of other people and nowhere is this more the case than in cancer. Family and friends, other patients, and healthcare professionals all have a role in supporting the patient.

> Some nurses smiled or waved whenever they came to my end of the ward; to others I felt invisible. Sometimes the absence of a smile made me feel desolate, and I felt lonely and neglected when the nurses were busy elsewhere in the ward, even though I did not need anything and I knew that other patients had greater needs. I appreciated it when anyone found a few minutes to spend with me.

Of course, not everyone has access to sufficient support, but in the context of such dangerous uncertainty, emotional support in particular often enables people with cancer to feel cared for, loved and valued, as well as reassured that this support will be sustained in the future. Importantly, it also enables people to describe their experience of the unfolding catastrophe and have their feelings and thoughts validated. 'Telling the story' of what is happening, and has happened, to friends and loved ones enables new meaning and ideas to emerge, problems to be confronted and solved, and helps the person integrate the events into their 'life narrative'.[78]

Most people overcome and adjust to the challenges of cancer through talking with other people and expressing their feelings.[12] In Chapter 3 we explore why social support is probably our most valuable resource in facing catastrophic events. For one thing, the emotional support of others enables people to confront the emotionally upsetting implications of cancer that they may have previously avoided or denied.

Cancer is very much an individual story for each person who has the disease. In the process of finding words to depict recent events, people reconstruct an ever more coherent mental map of the world, integrating what has happened into their ongoing life story. The value of narrative (telling one's story), whether to a friend, healthcare professional, or therapist, or even writing it down, is that it enables people to 'organize

---

[12] Curiously, emotional expression has received something of a bad press in the literature on coping. Emotion-focused coping is thought to lead to poor psychological outcomes, though this may be largely because of conceptual confusion. There is more than enough empirical evidence to support the value of people expressing their emotions (e.g. Pennebaker 1995; Stanton *et al.* 2000) provided they are competent at expressing them, they believe it is helpful, and there are people in whom to confide (Surgenor and Joseph 2000).

Pennebaker JW. (ed.). (1995). *Emotion, disclosure and health.* Washington: American Psychological Association.

Stanton AL, Kirk SB, Cameron CL, and Danoff-Burg S. (2000). Coping through emotional approach: scale construction and validation. *Journal of Personality and Social Psychology* **78**:1150–69.

Surgenor T and Joseph S. (2000). Attitudes towards emotional expression, relational competence and psychological distress. *British Journal of Medical Psychology* **73**:139–42.

and represent experiences and/or events as meaningful wholes ... [to] bind and congeal an individual's behavior and experiences into meaningful unities'[79] (Russell and van den Broek 1992, 344).

All psychological therapies rely on the power of this process,[80] though historically some writers have seen emotional expression as merely a form of catharsis or discharge rather than an expression of something important within the person.[81] In fact, regardless of the medium (e.g. confession, atonement, talking to confidantes, writing, psychotherapy, etc.), it seems that the depiction of stressful event in words, and the identification of the associated emotions ('reliving the event') helps people integrate stressful experiences. Emotional disclosure is somehow fundamental to emotional health[82], even if cultural practices in the need, form, and effectiveness of emotional disclosure vary to some extent around the world.[83]

> Writing it down makes me look for the positive – I will continue on a daily basis.

> I want to legitimise my feelings by writing them down. I'm scribbling my thoughts in a secret notebook by my bed. I can't wait to get to the computer to sort them out.

Writing about traumatic events has been reliably found to improve physical and psychological health,[84] and there is even preliminary evidence that written emotional expression can produce symptom improvements in people with chronic illnesses, such as asthma and rheumatoid arthritis,[85] though on this point scepticism exists.[86] The depiction of experiences and feelings through personal creativity such as writing,[87] music,[88] and art[89] is another important way for people to make sense of events and integrate them into their lives. Creative activity not only enables people to express their feelings and ideas, it also allows them to feel a sense of purpose, resourcefulness, and achievement that can lift their whole spirit. This is how one cancer diarist put it:

> I found that keeping a diary helped me to organise my thoughts and feelings and to see things more objectively. I also found it useful to look back to remind myself how I had felt ... I found it a useful discipline to confront my feelings on a daily basis – it helps me to remain positive.

Finally, there is yet another way people manage the personal and social changes brought about by serious illness. Not everyone finds it easy to talk about their feelings and thoughts, let alone write about them, especially if emotional expression is regarded as a sign of weakness. But everyone thinks. Although it is not easy to study what people think about in private, most people would probably agree that they spend as much time reflecting privately on events, as they do articulating their thoughts and feelings to others. This has had obvious adaptive value in helping people take stock of changing conditions, make plans to overcome what is changeable, and adjust to what is not. The fact that we think, ruminate, and worry about ourselves, other people, and events in our lives can nonetheless lead to problems when these mental scenarios become intrusive on our thinking, leading to sustained distress and additional problems (constant worrying, anxiety, depression, insomnia).

Quality of life

A huge literature has developed around the idea of 'quality of life'. This interest in the effects of a person's health or illness on their overall well-being or happiness is a response to the concern that 'too often a patient's distress is narrowly defined by the healthcare system and their illness is described in terms of the biology of disease ... while the associated suffering of the patient is ignored'.[90] (Cohen *et al.* 1996, p. 753.) As a construct, quality of life naturally follows from the World Health Organization's definition of health as complete physical, mental and social well-being, not merely the absence of disease or infirmity.[91] So in recent years, albeit still in far too few studies, medical research has increasingly measured the comparative effects of cancer treatments on aspects of the patient's experiences, not simply tumour regression or length of survival. Cancer clinicians have long recognized that their treatments must strike a balance between quantity and quality of life.

The difficulty, however, is that while tumour size and survival times are relatively easy to measure, quality of life outcomes are not. Nonetheless, many reliable and valid measures of quality of life are now available though to evaluate them is beyond the scope and remit of this book. A brief description of several of the main ones currently used can be found in Appendix 1.

There is no universally appropriate quality of life tool. In the same way that the construct 'intelligence' is defined by what intelligence tests measure, quality of life tends to mean whatever is measured by quality of life instruments. Researchers must choose the best tool for whatever aspect of quality of life they are trying to measure. Gone are the days when quality of life was measured using a one-dimensional scale such as the Karnofsky Performance Scale.[92] This may still be a useful measure if one is primarily interested in self-care and ambulation, but few people would regard it as an adequate measure of 'quality of life' (though interestingly patients themselves, and presumably everyone, tends to understand quality of life as a 'summary impression of their experience').[93] These days a number of multidimensional scales exist that attempt to cover some of the main facets of what people generally value in their lives; one method even allows the patient to nominate the areas of their life they regard as most important before these are measured (*see* Appendix 1). Factor analyses have identified seven distinct domains,[94] though one might wish to add a spiritual–existential dimension to this list.

Core components of quality of life:

1 physical concerns (pain and other symptoms)

2 functional ability (mobility, self-care, activity level, etc.)

3 family well-being

4 emotional well-being

5 treatment satisfaction

6   sexuality/intimacy (including body image)

7   social functioning

Unfortunately, while useful in research, in clinical *practice* quality of life questionnaires can seem pretty remote and impersonal. They are also impractical for those who are seriously ill, have cognitive impairments or communication difficulties, or who are severely distressed—in other words, precisely those patients for whom it would be most helpful to have quality of life information to inform decision-making.[95]

So this book is concerned with all these themes because these are the key factors in providing best supportive care. To maximize quality of life one must ascertain what an individual values in their life and how these 'valuables' can be affected by a particular treatment or symptom. Understanding what a person values is therefore often pivotal to helping them achieve an optimal quality of life.

Context

Some patients are prepared to sacrifice quality of life in exchange for even the slightest chance of cure.[96] People in chronic pain may choose complete analgesia at the expense of heavy sedation or, conversely, greater wakefulness at the expense of higher levels of pain. What is clear is that quality of life is an individual, subjective, and unique construction that comprises many facets. It depends on the specific context of the particular individual, rather than some universally valued 'thing' that everyone shares to varying extents.

Over 2000 years ago Aristotle made the point that what people value in life is often only apparent when they don't have it, or have lost it. What people value is based on implicit expectations and these vary according to the context:

> With regard to what happiness is people differ, and the many do not give the same account as the wise. For the former think it is some plain and obvious thing, like pleasure, wealth, or honour; they differ, however, from one another – and often even the same man identifies it with different things, with health when he is ill, with wealth when he is poor.[97]
>
> (Aristotle: *Nicomachean*)

A more modern definition similarly holds that quality of life is always relative to one's expectations and 'depends on present lifestyle, past experiences, hopes for the future, dreams, and ambitions':

> Quality of life measures the difference, or gap, at a particular period of time between the hopes and expectations of the individual and that individual's present experiences.[98]
>
> (Calman 1984, p.124)

As we have explored earlier in this chapter, people's assumptions and expectations are formed by their previous and current experiences in life. Of course they reflect 'shared views about how one ought to be able to live' (Culyer 1990, p. 21) and these views vary over time and place.[99] Just as measures of quality of life strive for cross-cultural validity, an individual patient's quality of life can only be *understood* within the context of their particular culture and social situation. Taking the time to understand cultural differences is vital to the way clinicians can maximize their patients' quality of life. Quality of life is not only subjective but also culturally bound.[100]

A person's quality of life is also like shifting sand, as expectations 'catch up' with prevailing reality (level of pain, family distress, extent of fatigue, etc.). This is not to say that people can always learn to put up with unpleasant conditions. People with cancer do their best to adjust their lives and expectations so as to work around, overcome or tolerate the problems they face, but people can only lower their expectations so far. Some symptoms are simply intolerable to endure, especially if they are perceived as permanent and unchangeable. But thanks largely to the hospice movement and advances in palliative medicine, these situations are becoming increasingly rare in countries where such services are developed. However, it is certainly misleading to talk of a 'return' to premorbid quality of life; objective conditions and expectations change, and can never be the same as they were.

> Since my diagnosis, everything has changed. Everything feels upside down – I'm no longer the same person, I seem to have no control over my life, and I just don't know what to expect anymore …. I want to go back to the person I used to be, but I can't.[20]

Summary

This chapter has tried to show that human beings are resourceful and adaptive creatures whose innate mental architecture enables them to transcend the most formidable of problems. Above all, we learn from our experiences and we depend upon one another for our safety and survival.

We argue that throughout their lives human beings develop assumptions and expectations about the world around them ('mental maps' of the physical and social world, including the self), drawn from the social world around them. All of us apply these expectations so that we can understand the unfolding events of our lives. In turn, our experience of life alters our assumptions and expectations about the world. Our 'mental maps' involve assumptions that are drawn from everything we have learned about how to live in the culture that surrounds us. Although we are not aware of many of the things we have learned during our lives, these mental maps enable us to experience each unfolding moment as part of a more-or-less coherent and continuous whole.

Everyone carries with them a story of their life, their 'life narrative or autobiographical memory'. Although there is an innate drive within everyone to draw conclusions from our experiences (so as to adjust our mental maps) there is also resistance to changing our most fundamental or 'core' assumptions, because this would entail a full-scale reorganization of our mental maps of the world.

Yet, this is precisely what psychologically traumatic events like cancer demand. When a catastrophic event occurs, people's most deep-seated assumptions about the world are violated and no long adequately make sense of the world. The unreal, dreamlike state of shock following the diagnosis of cancer is a powerful case in point.

A period of adjustment is required, and not just psychological adjustment. In the case of cancer it is people's employment and domestic arrangements, their social conditions, their relationships with other people and their spiritual beliefs that are also often tested and changed. Not to mention reacting to the demands of notoriously harsh treatments. People manage the stressful adjustments to the core assumptions of their lives in many different ways, but there is often a push–pull quality to the way people process and integrate dramatic events like cancer: e.g. wanting to avoid or deny the frightening implications while, at the same time, needing to make sense of them.

Ultimately, the key task of psychosocial adjustment to cancer is for each person affected to thread their alarming new experiences into the fabric of their continuing life story, so that they can re-engage productively with their life. Appendix 2 translates many of these ideas into the form of a psychosocial booklet, which was designed to normalize people's emotional reactions and experiences in response to cancer, and help them engage with these processes of adjustment.

In the context of the turmoil of cancer, healthcare staff are pivotal in shaping their patients' expectations and actual experiences. By providing guidance and hope and by being sensitive and responsive to the unique needs of each and *every* person, healthcare staff can ensure that people with cancer, whatever their situation, are able to maximize their quality of life.

References

1. American Society of Clinical Oncology (1998). Cancer care during the last phase of life. *Journal of Clinical Oncology* **16**:1986–96.
2. Geraghty JG, Zbar A, and Costa A. (2002). Informing the public about advances in cancer therapy. *European Journal of Cancer Care* **11**:25–32.
3. Wilson EO. (1998). *Consilience.* London: Abacus, Little Brown and Co.
4. Taylor SE. (1983). Adjustment to threatening events: a theory of cognitive adaptation. *American Psychologist* **38**:1161–73.
5. Donald M. (1998). Hominid enculturation and cognitive evolution. In: C Renfrew and C Scarre (ed.), *Cognition and material culture: the archaeology of symbolic storage,* Cambridge: McDonald Institute for Archaeological Research.
6. Dawkins R. (1989). *The selfish gene,* 2nd edn. Oxford: Oxford University Press.
7. Frijda NH. (1988). The laws of emotion. *American Psychologist* **43**:349–58.
8. Power M and Dalgleish T. (1997). *Cognition and emotion: from order to disorder.* Psychology Press: Hove, East Sussex.
9. Plotkin H. (1997). *Evolution in mind – an introduction to evolutionary psychology.* London: Penguin.
10. Zimmer C. (2001). *Evolution: the triumph of an idea.* New York: Harper Collins.
11. Pinker S. (1997). *How the mind works.* New York: W.W. Norton.
12. Lowe EJ. (1998). Personal experience and belief: the significance of external symbolic storage for the emergence of modern human cognition. In: C Renfrew and C Scarre (ed.), *Cognition and material culture: the archaeology of symbolic storage,* Cambridge: McDonald Institute for Archaeological Research.

13. Gibson EJ and Walk RD. (1960). The visual cliff. *Scientific American*, **202**:64–71.

14. Bowlby J. (1971). Attachment and loss, Vol. 1. *Attachment*, London: Hogarth Press.

15. Isen AM. (1990). The influence of positive and negative affect on cognitive organisation: some implications for development. In: NL Stein, B Leventhal, and T Trabasco (ed.), *Psychological and biological approaches to emotion*, Hillsdale: Erlbaum.

16. Damon W and Hart D. (1980). *Self-understanding in childhood and adolescence*. Cambridge: Cambridge University Press.

17. Claxton G. (1998). *Hare brain tortoise mind: why intelligence increases when you think less.* London: Fourth Estate, p. 21.

18. Fonagy P, Steele M, Steele H, Leigh T, Kennedy R, and Target M. (1993). The predictive specificity of Mary Main's adult attachment interview: implications for psychodynamic theories of emotional development. Paper presented at conference: John Bowlby's attachment theory: historical, clinical and social significance. Toronto, Ontario. Cited in West ML (1997). Reflective capacity and its significance to the attachment concept of the self. *British Journal of Medical Psychology* **70**:17–25.

19. Midgley M. (2001). The many maps model. Abstract of paper presented at the consciousness and experiential psychology 5th conference: awareness. *Consciousness and experiential psychology newsletter*. Leicester: British Psychological Society.

20. Brennan J. (2001). Adjustment to cancer – coping or psychosocial transition? *Psycho-Oncology* **10**:1–18.

21. Hamilton DL and Rose TL. (1980). Illusory correlation and the maintenance of stereotypic beliefs. *Journal of Personality and Social Psychology* **39**:832–45.

22. Kanizsa G. (1976). Subjective contours. *Scientific American* **234**:48–52.

23. Case R. (1999). Conceptual development. In: M Bennett (ed.), *Developmental psychology: achievements and prospects*, London: Psychology Press.

24. Keil FC. (1999). Cognition, content and development. In: M Bennett (ed.), *Developmental psychology: achievements and prospects*, London: Psychology Press.

25. Janoff-Bulman R. (1992). *Shattered assumptions: towards a new psychology of trauma*. New York: The Free Press.

26. Rachman S. (1980). Emotional processing. *Behaviour Research & Therapy* **18**:51–60.

27. Freud S. (1971). *New introductory lectures on psychoanalysis.* (Pelican Freud Library, Vol. 2) Harmondsworth: Penguin (Orginally published 1933).

28. Ehlers A and Steil R. (1995). Maintenance of intrusive memories in posttraumatic stress disorder: a cognitive approach. *Behavioural and Cognitive Psychotherapy* **23**:217–49.

29. Foa EB, Steketee G, and Rothbaum BO. (1989). Behavioral/cognitive conceptualizations of post-traumatic stress disorder. *Behaviour Therapy*, **20**:155–76.

30. Horowitz MJ. (1986). *Stress response syndromes*, 2nd edn. New York: Jason Aronson.

31. Parkes CM. (1988). Bereavement as a psychosocial transition: processes of adaptation to change. *Journal of Social Issues* **44**:53–65.

32. American Psychiatric Association (1994). *Diagnostic and statistical manual of mental disorders: DSM-IV*, 4th edn. Washington, DC: American Psychiatric Association.

33. Baider L and Kaplan De-Nour A. (1997). Psychological distress and intrusive thoughts in cancer patients. *Journal of Nervous and Mental Disease* **185**:346–48.

34. Baum A and Posluszny DM. (2001). Traumatic stress as a target for intervention with cancer patients. In: A Baum and BL Anderson (ed.), *Psychosocial interventions for cancer*, Washington, DC: American Psychological Association.

35. Deimling GT, Kahana B, Bowman KF, and Schaeffer ML. (2002). Cancer survivorship and psychological distress in later life. *Psycho-Oncology* **11**:479–94.

36. Tedeschi RG, Park CL, and Calhoun LG. (ed.) (1998). *Posttraumatic growth: positive changes in the aftermath of crisis.* Mahwah, NJ: Lawrence Erlbaum Associates.

37. Guibert H. (1991). *A l'Ami qui ne m'a pas Sauve la Vie* (To the friend who did not save my Life). Paris: Editions Flammarion.

38. Cella DF, Mahon SM, and Donovan MI. (1990). Cancer recurrence as a traumatic event. *Behavioral Medicine* **13**:15–22.

39. Leventhal H, Meyer D, and Nerenz D. (1980). The common-sense representation of illness danger. In: S Rachman (ed.), *Contributions to medical psychology*, Vol. 2, New York: Pergamon Press, pp. 7–30.

40. Baider L, Peretz T, and Kaplan De-Nour A. (1993). Holocaust cancer patients: a comparative study. *Psychiatry* **56**:349–55.

41. Lazarus RS and Folkman S. (1984). *Stress appraisal and coping.* New York: Springer.

42. Carver CS, Pozo C, Harris SD, Noriega V, Scheier MF, Robinson DS, *et al.* (1993). How coping mediates the effects of optimism on distress: a study of women with early stage breast cancer. *Journal of Personality and Social Psychological* **65**:375–90.

43. Watson M, Greer S, Rowden L, Gorman C, Robertson B, Bliss J, *et al.* (1991). Relationships between emotional control, adjustment to cancer and depression and anxiety in breast cancer patients. *Psychological Medicine* **21**:51–7.

44. Parle M, Jones B, and Maguire P. (1996). Maladaptive coping and affective disorders among cancer patients. *Psychological Medicine* **26**:735–44.

45. Lam WW and Fielding R. (2003). The evolving experience of illness for Chinese women with breast cancer: a qualitative study. *Psycho-Oncology* **12**:127–140.

46. Noyes R and Holt CS and Massie MJ. (1998). Anxiety disorders. In: JC Holland (ed.), *Psychooncology*, Oxford: Oxford University Press.

47. Stark GPH and House A. (2000). Anxiety in cancer patients. *British Journal of Cancer* **83**:1261–7.

48. Chaturvedi SK. (1991). What's important for quality of life to Indians – in relation to cancer. *Social Science and Medicine* **33**:91–4.

49. Heaven C and Maguire P. (2003). Communication issues. In: M Lloyd-Williams (ed.), *Psychosocial issues in palliative care*, Oxford: Oxford University Press.

50. Sue DW and Sue D. (1990). *Counseling the culturally different: theory and practice*, 2nd edn. New York: Wiley. Cited in Enelow AJ, Forde DL, Brummel-Smith K. (1996). *Interviewing and patient Care*, 4th edn, Oxford: Oxford University Press.

51. Cox GR. (2002). North American native care of the dying and grieving. In: JD Morgan and P Laungani (ed.), *Death and bereavement around the world volume 1: major religious traditions*, Amityville, NY: Baywood Publishing Co.

52. Austin JT and Vancouver JB. (1996). Goal constructs in psychology: structure, process, and content. *Psychological Bulletin* **120**:338–75.

53. Tennen H and Affleck G. (1998). Personality and transformation. In: RG Tedeschi, CL Park, and LG Calhoun (ed.), *Posttraumatic growth: positive changes in the aftermath of crisis.* Mahwah, NJ: Lawrence Erlbaum Associates.

54. Nerenz DR and Leventhal H. (1983). Self-regulation theory in chronic illness. In: TG Burish and LA Bradley (ed.), *Coping with chronic disease: research and applications*, London: Academic Press.

55. Frank-Stromberg M, Wright PS, Segalla M, and Diekmann J. (1984). Psychological impact of the "cancer" diagnosis. *Oncology Nursing Forum,* **11**:16–22.

56. Dunkel-Schetter C, Feinstein L, Taylor SE, and Falke RL .(1992). Patterns of coping with cancer. *Health Psychology* **11**:79–87.

57. Beck AT. (1967). *Depression: clinical, experimental, and theoretical aspects.* New York: Harper and Row.

58. Nunn K. (1996). Personal hopefulness: a conceptual review of the relevance of the perceived future to psychiatry. *British Journal of Medical Psychology,* **69**:227–45.

59. Csikszentmihalyi M and Csikszentmihalyi IS. (1988). *Optimal experience: psychological studies of flow in consciousness.* Cambridge: Cambridge University Press.

60. Dew AM, Bromet EJ, and Penkower L. (1992). Mental health effects of job loss in women. *Psychological Medicine* **22**:751–64.

61. Street H. (2003). The psychosocial impact of cancer: exploring relationships between conditional goal setting and depression. *Psycho-Oncology* **12**:580–9.

62. Zemore R, Rinholm J, Shepel LF, and Richards M. (1989). Some social and emotional consequences of breast cancer and mastectomy: a content analysis of 87 interviews. *Journal of Psychosocial Oncology* **7**:33–45.

63. Wallston BS, Alagna SW, DeVellis BM, and DeVellis RF. (1983). Social support and physical health. *Health Psychology* **2**:367–91.

64. Helgeson VS and Cohen S. (1996). Social support and adjustment to cancer. *Health Psychology* **15**:135–48.

65. Northouse LL, Dorris G, and Charron-Moore C. (1995). Factors affecting couples' adjustment to recurrent breast cancer. *Social Science and Medicine* **42**:69–76.

66. Gritz ER, Wellisch DK, Siau J, and Wang H-J. (1990). Long-term effects of testicular cancer on marital relationships. *Psychosomatics* **31**:301–12.

67. Andrykowski MA, Brady MJ, and Hunt JW. (1993). Positive psychological adjustment in potential bone marrow transplant recipients: cancer as a psychosocial transition. *Psycho-Oncology* **2**:261–76.

68. Pistrang N and Barker C. (1995). The partner relationship in psychological response to breast cancer. *Social Science and Medicine* **40**:789–97.

69. Curbow B, Somerfield M, Legro M, and Sonnega J. (1990). Self-concept and cancer in adults: theoretical and methodological issues. *Social Science and Medicine* **31**:115–28.

70. Mirowsky J and Ross CE. (1989). *Social causes of psychological distress.* New York: Aldine de Gruyter.

71. Janis IL, Rodin J. (1979). Attribution, control, and decision making: social psychology and health care. In: GC Stone, F Cohen, and NE Adler (ed.), *Health psychology*, San Francisco: Jossey-Bass.

72. Williams J and Koocher GP. (1998). Addressing loss of control in chronic illness: theory and practice. *Psychotherapy* **35**:325–35.

73. Bowlby J. (1979). *The making and breaking of affectional bonds.* London: Tavistock Publications.

74. Moos RH. (1986). *Coping with life crisis: an integrated approach.* New York: Plenum Press.

75. Taylor SE and Brown JD. (1988). Illusion and well-being: a social psychological perspective on mental health. *Psychological Bulletin,* **103**:193–210.

76. Somerfield MR, Stefanek ME, Smith TJ, and Padberg JJ. (1999). A systems model for adaptation to somatic distress among cancer survivors. *Psycho-oncology* **8**:334–43.

77. Maltby J, Lewis CA, and Day L. (1999). Religious orientation and psychological well-being: the role of the frequency of personal prayer. *British Journal of Health Psychology* **4**:363–78.

78. Reissman CK. (1990). Strategic uses of narrative in the presentation of self and illness: a research note. S*ocial Science and Medicine* **30**:1195–200.

79. Russell RL and van den Broek P. (1992). Changing narrative schemas in psychotherapy. *Psychotherapy* **29**:344–54.

80. Holmes J. (1998). Narrative in psychotherapy. In: T Greenhalgh and B Hurwitz. (ed.), *Narrative based medicine: dialogue and discourse in clinical practice*, London: BMJ Books.

81. Mahoney MJ. (1995). Emotionality and health: lessons from and for psychotherapy. In: JW Pennebaker (ed.), *Emotion, disclosure and health*, Washington: American Psychological Association.

82. Pennebaker JW. (ed.)(1995). *Emotion, disclosure and health*. Washington: American Psychological Association.

83. Wellenkamp J. (1995). Cultural similarities and differences regarding emotional disclosure: some examples from Indonesia and the Pacific. In: JW Pennebaker (ed.), *Emotion, disclosure and health*, Washington: American Psychological Association.

84. Pennebaker JW. (1993). Putting stress into words: health, linguistic, and therapeutic implications. *Behaviour Research and Therapy* **31**:539–48.

85. Smyth JM, Stone AA, Hurewitz A, and Kaell A. (1999). Effects of writing about stressful experiences on symptom reduction in patients with asthma or rheumatoid arthritis. *Journal of the American Medical Association* **281**:1304–9.

86. Greenhalgh T. (1999). Writing as therapy. *British Medical Journal* **319**:270–1.

87. Sampson F. (1999). *The healing word – a practical guide to poetry and personal development activities*. Milton Keynes: The Poetry Society.

88. Porchet-Munro S. (1998). Music therapy. In: D Doyle, GWC Hanks, and N MacDonald (ed.), *Oxford textbook of palliative medicine*, 2nd edn, Oxford: Oxford University Press.

89. Ziesler AA. (1993). Art therapy – a meaningful part of cancer care. *Journal of Cancer Care* **2**:107–11.

90. Cohen SR, Mount BM, and MacDonald N. (1996). Defining quality of life. *European Journal of Cancer Care* **32A**:753–4.

91. World Health Organization. (1946). *Preamble of the constitution of the World Health Organization*. Geneva: WHO.

92. Yates JW, Chalmer B, and McKegney FP. (1980). Evaluation of patients with advanced cancer using the Karnofsky performance status. *Cancer* **45**:2220–4.

93. Donnelly S. (1996). Quality of life assessment in advanced cancer. *Palliative Medicine* **10**:275–83.

94. Cella D. (1998). Quality of life. In: JC Holland (ed.), *Psychooncology*. Oxford: Oxford University Press.

95. Addington-Hall J, and Kalra L. (2001). Who should measure quality of life? *British Medical Journal* **322**:1417–20.

96. Fallowfield L. (1990). *The quality of life*. London: Souvenir Books.

97. Aristotle. (1984). *Nicomachean. Ethics Book 1 Ch.4 1095a, 20–25. In: J Barnes (ed.), *Complete works of Aristotle*, The Revised Oxford Translation, Princeton: OUP.

98. Calman K. (1984). Quality of life in cancer patients – an hypothesis. *Journal of Medical Ethics* **10**:124–27.

99. Culyer AJ. (1990). Commodities, characteristics of commodities, characteristics of people, utilities, and the quality of life. In: S Baldwin, C Godfrey, and C Propper (ed.), *Quality of life: perspectives and policies*, London: Routledge.

100. Kleinman A. (1988). *The illness narratives: suffering, healing and the human condition*. New York: Basic Books.

Chapter 2

Personal context

Changed lives 47
Expectations about Illness. 49
Shock of diagnosis. 51
Denial and avoidance 53
Delays to diagnosis 56
'Why me?'—the meaning of cancer. 57
Coping with treatment 60
Relationship with the healthcare team. 61
Practical concerns 63
Relationships with family and friends. 65
Impact on self. 68
Hope. 71
The body 73
Existential beliefs. 77
Ending treatment. 80
Living with uncertainty 82
References 84

Changed lives

If someone had told me that this time last year I would discover I had breast cancer, I would have thrown up my hands in horror and have said smugly, "Don't be ridiculous. I'm fit and healthy, I'm vegetarian, I don't smoke and only drink the recommended weekly allowance of wine! I run, I have a good job and have done well in my career, I have a family and my outlook on life is positive and it will, well, never happen to me. People like me don't get cancer".

It was a kick in the teeth to discover that in July 1992 I had a malignant lump in my breast – a week later I was experiencing a lumpectomy and the removal of malignant lymph nodes under my arm. Since then when the lump was discovered until now I have been to hell and back and for a long time during chemotherapy I thought that I never would be back. But I am. Well, almost. I am starting work again next week and am at last beginning to live my life once more.

I think that one of the worst aspects of the diagnosis, the operation, chemotherapy, radiotherapy, and convalescence is the feeling that one's life has become out of control. Suddenly, from being a woman who felt so much in control, I became a wreck, with an inability to see the point in anything; out of the blue I wasn't the caring mother, or well-organized teacher, or the person that used to endeavour to be all things to everyone – I was useless, of no use to anyone. I would lie in bed listening to the world carrying on without me, doing the things I used to do, and someone else being the person I used to be. I would scream and scream inside with panic that people should see me now as nothing: wrecked and crippled by cancer, not only in body but in mind too. I became so afraid of dying that it plagued me constantly, but the next minute I would be feeling that I wanted to kill myself. At least if I killed myself then I would be in control of whether I lived or died. As with any life-threatening illness, facing so suddenly the fact that you are not immortal is simply a terrible shock especially when I felt that my life was 'so great!'

But more recently I've realized that my life wasn't actually so great after all. It was to a large extent awful. There I was trying so hard to be super-Mum, super-wife, superwoman in fact. And I realized how addicted I had become to my work – partly because I needed my own identity away from my family but also because I had to prove to someone somewhere that I could do all these things and cope as well. That 'someone somewhere' has turned out to be me, and by getting cancer I felt that I had let myself down and that I really couldn't cope at all.

I know now that I am not going to pretend anymore, and I'm not going to hide my shortcomings or my capabilities but start living my life, however short or long that may be. The thing is not to look back, but to say to oneself:

Don't be afraid your life will end; be afraid it will never begin.[1]

Lucy, Bristol, UK

This chapter looks at the psychosocial impact of cancer from the patient's perspective, and its implications for how healthcare staff can provide optimal supportive care. People have complicated lives, and cancer can intrude on every corner of them. It certainly does not just affect people while they are attending hospitals, although their contact with healthcare professionals is critical to how people with cancer make sense of what is happening to them and how safe they feel. Healthcare staff must therefore have a firm grasp of some of the key concerns and challenges experienced by people with cancer.

Probably the biggest challenge for people with cancer is having to adjust to too many changes at once: the frightening reality of a life-threatening illness, the notoriously exhausting demands of treatment, and the many worrying disruptions to their personal and social lives. As we explored in Chapter 1, having to deal with multiple changes is inherently stressful.

Healthcare environments and procedures are unfamiliar to most people. Thus, one of the most important supportive care roles of all healthcare professionals is to help people make sense of the many confusing and uncertain elements of their medical treatment. By providing patients and their families with preparation, orientation, guidance, information, support, and a coherent 'road map' of their journey through treatment, healthcare staff can enable their patients to reassert control over what is happening to them.

---

[1]This is from a letter, written to the author, by a 40-year-old woman several months after finishing her treatment for cancer.

Throughout the treatment of cancer there is often a balance or tension between different forces within people. For example:

- wanting to keep life the same, as opposed to becoming immersed in the world of one's treatment;
- needing to face the full implications of the diagnosis and prognosis, as opposed to wanting to keep these thoughts at bay;
- needing to depend on others, as opposed to wanting to feel self-reliant and in control;

Every person is a unique combination of these many tensions so to draw anything but general conclusions about 'cancer patients', or to use crude classification systems, runs the risk of simplifying, even diminishing, what is distinctive and exceptional about each person. A more helpful approach we believe is to understand how people adapt to and manage catastrophic change in their lives, the subject of Chapter 1. In this chapter we consider some of the changes and challenges that people with cancer are confronted with.

Everyone approaches cancer with particular beliefs about the illness that they have drawn from the society around them. We therefore start by examining some of the more widely held assumptions that shape people's reactions to cancer. Many of these ideas may be based on out-dated knowledge or 'folklore', but this makes them no less powerful in influencing how people approach their illness.

Expectations about illness

People come to cancer with their own associations and ideas about the disease. Some of these ideas are accurate, and some inaccurate. Some people overvalue and overstate the dangers of cancer, some understate them. But one thing is sure, cancer is understood in varied ways, some of which magnify the patient's distress.

Ironically, the title of this book reflects a common misconception about cancer. The public generally perceives cancer as a single homogenous disease. In reality, there are over 200 classifiable cancers and as many treatment options; moreover, some cancers are much more easily and successfully treated than others. Although it is thought to be highly unlikely that a single answer or magic pill will be found, much of the public is waiting for 'a cure for cancer'.[1]

Cancer is seen as a particularly nasty disease within most cultures, and the very word 'cancer' is unspeakably frightening to many people. It has certainly attracted some unpleasant imagery. Common images of cancer—a growth within the body, a long wasting disease, one's own body destroying itself, a painful end—are echoes of the origins of the word 'cancer'. Derived from the Latin word for crab, from the ancient Greeks onward, cancer was believed to creep up sideways through the body, holding on tenaciously to its victim. Diseases that have had no obvious identifiable cause (e.g. leprosy, tuberculosis, bubonic plague) have historically provoked mystery, not to say mysticism, among the population, as people have attempted to attribute a cause.[2] Sin has been one such cause within Judeo-Christian culture; illness has often been viewed as a punishment (divine retribution) for sinful behaviour or sinful thoughts,[3] shame being the primary mark of stigma. These days, popular culture in the West tends to ascribe more secular causes for cancer, but often on the basis of no better evidence: sugar substitutes, bruises, microwave ovens, stress, spicy food, breast-feeding, germs, etc.

Even as recently as the beginning of the twentieth century, the diagnosis of cancer was a definitive death sentence and caused the person to be 'stigmatized, isolated, and humiliated, a fate similar to that of persons with leprosy and syphilis. Most people feared that cancer was contagious also,[4] (Holland 1998, p. 4). It is little wonder that cancer was rarely discussed in public (except by euphemism—a 'lingering illness'), and frank diagnoses were rarely given (again, except by euphemism—'a growth'). In many parts of the world this continues to be the norm, perhaps reflecting the quality of available healthcare. Some of the varied social conditions through which cancer is experienced are discussed in Chapter 4.

Public perception also changes with the age of the person who has cancer. Although around half of the people who die of cancer in the UK are over 75 years old, the proportion of all deaths is more conspicuous among those who are younger. Among women aged 45, for example, roughly 50 per cent of all deaths are from cancer. By the time women are 60, this proportion has dropped to under 30 per cent.[5] These younger deaths are often perceived to be more tragic because of the years of life lost and because of the role of these women within their family, where there will often be dependant children. At any rate, the public tends to overestimate the deaths that cancer does cause.[6]

In summary, the culture in which people spend their lives is fundamental to how they make sense of serious illnesses like cancer. For example, the common anxiety among older people in the West about becoming 'a burden' and losing one's autonomy is less pronounced in cultures where older people are more valued and where the family holds more significance than the individual.[7] Consider a few cultural views about illness (while remembering that a general tendency within a culture does not mean that a particular individual within it necessarily conforms to its 'norms'):

The indigenous Aboriginal people of Australia greatly fear illness of any sort and believe it to be the result of a spell cast by a medicine man in retribution for a slight or wrong-doing. The diagnosis of illness therefore carries the implication of sorcery for the individual and their family. The majority of indigenous people however, prefer to die in hospital since it is customary for the family to have to move away from the place where the death occurred. Hospitalization therefore averts this huge upheaval for the rest of the family[8].

In Japan, where revealing the diagnosis of cancer is not usual practice,[9] patients often receive active treatment up to the end of their lives. In one survey, 80% of patients who became suspicious of the diagnosis they had been given chose not to ask further questions. The remaining 20% who did ask questions often became irritated by the evasiveness of the answers they received.[10] In 1992 over 93% of cancer patients in Japan died in an institution.

Among traditional sub-Saharan Africans, someone who is guilty of misbehaviour is thought to have become vulnerable to evil forces (and consequently illness) because they lose the protection of their disappointed ancestors. However, the entire village community is expected to visit the sick patient, not just the patient's extended family. Hospitals are associated with places where people die and most traditional people will only accept admission after first consulting their traditional healer.[11]

A telephone survey of over 1000 households in southeastern United States found that nearly 90% believed in religious miracles, 80% believed that God acts through medical doctors to cure sickness, and almost 60% believed that God's will was a factor in the healing process when they are ill. Nonetheless, despite doctors being seen as instruments of God's will, American doctors rarely engage in spiritual discussions with their patients.[12]

Among Hong Kong Chinese women the loss of a breast from cancer is often less stigmatizing than the loss of hair, weight gain, or facial changes, largely because the former can be hidden while the latter cannot. The social pressure in Chinese communities, steeped in Confucianism, to avoid being seen as different is matched by a corresponding obligation to stay healthy and keep the body undamaged, lest it bring bad luck to the family. Disease thus carries a moral imperative and the threat of social exclusion.[13]

Shock of diagnosis

> No news, however awful it may be, will ever give me the dreadful fright I got when I was told I had cancer. Something in the depths of my heart has turned into stone.

The diagnosis of cancer may be expected. It may have been the result of routine cancer screening or the investigation of some other ailment. After some months of uncertainty, it may even represent something of a relief to have a diagnosis. For some patients there may be no apparent symptoms at all. But, regardless of how it comes about, cancer continues to represent a probable death sentence in the minds of most people. The meaning of a cancer diagnosis is therefore inextricably bound up for the patient and family with issues of prognosis. This is even more likely to be the case when a recurrence of the condition is diagnosed, an event that is rated by patients as even more upsetting than the initial diagnosis.[14] But unless the person is fully expecting it to be cancer, the diagnosis is almost always a chilling shock.

On hearing the word 'cancer', most people seem to hear the word 'death'. Even where a person can be reassured that a cure or long-term remission is likely, death is no longer an abstract moment to be faced on some distant future day, it becomes a very real and imminent possibility. The spectre of one's mortality can cause such shock as to shove predictable, everyday reality to the side.

> It felt like a bad dream. One minute life was chuntering on. The next – well, someone switched the reels, the road forked and I didn't notice. Somewhere, in some parallel universe, life was continuing to chunter on…

The words 'surreal', 'nightmare', or 'bad dream' often arise when people describe the day of their diagnosis. The other common word is 'fear'. All the assumptions and expectations about cancer that the person has acquired become active. Here's how the American Tour-de-France multiple-winner Lance Armstrong described it:

> I thought I knew what fear was, until I heard the words You have cancer. Real fear came with an unmistakable sensation: it was as though all my blood started flowing in the wrong direction. My previous fears, fear of not being liked, fear of being laughed at, fear of losing my money, suddenly seemed like small cowardices.
>
>   Everything now stacked up differently: the anxieties of life – a flat tire, losing my career, a traffic jam – were reprioritized into need versus want, real problem as opposed to minor scare. A bumpy plane ride was just a bumpy plane ride, it wasn't cancer.[15]
>
> (Armstrong 2001, p. 73)

These quotes poignantly convey how the diagnosis of cancer can often be psychologically and socially traumatizing. By using the term 'traumatic', however, we are not implying a diagnosis of post-traumatic stress disorder (PTSD), though increasingly this label is being applied to people with cancer.[16] But we are suggesting that similar processes are at work, whether or not the person is diagnosed with PTSD (*see* Chapter 1).

Traumatic events are traumatic not just because they are sudden and unexpected and result in a dramatic loss of control and safety. Traumatic experiences also involve a form of mental disorientation—the failure of existing assumptions about the world to make sense of what is happening. There is an unreal, dreamlike quality to unfolding reality. Worst-case nightmare scenarios are *actually* happening and none of the assumptions of one's mental maps seem adequate to predict what will happen next or how one should behave. There is often a psychological 'distance' (dissociation) from what seems to be happening. The road of predictable daily life 'forks', and the person is thrown into 'a parallel universe' where little seems to be the same or predictable. An intense rush of fear floods through the individual as they contemplate a very real threat to their lives and to the lives of loved ones. All of a sudden, everything 'stacks up differently'.

In situations of high stress, short-term memory and concentration become poor and people have difficulty absorbing new information. People often remember words that hold particular meaning for them.

> Some words are etched on your gut as you hear them, others you simply can't take in. It is good and necessary advice to have someone with you at moments like this, just so they can tell you what you heard.

Most people soon release some of the shock through crying. Yet for others, shock can lead to an apparent shutting down of emotion—the person feels numb and cut off from their feelings, even surprized by their own calmly rational response. This is a form of psychological distancing from the full impact of the news, keeping the overwhelming information at bay until the person is ready to absorb it. Another common response to serious shock is for people to become apathetic and compliant with a child-like dependency on others.[17] Indeed, various authors have noted that at times of crisis people are more likely to turn to 'parental' figures of authority for safety and guidance.[18, 19]

Here is how a 22-year-old woman remembered her brain cancer diagnosis earlier in the year:

> The worst thing was turning to my mother and saying 'I don't want this to be happening' and seeing her crying and realising she was feeling completely helpless to do anything.

These initial alarm reactions can last minutes or hours, though the dissociated dream-like state can sometimes go on for days as the person acclimatizes to their new 'parallel universe'. The intense fear felt by patients and their families, however, abates more slowly, mostly in response to the information and care they receive from the medical team.

The process of diagnosis, moreover, is not always a smooth or linear process. It can often be a chaotic time and involve a number of uncomfortable and intrusive tests, some of which have to be repeated. Diagnosis becomes especially complex and protracted when there are several different professionals involved, different hospital departments and even different institutions.[20] A roller-coaster of good and bad news, or a demoralizing sequence of 'more bad news', seems to define the early days of some patients' cancer experience.

Throughout, the patient and their loved ones are adjusting to the changing reality of their situation, the uncertainty of the prognosis, the demands of treatment and the many other changes that have to be confronted during the months which follow. The rest of this chapter is about some of these changes.

Denial and avoidance

> I try not to think too much about the situation, and I find that when I read a book about the specific subject I tend to find that my sprits fall significantly. I can only conclude that the more I discover about it, the less confident I feel about making a full recovery. Sometimes ignorance is bliss. A couple of weeks ago G. [husband] got quite angry with me because it transpired that I had not absorbed some very important details that Mr. W. [surgeon] had told me in the hospital i.e. that I had grade 3 cancer (the most aggressive strain). G. was telling me off for not asking more questions etc, but it occurred to me afterwards that perhaps I had somehow chosen not to acknowledge the information, or perhaps I had not realized the significance of it, as if my mind was putting up some kind of defence in a subconscious manner.

The diagnosis of cancer has so many implications and violates so many deeply held assumptions that a retreat into some form of temporary denial and avoidance is normal and adaptive. Preferring not to talk about it, read about, or even think about cancer is a way of keeping it at bay. Knowing that one's illness is incurable, or that life-expectancy is probably shorter than one assumed, is difficult news for anyone to absorb. It is therefore essential that healthcare staff do not automatically assume that denial is pathological. Psychological defences are always there for a reason.

As described in Chapter 1, denial and avoidance are common mental defences towards information that is unacceptably different from the expectations or assumptions that people hold about the world. Denial and avoidance and other defence mechanisms allow information to be filtered more slowly so that the person can maintain a coherent picture of the world around them while they slowly absorb the new information. This may even temporarily keep distress and anxiety at relatively low levels. Some authors have argued that denial, or perhaps more accurately disavowal, acts like a 'cover story'[21] to take the place of the traumatic information that is being gradually and privately absorbed. Avery Weisman expressed it like this:

> Denial is how one simplifies the complexity of life … It revises or reinterprets a portion of painful reality, avoiding what it threatens to be, and holding fast to the image of what has been.[22]
> (Weisman, 1979, p. 44)

There is a paradoxical quality to denial—to deny something implies that it carries a threat and is therefore already 'known'. In fact, some people are curiously aware of their own mental avoidance strategies. For example, one woman attended the hospital alone thinking she had simply cracked a rib when bending down. She was shocked to be diagnosed with bone metastases from an unknown primary. She later said:

> The first couple of days I suppose I knew I was in denial. I talked about it as if it was someone else; I didn't really feel much.

Note that she states that she 'knew' she was 'in denial', and not feeling anything, and implies that she knew this response was somehow inappropriate to the situation. In fact, she was more concerned about her husband who had had a heart attack the previous year. She left the clinic and calmly phoned her husband's supervisor at work, explained the situation to him and arranged for her husband to be driven home. She became aware of her feelings two days later at around 4.00 am when she awoke in terror from dreams of funerals and people crying.

Denial is rarely an all-or-nothing behaviour, even when it persists. There are often fluctuations between acceptance of the diagnosis or prognosis and denial of it, a situation that has been called 'middle knowledge'.[22] Thus, people often hold contradictory beliefs. For example, a patient in hospital who has been told he has only a few weeks to live may appear to be in denial when he tells the nurse that he is looking forward to getting back to work in his treasured garden. But a few minutes later, given a different context, he may be prepared to talk about his fears of dying. Similarly, a person may refuse to accept the fact that they have cancer, or they may accept the diagnosis but deny its implications, or they may be dissociated from their own distress.

> Results next week, plus x rays, bone scan … the wheels are in motion and we are being swept along. When will it end? I'm shaking all over again and my heart is about to burst out of

my rib cage. Why am I like this? I still can't honestly believe that I have cancer. It is like being in a bubble. I am floating along in my protected, remote environment whilst all these things are happening in another dimension, called reality.

Denial and avoidance become a problem largely when they complicate communication with other people. When a patient or any other member of the family avoids talking about the illness, others become concerned that he or she may be suffering in silence, and other family members may become worried about saying the wrong thing. As a result, family communication can become strained and inhibited. Likewise, healthcare staff who wish to progress their treatment plans, may feel disabled or awkward in their communication with a patient in denial. Perhaps most difficult are the occasions when a patient's life is coming to an end and the family are unable to discuss important issues affecting all of them.

There are times when denial causes significant difficulties and compromizes the best interests of the patient. When a patient's denial leads them to neglect their illness such that it compromizes their prognosis, or when it serves to alienate people to the extent that the patient becomes socially isolated, then some form of intervention is desirable (*see* Chapter 6—Working with Someone in Denial).

Finally, there are many forms of denial and avoidance. For example, 'being positive' is obviously a valid and helpful strategy for dealing with cancer, *provided* it is sufficiently permeable. However, unwavering 'positive thinking' is often a way of avoiding certain thoughts and feelings, and can cause communication difficulties for loved ones who may need to discuss possible outcomes in the future. The reason for its popularity lies in the comfort it provides. Like any faith, 'positive thinking' gives people a source of hope and structure, as well as something they can actively do to increase their chances of salvation. Above all, the culture of 'positive thinking' prevents the discussion of unpleasant 'what-if' scenarios set in the future—in fact, the act of making contingency plans is characterized as 'thinking negatively'. Positive thinking, when taken too far, prevents the expression of legitimate feelings such as sadness and anger, unhelpfully burying these important emotions.

Healthcare implications

- For most people, denial and avoidance are temporary ways of reducing the distress of bad news. They serve to filter new information by slowing down its absorption. They should therefore be thought of as largely normal defence mechanisms that will diminish in time.

- Psychological defence mechanisms are there for a good reason and should not be challenged directly. Rather, one should start by asking the patient what they understand about their current situation, offering opportunities for them to examine different feelings or thoughts they may be having about it. If people feel they are being listened to by someone who cares, they are more likely to explore a wider range of concerns and possibilities.

- When denial persists and interferes with the patient's health or relationships, some form of intervention may be necessary (*see* Chapter 6).

Delays to diagnosis

People's assumptions about illnesses such as cancer influence how they react to 'symptoms' and the meaning they give to them. Although not a widely researched topic, many people spend a lot of time thinking about how their cancer came to light. Finding a lump on the body while washing; feeling a persistent pain; having a dry cough; feeling perfectly well but attending a cancer screening clinic—these are all very different pathways to the shock of diagnosis. A lump in the breast may alarm some women enough to consult a doctor, but for others it may mean nothing. Alternatively, the lump may be so threatening for some women as to leave them paralysed with fear, causing them to delay seeking any form of medical advice until they are forced to. Likewise, our feelings about various parts of the body (lung, breast, stomach, prostate) influence how we view illness or damage to such organs and the way we expect them to be medically treated.[23]

> The terror was the constant return to mind of the memories of the three months preceding the diagnosis and the utterly obsessive and compulsive trap they set me, as I would revisit, time and time again, what I could have done differently to speed up my diagnosis and so get the cancer [diagnosis] earlier.

Many patients feel regret, anger, and guilt about delays to the diagnosis, whether because they ignored the symptoms, did not notice them, or were too frightened to respond to them. 'Why didn't I go to the doctor earlier?' is a common source of anguish. But in many instances the delay is not caused by the patient but by the healthcare service. General practitioners see thousands of patients a year and act as gatekeepers to hospital-based specialists. In the UK, for example, between 10% and 15% of GP consultations result in a referral to a specialist. Inevitably their gate-keeping can sometimes be too stringent and the consequence of this is that patients are not referred to specialists as quickly as they should be. Moreover, some cancers are difficult to diagnose either because they masquerade as other diseases, are particularly rare, or the patient has other medical conditions that complicate the picture. Diagnostic delays caused by family doctors or hospitals in the UK are largely undocumented though in one interview study of more than 400 cancer patients over 30 per cent reported delays.[24]

Although short delays in the commencement of treatment may often be *clinically* unimportant in the view of healthcare personnel, they are often *experienced* by patients as diminishing their chances of survival. Anger towards family and hospital doctors may not be surprising, but it should not be dismissed as 'understandable.' Some delays are indeed due to medical negligence.

Finally, as already mentioned, the diagnosis of some cancers can be difficult to establish and the process becomes protracted. Patients and their families describe this as being like an emotional roller-coaster, usually with emotional exhaustion and hopelessness being the end of the ride:

> Why is it all happening to us? When life can't seem to get any worse, it does. One day it seems like good news and the next it's bad. I don't think we can take much more of this.

Healthcare implications

- Patients who are concerned about their own delay in reporting symptoms may find it helpful to talk through these concerns with someone knowledgeable who can correct any misconceptions regarding the significance of short delays.

- Where there has been a significant delay, the healthcare professional should listen and acknowledge the patient's concern and provide them with information concerning common avenues of complaint and litigation, as required. At the same time they should be helping to reorient the patient towards positive treatment goals.

- Patients and their families should be given opportunities, if desired, to question their doctors regarding the events leading to their diagnosis. While doctors may fear litigation, many patients appreciate openness and honesty about the reasons for delays (*see* Chapter Six—Angry, Difficult, or Disliked Patients).

- Those who have been through any form of protracted process of diagnosis are likely to become emotionally exhausted. Additional emotional support should be offered wherever possible.

- People with persistent intrusive guilty ruminations about delays may require assessment by a psychosocial specialist.

'Why me?'—the meaning of cancer

Wanting to find a cause for things that happen to us is part of our instinctive need to learn from experience[25] (*see* Chapter 1). If a plane crashes, accident investigators go to extraordinary lengths to find the cause, with the obvious aim of preventing it from happening again. So it is with people generally. Catastrophic events require an explanation, and people invariably find them. In one study, 95% of the breast cancer patients interviewed offered an explanation for why their cancer had occurred,[26] (though other studies have reported lower figures.[27]) Such attributions have been shown to lead people to change their behaviour (e.g. a healthier diet) in order to achieve a sense of control over the disease, and a *break* with what is perceived to have been unhealthy about their past lifestyle.[26]

> A lot of the summer was spent with questions. For example, was my cancer meaningful? (I mean given to me. The effect of a cause. In which case was it my fault? What if it were a punishment, or simply the inevitable end of my lifestyle ... Had I really been so much more

out of line than other people?) Or was it meaningless? In which case, what was the point in anything?

The difficulty with cancer is that, unless someone has clearly engaged in risky behaviour (e.g. smoking), been exposed to a known carcinogen, or has a genetic risk that can be established, there is very little that medicine can tell them about why they developed their particular cancer. Clinical medicine is probably less interested in discussing the causes of chronic illness than in what it can do to treat the particular condition.[20] General explanations to do with accumulative genetic damage, oncogenes, mutations, etc. rarely suffice. Most people are looking for precise explanations that relate to themselves personally, and when doctors are unable to furnish these reasons, patients often look elsewhere. And in the context of ambiguity and uncertainty, people are particularly susceptible to believing what they find.[18]

Every society abounds with folklore concerning the causes of illness, and these ideas vary from culture to culture. The West has seen a myriad popular theories for cancer, including stress, personality, diet, emotional repression, weakened immune system, bad or negative thinking, and so on. Coupled with the view that 90% of cancers are caused by factors under people's direct control,[28] such theories put the burden of responsibility for getting cancer squarely on the patient. The culture of the West perhaps 'encourages us to think that the correct attitude of mind, diet, or exercise gives us control over our bodies, to remain healthy and alive[23] (Altschuler 1997, p. 10). In the context of these social beliefs in personal responsibility, self-questioning can easily result in self-blame. Guilt is a precursor to depressed mood. Little wonder that 'Why me?' questions have been linked to greater distress, at least among women with breast cancer soon after their diagnosis.[27]

> That one might die because of – say, moving house and therefore to a new GP surgery and landing accidentally amidst crap doctors didn't really fit in with my idea of a meaningful life. How haphazard and risky did that make things? Your life hanging on such arbitrary threads. That a missed chance to see a consultant or a failure to describe my pain well enough might be the reason I would die …

Asking 'Why me?' assumes a rational cause-and-effect world in which catastrophes do not fall arbitrarily on victims. It is a question that, in the light of no answers, becomes a rhetorical statement of protest, an existential injustice. However, while people with cancer often suppress these feelings of fury, they are commonly exhorted to 'fight' their cancer as a way of surviving it. For many the fight against their illness does become the central motif of their cancer story. But not everyone wants to be in a fighting mood to cope with cancer.

> M. [daughter] directed me to an article in the Sunday Times magazine yesterday. It was about a woman who had had a lumpectomy. The title of the article was something like 'Fighting Fit'. This business of Fighting is something I cannot take on. I am not in the mood for a fight. Equally I do not hope to go under with cancer particularly. I feel gentle towards myself – I have no anger, not at the cancer, not at anything really. The cancer is part of me and as such must be dealt with.

Many people attribute their cancer to stressful events in their recent past, such as a bereavement though, despite its intuitive appeal, there is little scientific evidence linking stressful life events with cancer or disease progression.[29, 30] Likewise, despite claims that personality can contribute to the development of breast cancer, the evidence strongly suggests that it does not.[31, 32] Some people attribute the cause of their cancer to a form of punishment, or divine retribution, for past misdeeds (as we have seen, this may be the prevailing view within some cultures). For others, cancer may be a catalyst to re-examine guilty feelings from the past, but in any event, ruminating about such causes can result in regret, guilt, and despair. Guilt, of course, extends to behaviour that may indeed have contributed to the cancer (smoking being the obvious example) so it is important that healthcare professionals are careful to avoid contributing to the patient's sense of self-blame.

> I hate not being in control of my health, having always tried to live healthily and keep fit. I resent that it didn't prevent this happening, even though I know it is probably just bad luck.

In summary, searching for causes is a normal response in the face of catastrophic events, such as cancer. However, this search for meaning can lead people to draw unhelpful or self-destructive conclusions: e.g. guilt and regret regarding one's past life. On the other hand, the purpose of questions like 'Why me?' is to regain a sense of control over one's life, especially the disease, and this process can sometimes lead to positive personal changes (*see* Chapter 1).

Healthcare implications

- Research suggests that the majority of people with cancer want to understand why they developed the disease. Clear information as to the causes of cancer, such as there is, may help prevent people from reaching unhelpful conclusions which can cause entirely unnecessary distress. It also serves to rectify popular misconceptions about cancer causation (e.g. that stress causes cancer).

- However unjustified they may seem to others, people's attributions for having developed cancer can cause significant distress (e.g. suppressed anger, guilt, depression). An opportunity to explore these thoughts and feelings can help people derive a more constructive meaning from their cancer, such as a chance for personal development or a healthier lifestyle.

- Healthcare staff should be sensitive to any guilt that patients may be feeling regarding previous behaviour which may have put them at increased risk of cancer (e.g. smoking), and not add to it by implying any level of blame.

- Providing patients with practical ways (healthy eating, relaxation, gentle exercise, etc.) in which they can contribute to their own treatment and recovery enables people with cancer to assume a sense of control over their lives (without necessarily having to assume a 'fighting' posture).

Coping with treatment

The period between diagnosis and the start of treatment is a hugely stressful time for many people with cancer.[33] However, patients and their families have barely had time to absorb the implications of the diagnosis, before they are plunged into their cancer treatment. In fact, surgery is sometimes offered before a definitive diagnosis is established, and the start of treatment can become enmeshed with and complicated by the process of diagnosis.[20]

The rapid start of treatment is a mixed blessing, for while most people are relieved to get their treatment underway (and their cancer 'out'), the rapidity of the changes can be overwhelming. For example, a preliminary study has found that women who obtained their breast cancer diagnosis on the same day as their diagnostic investigations become more depressed two months later than those who were forced to wait six days for their diagnosis.[34] Thus, the clinician's well-meaning desire to start treatment as soon as possible should be tempered by the need for patients and their families to feel ready, prepared, and in control of unfolding events. When events are perceived to be uncontrollable, they are more likely to be experienced as stressful.[35]

> My main distress came from the feeling that I was trapped by events and that nothing could give me back my physical integrity as a person or speed my recovery – I just had to accept help and my frailty, and be patient.

The start of treatment represents a comprehensive break with the normal routines of everyday life. Ordinary expectations of daily life are replaced with anxious uncertainty, and trying not to worry about the unthinkable. All that the patient knows is that months of notoriously demanding cancer treatment are about to begin, but without any certainty of cure. For those with recurrent illness, restarting treatment represents even more uncertainty at a time when they may be feeling despair and disappointment. Hospitalization is particularly stressful: the individual is away from home, is forced to meet many new people, has to eat and sleep in an unfamiliar environment without much privacy, and faces the uncertain prospect of painful, unpleasant, or even life-threatening procedures. The public's beliefs about some of these treatments (e.g. chemotherapy) tend to be more negative than those of people who have actually experienced them.[36] However, if information is offered in a caring and supportive way, the individual can begin to predict more accurately what is about to happen, uncertainties can be reduced, and anxiety diminished. Information provides some measure of control, as does active collaboration in treatment plans, though people vary to as to how much information or collaboration they want.

Surgery, radiotherapy, chemotherapy, and hormone therapies are the main treatments offered to cancer patients. All of these are associated with unpleasant side-effects and other implications and these are discussed in Chapter 5.

Healthcare implications

- Medical treatment should always be *offered* to patients, rather than imposed upon them (*see* Chapter 6). This entails careful explanation and guidance through each step of the proposed treatment. The process should be experienced as a negotiation (i.e. two-way communication) which does not leave the patient feeling they must 'take it or leave it', but enables the patient to retain as much control over decisions as they wish. Too often treatment calendars (e.g. a course of radiotherapy) are made to suit the needs of institutions and professionals rather than the needs of individuals. Again, this should ideally be a process of negotiation rather than imposition.

- It is easy for professionals who work in medical settings to forget just how unfamiliar and daunting these settings are to people who may never have been seriously ill before in their lives. Health professionals are often perceived to be intimidating yet it is they who create the context for the treatment that is to follow. Sensitive communication and awareness of the patient's apprehensions should be routine practice in preparing people for treatment.

- If patients have a clear rationale and understanding of why they are being offered a particular treatment, why it needs to be delivered in the way it is, and what it is likely to feel like, they are more likely to feel a sense of control over future events and be less stressed by them. Although patients differ in terms of how much information they desire, easy *access* to intelligible information is the key issue.

- A key worker (such as a specialist nurse), or a trained volunteer, should provide an orientation for new patients. A process of orientation to new hospital settings (wards, departments, treatment settings) is essential in order to reduce ambiguity and the awkwardness of not knowing what one is supposed to do or where to go.

Relationship with the healthcare team

(see Chapter 6—Staff–Patient Relationships)

People are not patients except to healthcare professionals. However, terms like 'patient' and 'doctor' carry with them widely-held assumptions about who does what to whom, who is the provider and who the recipient, who has authority and power, and who does not. People internalize these assumptions from the society around them and bring them to their consultations with doctors or patients. Furthermore, patients usually meet professionals on 'professional territory' (e.g. hospital) that is unfamiliar and intimidating and this reinforces their lack of control.

In the world of cancer care, patients rightly see doctors and other healthcare staff as being potential life-savers and such professionals are generally given due respect for this. But there is more to this relationship. At times of crisis and uncertainty, people are particularly receptive to outside influences,[18] and tend to turn to people who, like parents, can provide guidance and safety.[19] Patients consciously and unconsciously *depend* upon medical staff to care for them, alleviate their symptoms, and save their lives. Professionals provide patients with safety by appearing to be in control of the situation.[37] For some people, however, this dependency on healthcare staff can lead to passivity and compliance. Conversely, as recently as the 1970s clinicians rated 'good' patients as those who are indeed passive and accepting, while 'bad' patients tend to be those who wish to become more involved and informed,[38] so the relationship may be more reciprocal than it first appears.

> I do NOT understand why clothes – all of them – are unceremoniously whipped off the moment ANY treatment is required. I find it so annoying as I clutch feebly at the flapping, vanishing sheets! It seems so absolutely unimportant to everyone else and indicates a complete absence of any wish to empathize.

The very act of presenting oneself as a 'cancer patient' carries the risk of losing one's identity as a normal person with rights and responsibilities. The cost of greater dependence on others is the risk of feeling more helpless and less able to exert control over one's own life. A belief in personal control is vital to an adult's sense of safety, dignity, and self-esteem, and where it is compromized there is more likely to be anxiety and depression.[39] Moreover, some people have a strong need to be active and independent at all times. For such people, the experience of being cared for as a hospital patient can feel intolerable.[40]

   The doctor must be constantly exploring this tension between the patient's need to depend on them for their safety and the patient's need to be in control over their lives. Not all patients want to exercize control over medical decision-making and, similarly, not all patients want to be fully informed about their prognosis, preferring to leave these aspects of control with the medical team. But many do. However, during medical consultations, between half and three-quarters of medical patients who want more information simply do not ask for it,[41] while patients often tell members of the healthcare team different things depending on the interest shown by the staff in the past.[42] Therefore, unless healthcare staff encourage open communication, their patients are unlikely to share their views and concerns.

Healthcare implications

- Patients begin their cancer treatment at a time of high stress and uncertainty. They look to the healthcare team to save or prolong their lives, and therefore have a dependent relationship with them. This places a responsibility on healthcare staff to 'contain' (i.e. hold onto and respond to) these feelings while using every opportunity to share control and information with the patient, as and when they are willing to take it.

- Doctors can provide a sense of safety and hope by showing that they have the resources (knowledge, expertize, a clear treatment plan, etc.) to respond to the illness, and will be an unwavering source of support during this frightening and uncertain time. But this 'strength' of leadership must not be at the expense of patients feeling they have lost control over what is happening to them. This tension over who assumes control differs from patient to patient, and changes over the course of the treatment (i.e. as patients feel less, or more, threatened by the illness).

- Patients can exercise control in different ways. Where there are genuine treatment choices to be made, many but not all patients will want to make them. A sense of collaboration with the medical team from the start enables people to feel that they are not merely passive recipients of treatment, but are respected for their own views and participation.

- Being given an active role (e.g. healthy diet, exercise, stress management techniques) in their treatment is another way for patients to assume a sense of control. This approach has been sorely lacking in conventional medicine and is thought to be one of the key attractions of complementary therapies.[43] Accordingly, it has been speculated that taking tamoxifen may serve to protect women from symptoms of post-traumatic stress[44] by giving them something active to do for themselves.

- Providing information about patient rights and responsibilities is yet another method of ensuring that healthcare does not encourage passivity. Leaflets which encourage people to prepare questions prior to consultations with their doctors (Chapter 6), with tips on how to be assertive, may help people regain a sense of control. Models of patient advocacy are also designed to achieve this end (*see* Chapter 7).

Practical concerns

Along the coast of the southern Indian state of Kerala, mouth cancer is the leading form of cancer among men and is particularly common among men who fish the Indian Ocean. Many of them chew betel nut (a stimulant) wrapped in a tobacco leaf (a carcinogen) in order to stay awake at night while tending their nets.[45] At present, because of limited resources, Keralan families are often required to travel many miles to stay with their sick relative in order to cook and provide for them, and until very recently morphine could only be obtained daily by the patient in person from centralized regional cancer centres, causing huge family disruption.[46] Given this social context, the practical implications of cancer are a distant echo of those found in more affluent countries, even if many of the psychosocial concerns of patients and their families remain similar.

Most of what goes on in the lives of people with cancer occurs outside the hospital or consulting room. Patients have to fit their cancer and its treatment into their already complex social lives. People's lives are filled with countless commitments to people and institutions, and cancer is not the only source of stress for them even if it quickly becomes paramount. Thus, the treatment calendar (i.e. length of treatment, appointment times, etc.) often has a greater psychosocial impact on people's lives than either the illness or its treatment.[20] This is especially the case for people on low incomes, or who are self-employed, for whom the loss of pay and the threat to family income can be a major source of stress and worry. Those who are single parents, unemployed, or facing poverty are almost certainly experiencing a number of other concurrent stresses.

In one recent UK survey of 402 mixed cancer patients, 23% rated practical help with financial matters as being 'important' or 'very important' to them and, of these people, 35% reported that this need was not being met by existing services.[24] Significantly, of those who rated help with filling out forms to be important, 24% reported that this need had not been met. Nearly half the sample rated practical help with transport to and from the hospital as being important or very important. Note that this survey was undertaken in Britain, a geographically small but relatively rich country. The transport requirements of getting to and from treatment centres in many larger and poorer countries such as India, are considerable. American studies indicate that transport difficulties are more likely among people who are older, African-American, or Hispanic, and among people on low incomes, and that transport difficulties clearly jeopardize people's access to cancer treatment.[47]

The disruption to normal social roles and responsibilities (e.g. employment, housework) caused by long, demanding treatments, the difficulty in meeting mortgage payments and other financial commitments, the responsibility for the care of dependents (e.g. elderly relatives and/or young children), and the difficulty in maintaining adequate medical insurance cover in some countries, are practical social concerns for almost any patient. People with cancer rarely mention these concerns to healthcare staff because they frequently feel shame in revealing financial or other social concerns. However, it has been shown that cancer patients who have multiple psychosocial concerns are more likely to feel helpless, and more likely to report anxiety and depression.[48, 49]

When cancer is advanced and the prospect of death becomes imminent, other practical concerns become prominent. Help with domestic tasks (laundry and cleaning, shopping and preparing meals) or additional equipment in the home (commodes, mattresses, incontinence pads, etc.) may be needed, but carers do not always express these needs or may be simply unaware that help is available.[50] The need to write a will and dispose of one's estate, to discuss one's personal wishes regarding the care of children, or to record one's thoughts regarding the funeral, are significant considerations. However, family and friends sometimes feel apprehensive about raising these issues lest they upset the patient and be perceived as losing hope. But if the patient has been fully informed about their prognosis and has begun to adjust to it, they usually welcome the opportunity of tackling these practical concerns (*see* Chapter 5—Palliative Care).

Healthcare implications

- Information about financial and other forms of social welfare, as well as financial and practical advice, must be easily accessible. Help with the completion of forms is often overlooked but is a much-needed form of practical support.

- The practical and social needs of people with cancer should be rigorously and routinely addressed. However, in view of the stigma and shame people sometimes feel in revealing these needs, help should be offered in ways that do not provoke indignity or humiliation.

- Access to adequate social work support is an essential component of any cancer service. Social and practical care are particularly important in the context of advanced illness.

Relationships with family and friends

When faced with a crisis or uncertainty, people turn to their family and friends for support. This natural tendency occurs whether one is three years old, forty-three, or eighty-three. We look to others to sustain us through the crisis, listen to our fears, and encourage us through hard times. This is known as 'social support' and can be thought of as a psychological 'shock absorber', buffering people from the stressful effects of life's difficulties (*see* Chapter 3).

As described in Chapter 1, human beings are an inherently social species who turn to others for their protection and safety. At times of crisis other people provide a safe environment in which people can explore the meaning of stressful events, and make changes to their deeply-held assumptions about the world. For example, studies have shown that when people have an emotional concern they are most likely to turn for support to their spouse or partner, if they have one.[51] Moreover, a confiding relationship has long been regarded as a protection or buffer against depression for those who are at a high risk of it.[52] Where people lack the support of other people they are more vulnerable to the emotional effects of chronic stress, notably anxiety and depression. Thus, people who are socially isolated or socially marginalized are at particular risk.

This general picture certainly holds true for the crisis of cancer. Numerous studies have testified to the importance of emotional support from trusted partners, relatives, or friends. People who have opportunities to express their fears and anxieties are generally less psychologically distressed.[53–55] Putting one's feelings and thoughts into words helps to give them shape and structure, and this enables one to feel more in control of events.

However, there are cultural and individual differences as to how acceptable it is to voice one's needs and from whom it is acceptable to seek support. For example, one study found that help-seeking behaviour within the immediate family tended to be seen as embarrassing to Japanese-American women with breast cancer due to the cultural belief that it is preferable to exert self-control rather than inconvenience others and become indebted. Chinese-American women, by contrast, tended to depend almost exclusively on support from nuclear family members. Of the three groups, Anglo-American women had the largest support network which spanned across family and friends.[56]

But although friends and family are often a vitally important source of support, they can also be a source of stress in themselves. For one thing, friends and family are frequently as distressed and shocked as the patient themselves.[57, 58] Consequently patients can find themselves providing as much support as they receive. Whatever the prognosis, the diagnosis of cancer confronts people with the prospect of permanent separation from loved ones that will inevitably occur at the moment of death. The examination of this stark reality is profoundly distressing, not only because of our own fear of leaving the world alone, but also because we anticipate the grief reaction of our survivors. The first thoughts in the minds of newly diagnosed parents of young children are usually less to do with themselves than with the plight of their children: What will happen to them if I die? What do I tell them? How do I tell them? The distress of these concerns cannot be overstated. Anxious rumination, about the fate of one's children or other important relationships, can become a discrete problem in itself (*see* Chapter 3).

> First saw the registrar who said that they were 99% certain there was cancer of the left kidney and secondary infection in the lungs. The normal procedure was to remove the kidney and follow it up with a course of interferon. Only 25% were successful with interferon. L. [specialist nurse] had some information on the side-effects of interferon. The world was starting to seem unreal. Dr P. came in and reiterated what his registrar had said. When asked the prognosis he suggested twelve months. All colour had gone from the world and I could not think properly. I felt I could give no support to J. and that I was leaving her in a way that I had not expected.

After knowing someone for years we develop implicit expectations about our relationship with them; we make assumptions about how they would respond if we needed them. However, when the crisis hits, other people do not always react in the way we expect them to, and whilst this can sometimes be a pleasant surprise if others exceed our expectations, it can often be a source of disappointment if they fail to meet them. Other people's attempts at being supportive can be misguided and unhelpful if patients are left feeling that their loved ones have minimized the seriousness of the cancer or been overly positive about the prognosis.[59] These attempts may be more beneficial to the 'supporter' than they are to the patient, who may feel that their genuine concerns have not been acknowledged.

People's relationships are always complicated because of individual and shared histories that shape them. One source of conflict can be in feelings about the wish or need to confide and discuss difficult issues or concerns. Sometimes when someone with cancer withdraws, it can be a caring but misguided desire to begin the process of separation early, so as to prevent profound feelings of loss in loved ones should one die. For other people, the need for their own support competes with their need to protect:

> When I saw my parents again I wasn't sure how to behave. Some part of me wanted to sit on their laps and cry like a child. Yet at the same time I wanted to be strong and adult and protect them from it – I knew it would distress them.

Finally, there tend to be gender differences in how people respond to the distress of cancer, and the use they make of other people's support. Women with cancer are often disappointed by their male partners if they withdraw or seem unable to respond to their distress.[60–62] On the other hand, men with cancer sometimes prefer to withhold their emotions as a way of feeling more in control, thus avoiding the perception that they are 'not coping'.[63] Although expressing emotions is widely regarded as psychologically healthy, there may be costs in doing so for some people (*see* Chapter 3—Gender Differences).

Healthcare implications

- Social support is the single most important resource most people have in coping with life stresses and difficulties. Talking through our thoughts and feelings enables us to 'make sense' of new experiences so that they can be more easily integrated into our mental maps of the world. This is true of the stress of cancer where emotional support has been shown to protect people from developing psychological problems. Healthcare staff provide an important element of this support through their interactions with the patient and their carers.

- Healthcare staff should be cautious in assuming that patients have sufficient support in their lives. There are numerous reasons why it may be absent. There may be cultural differences as to where and how much people expect to access support. In addition, those who are socially isolated or marginalized are especially vulnerable to the stresses of cancer, and should be offered ongoing emotional support by trained personnel.

- Although people with cancer may superficially appear to have good support systems, this may be an illusion. Potential supporters may be perceived by the patient to be too distressed themselves, incompetent at support, or too vulnerable to be a source of support. Alternatively, the patient may abhor the thought of being 'a burden' on others and consequently fail to make use of the support at hand. Access to additional emotional support should therefore be available for all who wish to use it (e.g. support and information centres, counselling).

- The fear of being a 'burden' on others is keenly felt by people who are used to others depending on them. One might try asking people who feel guilty about asking for support to imagine 'the shoe being on the other foot': *'How would you feel if [the particular friend or relative] had the cancer and approached you for your support? Would you feel they were being a burden on you?'* This simple formula reminds people that it is an honour to be asked for one's support.

- While expressing one's emotions may be generally helpful, pressure to do so may compromize other important needs, such as the dignity of being seen to be 'coping on one's own'.

- The open expression of feelings is sometimes equated with 'not coping'. It can be helpful to remind patients and carers that their emotions are quite understandable, given the stress they have been under. Crying, for example, is a capacity that is wired into the species and can be a useful means of releasing pent-up emotion. However, one must be wary that, in normalizing people's emotions, one is not inadvertently blocking them by appearing to trivialize them (*see* Chapter 6).

- Friends and family members will be making their own adjustments to the patient's illness and all its implications. Research has shown that partners are sometimes as distressed as patients and therefore may require additional support. Serious illness leads people to confront aspects of their relationships that had hitherto been neglected or assumed. This process can create waves of change throughout the family system, sometimes leading to a healthy re-examination and realignment of personal relationships, and sometimes exposing dysfunctional relationships and a need to separate.

Impact on self

The shock of diagnosis is followed by psychological and social disorientation, an abrupt hiatus of normal complicated life, as new priorities quickly establish themselves: the onset of treatment, reorganizing commitments to other people, rethinking plans and goals, and so on. Many people redefine themselves as a 'cancer patient', while staring at the implications of a more limited future than they had expected. In fact, the changes that follow a cancer diagnosis pile up so quickly upon one another that people can soon feel they have lost control over their lives.

Any serious illness, especially one that requires lengthy treatments or leads to chronic ill-health, inevitably affects the roles people perform and, consequently, how they view themselves. From the outset illness requires people to assume the role of 'patient' with its many connotations about how patients are expected to behave. This role transition can be hard enough. But some patients describe having 'crossed the line' from being a well person to being 'a cancer patient', with all its socially-loaded significance.

> I have decided to join the women who meet on Monday nights, but what a difficult step it has been – and still is – to acknowledge that, yes, I belong to the category of people who have been hit by cancer.

From being in control of their daily routines, patients have to conform to those of the hospital, their treatment calendar. From being independent 'free agents', patients are forced by their illness to depend on others for their health and well-being, getting around, or emotional buoyancy. Self-esteem and a sense of competence protect against depression because people feel it is their own actions that control what happens to them.[64] Little wonder many people with cancer feel so depressed at times.

> M. [breast care nurse] telephones at around midday to see how I am. I am honest for once and say that my emotions are everywhere. But why? It's not discomfort or the disfigurement that upsets me ... it is frustration of no longer feeling in control – of not having the immediate future planned, as I am prone to do, we decide.

Every person performs a large number of roles throughout their lives. Roles involve not only one's own but other people's expectations, indeed cultural expectations, about how one should behave. A single person may perform the role of daughter, sister, mother, wife, sexual partner, school teacher, student, football fan, fund raiser, business partner, and friend. Her identity (or self-concept) is constructed over time from all these different roles, and her self-esteem (how she values herself) is derived from how she performs in these different roles. She may regard herself as having been a *troublesome* daughter, a *caring* mother, a *firm* but *effective* teacher, a *thoughtful* friend, and so on. All these roles are shaped by the cultural expectations that surround the individual.

The social roles people perform give them daily feedback as to their capabilities and limitations, their own perceived value in the world, and their control over it. We are mostly unaware of the feedback we absorb about ourselves, but when this social feedback is suddenly unavailable (such as during hospitalization) it can have a savage impact on our confidence and mood. The effects of illness and prolonged and demanding treatments (e.g. fatigue, nausea, pain) can lead people to withdraw from roles, and thus social contacts, which were previously important to their self-worth. The village routines, work and marketplace, weekly bingo nights, religious ceremonies, and the drink in the pub—all may have to be shelved while the individual focuses on their illness and its treatment. Suspending these social roles also means suspending opportunities for feedback about oneself. No longer are people reminded that others think them funny, clever, talented, caring, respected, or needed. Patients begin to doubt themselves, their qualities, and their competence.

Unfortunately, low confidence and low mood can be a formula for psychological withdrawal and an escalation of the problem. Social discrimination and dislocation (e.g. employment difficulties,[65, 66] poverty, lack of insurance, homelessness, etc.) can bring additional feelings of helplessness and powerlessness.

> The times I cope best are when I am at work – I'm no different as far as others are concerned, and this is how I must see myself … I am still the same person – I have a serious problem to cope with and I must not become dominated by it. My aim is to let it make me a better person.

In short, the demands of treatment can quickly lead people to lose their confidence and self-esteem, making a return to 'normal life' more difficult at the end of treatment. There is a sense of dislocation with what normal life should be like:

> I just want to get my life back on track.

> Woke up weepy – not a good start to any day! I just wish that I could turn the clock back 6 weeks, to when life was 'normal'. I truly wish I could do that – just one ordinary day without the Big C being present.

Couples and families undergo countless changes over the course of cancer (*see* Chapter 3). Both the illness and its treatment place shifting demands on every member of the family, and the entire family system quickly has to accommodate rapid change. The sick person may feel under pressure to maintain whatever role they have traditionally performed within the family, but may find themselves unable to sustain it due to the symptoms of the disease or the treatment. For example, mothers may wish to retain their nurturing role yet feel in need of care for themselves; this can result in considerable guilt if they feel they are failing their family. Similarly, the need for family members to care for the patient, and take over their roles, may be interesting at first but can soon turn into frustration and a desire to return to 'the way things used to be'. Couples may be unable to sustain the sexual element of their relationship and mutual doubts and fears may creep into it. And so on. In the midst of such family turmoil it is easy for the patient to feel guilty and depressed that they have upset everyone and have become a burden on the family.

When cancer causes serious disability some social roles must be permanently given up. This can cause a protracted period of mourning as the individual attempts to adjust to a world in which previously valued activities are no longer available to them. Wherever possible, the task is one of substituting new activities and roles for old ones, but unless there is an acknowledgement of the loss and the importance of mourning it, such a suggestion can seem crass and insensitive.

If the disease becomes advanced there will be a more general closing down of social roles and responsibilities.[67] It has been suggested that some of the feelings of loss associated with relinquishing one's roles can be lessened if these roles can be passed on to other people.[68] Certainly, opportunities to review the various roles the patient has held in their life provides other people with a chance to acknowledge and celebrate their value and worth, and for the patient to derive a more coherent meaning from their lives (*see* Chapter 5—Palliative Care).

Finally, the withdrawal from certain social roles can sometimes represent a welcome break, leading people to reassess the value of roles they had taken for granted. Work may seem less important than spending time with the family, and addressing one's own needs and aspirations may suddenly seem long overdue. Indeed, this can lead to some positive lifestyle changes:

> Life is too short to be involved in things we don't really want to do!

Healthcare implications

- It is important to encourage patients and their families to stay engaged with their normal roles and responsibilities, in as far as they feel well enough to do so. The social roles people perform provide them with daily feedback as to their value in the world and their control over it. Without this feedback people quickly lose confidence in themselves and begin to question their competence and worth. Such feelings are a precursor to anxiety and depression, and make it more difficult for people to return to their normal social roles when treatment comes to an end.

- It is also essential for healthcare staff to warn patients that the illness and the side-effects of treatment may lead people to feel too sick or exhausted to maintain normal activity levels. However, patients should be warned as well that they risk losing their confidence and self-worth if they fail to resume their normal social roles (e.g. work, family, recreation, etc.) whenever they are ready and able to.

- The extent to which people are able to maintain control over their lives will impact on their self-esteem. Healthcare staff can influence the individual's new role of being a 'patient' by ensuring that all patients have access to as much information as they wish, and are invited to be active collaborators in their treatment to the extent that they want to be.

- Where roles have to be more permanently relinquished, due to disability or impending death, there will be a period of mourning. By acknowledging these losses and enabling the patient to reflect on them, healthcare staff can help patients derive a sense of meaning and self-worth.

Hope

Many people with cancer react to their diagnosis by preparing for the possibility of their death.[69] No matter what prognosis has been given, cancer forces people to examine the possibility that they may not live as long as they had assumed they would. Suddenly their hopes and dreams for the future are threatened. Long-standing implicit life-goals become clear and distinct yet, at the same time, their eventual attainment may seem unlikely and even unrealistic. The threat of cancer therefore leads people to re-examine these unspoken priorities (the assumptions underpinning their key goals in life).[70]

Goals are vital to our emotional well-being. Having a 'wished-for' future is one component of hope which has been defined as a 'general tendency to construct and respond to the perceived future positively'[71] (Nunn 1996, p. 228). Having things to look forward to and things to achieve is what motivates and structures our lives. Indeed, much of our sense of ourselves is bound up with our own personal 'life trajectory' (our life story) which includes goals and rewards in the future[72] (see Chapter 1).

So, how does hope fare when people perceive cancer to be an 'amputation of the future'?[73] If someone remains hopeful when everyone else concedes that the situation seems hopeless, is this person in denial or merely being optimistic? And is opting for the pessimistic view always a bad strategy?

There are many accounts in scientific and popular literature that show that a personal crisis can also be an opportunity for change.[74] Some life goals may be dismissed as trivial and no longer important, and a number of people report that their illness helped them develop entirely new goals and priorities.[26, 75] The revision of this part of our mental model of the world is what is often associated with a 'healthy' or 'positive' personal transition, but it can also reawaken unresolved problems from the past.

> This cancer scare has changed me radically. It has rocked me and shaken me up. It is bringing all sorts of hidden emotions to the surface and made me aware that there are still things that need attention from the past.

The demands and uncertainty of cancer lead some people to abandon goals that previously motivated them and gave them a sense of purpose and well-being. Some authors have described the contrast between individuals whose lives are entirely dominated by their disease and those who are able to 'encapsulate' it, and try to fit it into their otherwise busy lives.[76] In other words, the latter group are able to maintain the 'motivational structure' of their lives by not abandoning all their existing goals.

Of course, cancer treatments and the illness itself severely challenge people's ability to stay involved with activities that would normally motivate them. Pain, nausea, weakness, and fatigue, not to mention hospital appointments, make it draining or difficult to plan to meet a friend next week, or work at that long-standing project in the garage. Consequently, people with cancer often disengage from normally appealing activities and cease to make plans for the immediate and longer-term future.

Without goals to achieve or events to look forward to, people are at risk of feeling hopeless and depressed.[77] A similar process may occur, for example, in the context of long-term unemployment where there is a high incidence of depression.[78] In fact, there is growing evidence that people who attempt to commit suicide have fewer positive thoughts about the future than other people, but not necessarily more negative ones.[79]

> I write in my notebook by my bed what I hope to achieve each day. Very small accomplishable jobs but I still don't get through them but it's a nice way to start the day with a plan. You got a plan, you got a life.

Not surprisingly, cancer patients who show optimism are ultimately less distressed by the disease.[80] Some people with cancer engage in what has been termed 'defensive pessimism' by failing to make plans for the future (e.g. a holiday) lest they be disappointed (e.g. by a recurrence of their illness)[81] Others fail to make plans in the superstitious belief that by doing so they would be 'tempting fate' ('If I plan a trip for next summer, I really would be asking for something to go wrong'.)[82] These common reactions are understandable given the uncertainty of any cancer prognosis, but can lead people to live their lives 'one day at a time'. While this strategy may be useful in the short term, keeping uncertainty at bay, it also gets in the way of purpose and hope. With time, however, people often regain the confidence that their lives are not about to end imminently and that it may be safe once again to invest in the future.

> The first time I had cancer I didn't buy a new pair of shoes for three years.

However, if people disengage from activities (which provide them with the rewards of pleasure and achievement) they not only put themselves at risk of depression[83] but also leave themselves with extra time in which to ruminate and worry. People with cancer often complain that the hardest time of the day is when they find themselves at home with nothing to do but think. Solitary thinking can, of course, be constructive (e.g. personal reflection) though, equally, can lead to frightening catastrophic thoughts resulting in anxiety.

The lack of goals and plans may be a particular problem in advanced disease when there often seem to be diminishing opportunities to achieve them. In palliative care, however, there is widespread acknowledgement that maintaining hope is achieved by patients and staff working together to set realistic goals to achieve (*see* Chapter 5).

Healthcare implications

- Everyone needs a sense of hope. Even when a patient's illness objectively appears incurable, it is important for most people to retain a hope that a cure or remission may yet be found. Buying a lottery ticket does not mean you believe you will win. Challenging this element of hope is needlessly cruel.

- Hope involves more than merely the wish to be cured. Having goals and plans are vital to people's sense of hope and meaning.[84] Without motivations to structure life, people are at greater risk of feeling depressed and anxious.

- People often need opportunities to mourn the loss of important life goals when these are no longer realistic and to talk through their fears about the uncertain future.

- The process of re-examining the priorities of one's life goals is stressful, but can also lead to healthy personal development and a new sense of meaning.

- Patients should be encouraged to stay involved with activities that provide a sense of achievement and/or pleasure. People feel most fulfilled when they are engaged in activities which are intrinsically motivating (e.g. creative arts and crafts, work, etc.).[85]

- The treatment should be regarded as a necessary obligation that must be fitted into patients' otherwise busy lives, rather than something which becomes the dominant feature.

- Realistic planning for the immediate and longer-term future should be encouraged: setting attainable goals to achieve, and events to look forward to, promotes hope.

The body

The passage of my life is written on my body, the pockmarks, the little scars of everyday trauma, childbearing, excess weight, sports or lack of them. And now comes a new one, not only surgery but brown veins creeping up my arms from the chemo site. And each hit adds a little ridge to my nails.

People experience the world and their entire lives through their bodies. With cancer, the body has been 'invaded' and 'attacked' by a disease that threatens its integrity and survival—nowhere does the metaphor of the need to 'fight' back seem more apt. The small field of psychosocial oncology is replete with empirical studies documenting the many ways that cancer treatment, if not the illness itself, can lead to profound changes in people's physical capabilities (e.g. fertility), appearance (body image), and sensation (pain and other physical symptoms). Cancer undermines people's implicit assumptions about, indeed their *relationship* with, their bodies in many different ways.

The body is no longer predictable.[86] Many people who have long survived cancer are plagued by the residual suspicion that cancer may return. One study found that nearly 90% of breast cancer patients were still thinking about breast cancer recurrence eight years after their surgery for it.[87] For some people these worries become intrusive ruminations or compulsive urges to check the body for any signs that the disease has returned (see p. 83). For others the presence of cancer can lead to feelings of revulsion towards their own bodies:

> I've been feeling I'm rotting from the inside out

For the most part, we take for granted the appearance, sensation, and capabilities of our bodies. People vary, however, according to how much of their identity is invested in different parts of their bodies and this affects the impact of cancer and its treatment.[88] A young woman may find the hair loss associated with chemotherapy intolerable, whereas a young man may not mind so much, though this probably depends on their culture. The amputation of the penis in a young man may be more traumatic than it would be in an older man. Everyone is highly invested in their ability to communicate and anyone would be hugely affected by the loss of their larynx, but perhaps even more so if they are a singer or an actor. Some people explicitly invest a great deal of their identity in their bodies, while others may inadvertently depend upon them for their livelihoods. Athletes, dancers, musicians, and others who have worked hard to maintain their bodies in first-rate condition may find it catastrophic to have to perceive themselves as seriously ill. On the other hand, agricultural or other manual labourers may be no less traumatized by their illness, and may be equally vulnerable to a loss of income and self-worth caused by their disability.

Any form of disfiguring disease or mutilating surgery can lead to body image problems if the patient is unable to tolerate or adjust to their changed appearance. Even among people whose identity is not especially tied to their physical appearance, there is a process of adjustment and mourning for their changed body, often involving self-doubt, a loss of 'self-esteem' and, not surprisingly, feelings of depression.

> Have just had a shower and hair-wash. Gave a last glance to my left breast. I will certainly be relieved to know that I have got rid of this malignant tumour which is threatening my life, but the vision of my mutilated chest makes me feel very angry and sad. Since puberty, I have been used to having two breasts and now, one of them is to be chopped away.

Of course, changes to a person's appearance require other people to adjust too. People with cancer find themselves having to renegotiate their relationships with other people and this often leads to relationship and sexual difficulties. For example, patients and their partners sometimes try to 'mind-read' what the other partner is feeling and thinking (*see* Chapter 3).

On the other hand it would be a mistake to assume that a change in physical appearance has the same meaning for everyone. A qualitative study of Chinese women in Hong Kong found that none of the women were concerned about the effect of their mastectomies on their sexuality and none felt the surgery had had a detrimental effect on their marital relationships. They were more concerned to avoid looking different, fearing social exclusion in a society intolerant of differences and non-conformity.[13]

Disfiguring surgery, especially around the head and neck, requires the patient to adjust to the broader social world, a world that may seem unsympathetic and insensitive to their plight. Learning to re-enter the public world of streets and shops, apparently obsessed with physical beauty, is understandably daunting for people left with a visible facial disfigurement or an impairment of speech. Even when the disfigurement is more easily hidden (such as a mastectomy) people often report feeling conspicuously different or less attractive compared with others. The loss of self-esteem is also a sense of loss.

> The woman doctor is delightful – friendly, open-faced, matter of fact, but when she bends forward over the [consent] forms there's half an inch of healthy cleavage visible which seems to me tactless. But then everywhere I look I see breasts, pairs of breasts, beautiful breasts – my 13 year old putting on a light tee shirt, women of all shapes and sizes in the pool, bra ads plastering the streets and underground – all healthily normal, abnormally beautiful.

But body image, in the sense of perceptions and feelings about the body's appearance, is only one aspect of people's relationship with their bodies. There are many other ways in which cancer and its treatment affect the individual's sense of their physical integrity and personal dignity. Stomas are a replacement for a bodily function that is normally taken for granted. Not surprisingly, they are associated with more distress when those given them feel that the stoma rules their lives and they are no longer complete people.[89] Lymphoedema not only changes people's physical appearance, but can also cause pain and chronic disability (causing more distress, of course, when it affects the dominant arm).[90] Hormone treatments not only cause weight gain but can also lead to menopausal symptoms, impotence, and infertility. While some cancer treatment may have only temporary effects on the body (e.g. hair loss, nausea, insomnia, and fatigue) they may be no less distressing for the individual affected. However, many symptoms continue for months or years after active treatment has finished.[87]

> I've been feeling pretty miserable – I'm just putting on weight and feel unhappy about myself and how I look. I know the drugs are partly to blame, but I can't help thinking about how good I felt when I did lose weight, but the effort of achieving that at the moment is not a very pleasant prospect – you need to be in the right frame of mind – it's a vicious circle.

Cancer, of course, can lead to permanent disabilities that require the individual and their loved ones to change the way they relate to one another and the way they structure their lives. Brain tumours may lead to enduring, cognitive, perceptual, or personality changes. A limb amputation may require a prosthesis or a wheelchair. Head and neck cancers are particularly devastating because they often result in communication difficulties (e.g. removal of the larynx), combined with a facial disfigurement and the loss of taste and/or smell.[91] Losing a breast, penis, testicle, ovary, or any other part of the body can alter the individual's sense of their bodies and their sexuality, making them feel less feminine or masculine, as well as less attractive and sexually desirable.

> I am one day further into the realisation that I have lost a breast. Tomorrow some of the padding will be taken away and in another day or two I will have to face myself in the mirror. Where shall I find the courage? And what of J. [husband]?

Advanced illness is associated with particularly challenging symptoms. Pain, weight loss, weakness, incontinence, and breathlessness can all cause significant distress for the patient, but also affect the individual's sense of control over their bodies. Such symptoms involve an ever-greater dependence on other people to treat and care for the patient, and a diminishing time in which to adjust to them. It is perhaps little wonder that advanced illness is associated with greater psychological distress and psychiatric disorder.[92]

Healthcare implications

- A person's identity is intimately bound up with their feelings and thoughts about their body. Although we are constantly using our bodies to interact with the world around us, we are usually unaware of our dependence upon them until we are ill. In cancer, even though people's paramount concern is with survival, the overall integrity of their body may be crucial to the *quality* of their survival.

- While much has been written about body image, cancer also affects the *capabilities* of the body and the way it *feels* to the patient. People vary to the extent that their feelings are invested in different parts of their bodies. Changes to the appearance, function, or sensation of the body have different meanings for different people. It is therefore important that healthcare staff do not presume to know the impact of bodily changes simply on the basis of superficial clues (e.g. the extent of surgery, the person's age, gender, or marital status, etc.).

- Healthcare staff should prepare the patient carefully prior to treatments that are likely to cause a loss of dignity (e.g. stomas), disfigurements, disabilities (e.g. loss of sexual function, communication difficulties), or unpleasant symptoms (e.g. pain, nausea, fatigue). If information is presented sensitively it can help lessen the traumatic impact of changes when they occur.

- It is essential to reassure patients that healthcare staff will continue to be available during and after the medical treatment. Adjusting to physical changes and overcoming side-effects can take considerable time; the presence of ongoing medical and emotional support with the aim of maximizing rehabilitation would clearly facilitate this adjustment process.

- The availability and quality of emotional support available to the patient must be assessed. Healthcare workers should learn about how the illness and its treatment have affected the patient's relationships with other people in their lives and what, if any, professional help is required and desired. *'How do you feel you are getting on with other people in your life?' 'Do you feel it's affected your relationship with … ?'*

- People with cancer rarely spontaneously tell their doctors or nurses about their concerns. Studies have shown that patients worry about being perceived as neurotic or a burden on their already busy doctors and nurses, and believe that nothing can be done to alleviate their concerns anyway.[93] This general belief that 'good patients do not complain' holds true for pain[94] as it does for emotional concerns.[93]

- Continue to assess the impact of the cancer and its treatment on the individual's self-esteem and identity. For example, *'How do you feel now when you look at your chest? … What has it been like for you since your larynx was removed? … How have you been feeling about yourself since having your stoma?'*

- Body image disturbance may be severe and sometimes seemingly out of proportion to what other people see, but there is rarely a pronounced distortion of body size or body weight, as seen in anorexia.[95] People affected should be patiently encouraged to confront their physical changes and re-engage with social roles, while continuing to express their feelings and work towards overcoming difficulties that do emerge.

- The prospect of recurrence for those in remission often conjures up fears of the unknown and the fantasy that no more treatment will be offered. Similarly, where cancer has become incurable, fears of abandonment by the healthcare team are particularly common.[42] It is important that the emphasis on continuity of care is not exclusive to palliative care, but is central to the philosophy of cancer care generally.

Existential beliefs

> I feel so full of love at the moment, so different to six months ago, it is as if that experience has changed me fundamentally.

This chapter has been about the many ways in which cancer and its treatment impact on the individual and their relationship with the world. We have tried to convey how life-threatening illnesses, such as cancer, undermine the core assumptions (i.e. future, relationships, self, body, etc.) by which people have lived their lives. Not surprisingly, all these fundamental assumptions are intimately related to existential/spiritual beliefs about the world (*see* Chapter 1—Core Human Assumptions).

> Life without me is almost impossible to imagine. I think of it in terms of missing events – the children's marriages, grandchildren, or, more mundanely, next year's fireworks, next spring–but even that is difficult to imagine. Part of the disappointment in missing these things is because you are aware they are going on without you.

Existential beliefs refer to a person's most deeply held convictions about their existence. These include assumptions about the existence of natural or supernatural forces, the meaning of one's existence, the nature of the world at large, and what happens after we die. Some of these beliefs are formally embodied in spiritual faiths such as religions but this is not true of all.

For some people the experience of cancer appears to confirm their existing beliefs about the moral or rational nature of existence, but for others it challenges these assumptions.[96] Patients describe a sense of existential loneliness, the awareness that in experiencing unfolding events and the possibility or certainty of their death, they are ultimately alone. Catastrophic events like cancer can leave people feeling lost in a spiritual sea without reference points—it can take time to adjust one's internal picture of the world to be able to make sense of what is apparently unfair and meaningless. This loss of existential meaning leads individuals to ask themselves 'What is the point?', suggesting that they question the futility of struggling with the physical and psychological suffering associated with cancer. This loss of spiritual meaning, or existential despair, may be a precursor to depression.

In America, for example, surveys have shown that 95% believe in God[97] and 90% believe in prayer, prayer being a widely used method of coping with cancer and its treatment.[96] European figures of 'religiosity' are considerably lower, especially in Britain. Spiritual belief systems are thought to provide people with cancer with emotional support,[98] though it may be the frequency of personal prayer that has the largest effect on people's well-being.[99]

> Feel 'normal' today. Need to do as Jesus said and really live each day at a time – stop fretting, worrying, getting aggravated about tomorrow. The trees are all budding with fresh green leaves and there's a light drizzle, the birds are singing and life is good – today.

Spiritual beliefs help people regain meaning in their lives, and find peace and security by feeling a connection with, and surrendering their control to, a higher power that transcends biological existence.[100] However, among one ethnically diverse American sample, about 40 per cent of cancer patients reported wanting help with finding hope, meaning in life, spiritual resources, and someone to talk to about finding peace of mind.[101] So although spiritual and religious faith may help support people through the experience of cancer, others may be left feeling confused, disillusioned, and lost.

> Nothing I suffer, nor M. [husband], can equal what Christ must have suffered, so it ill becomes me to ask for everything. All I can do is hope and trust and lay myself and my loved ones and those who treat me before Him, I am so aware of my impotence and lack of control of my life, it is really a knife edge I live on just now. My emotional fragility scares me. My trust in God is growing because it is the only stable thing in this, my insecure world.

However, in spite of, or perhaps because of the existential questions raised by the threat to their mortality, many people discover that the crisis of cancer acts as a catalyst for positive change and personal growth.[84] This finding is no longer a matter of anecdotes and personal testimonies in the popular press. Studies have shown that, following cancer, patients feel more appreciation of life[102] and a more positive attitude towards living,[103, 104] they derive meaning and construe personal benefit from the experience[26] and a greater satisfaction with religious concerns,[105] and are less concerned about the 'nonessentials of life'.[106] Finally, personal relationships are often improved or strengthened.[105, 107] In short, the recalibration of one's most core assumptions, while stressful, does not always lead to negative consequences. The relationship between positive personal growth and longer-term distress is not yet clear[102] though it seems likely that the negative changes of cancer exert a more powerful influence than the positive ones.[108] Nonetheless, cancer can sometimes powerfully stimulate insight.

> Being ill has taught me
>
> To be more assertive
> To re-evaluate what's important to me
> To express my needs
> To limit what I will take on emotionally/physically
> To not take anything for granted especially time
> To enjoy the simple things
> That D. [husband] wants our baby
> How angry my mother makes me

People's cultural and religious background influences and often defines how people are expected to behave in relation to one another. People especially rely on these customs and habits at times of crisis, but although someone may profess to follow a religion, people will differ as to how strictly they adhere to its customs. Therefore healthcare staff should try to accommodate these needs by asking patients about any particular cultural or religious needs they may have rather than assume what these might be.

Healthcare implications

- Everyone has existential beliefs though not everyone practises a formal religion. These fundamental beliefs about the world frequently come into focus as patients contemplate the possibility of their death (*See* Chapter 5—Palliative Care). A person's 'religiosity' has been shown to be an important resource in reducing the distress of cancer,[98, 109] though even those without a formal religion may well be facing an existential crisis or feeling existential loneliness.

- Physicians often underestimate the importance of religion to patients coping with illness with the result that they neither assess existential concerns, nor refer those in spiritual crisis to those who may be able to help (spiritual and lay counsellors, religious leaders, etc.).[110] Yet it seems that patients frequently want their doctors to address their spiritual needs.[111] Healthcare staff may feel embarrassed to discuss existential concerns because they are seen as private matters though family doctors, who have a long-standing relationship with the patient, may feel more comfortable discussing these issues.

- Access to spiritual support should be clearly available throughout a patient's contact with the healthcare service. Addressing spiritual needs is not about finding answers for patients but, rather, allowing them to articulate their questions and conflicts so as to find their own answers. Simply listening to and acknowledging these concerns can be helpful and effective. It can be reassuring for patients to hear that others in their situation also sometimes question their faith, or have existential concerns. Where the issues are complex, or involve questions of doctrine, the healthcare professional should ask the patient if they would like to speak to a counsellor or religious leader. Canadian,[112] Australian,[113] and American[84] clinicians have established formal psycho-existential therapy programmes to address these concerns.

- Among those who say they have a religion there will be strict adherents, but also those who feel a part of their religious group without believing or practising its customs. It is important to be sensitive to these differences and not to assume that someone describing themselves as, for example, Jewish or Hindu will necessarily follow all or any of the customs associated with these religions.

- Health services, especially inpatient services, should strive to accommodate the cultural and religious needs of their users. Healthcare staff should get into the habit of asking patients about any such needs they may have, and be prepared to learn something from each patient. For example, a person's needs in relation to food and diet should be considered, as well as modesty (particularly with respect to physical examinations by people of the opposite sex), cleanliness, prayer, blood transfusions, and religious holidays.

Ending treatment

September is here and I'm lonely. The party's over and I'm in that limbo where my cancer is yesterday's news but I'm not quite well enough to take my place again in the normal scheme of things. A few people have said, not in so many words but to the effect that now my treatment is over that's it and I can go back to work, to life again. But there is no going back, only forward I suppose. Things will never be the same again.

The end of prolonged active treatment is yet another transition and, for many, a time of crisis. Even among those with a good prognosis there are often ambivalent feelings: relief that one may soon start to feel normal again, yet also the fear that one is being cast adrift from the 'safety net' of healthcare staff and active treatment. The prospect of a return to some sort of normality may be attractive, but the form this should take is rarely clear at first. Furthermore, the end of treatment invites the question: how long will it last? What does the future hold for me? Indeed, for those leaving hospital but *not* returning home (e.g. another hospital, nursing home, hospice), the situation may feel even more doubtful.

I'm not feeling much happier today. I'm tired and frustrated at not being able to 'get a grip'. I feel that now the treatment is over, that's it – cancer gone, problem gone – so why don't I just get back to 'normal'? I wish I could speak to someone who really understands – not just someone who listens sympathetically.

Over the many months of treatment most patients adapt to the routines of hospital visits, and become used to the support from healthcare staff and other patients. Active treatment may be unpleasant but at least it gives people the reassurance that they are 'doing something', in contrast to seeing what the future holds.[114] Hospitals provide a social milieu in which there are others in the same boat, people with whom the patient can speak openly about cancer; sometimes this is in sharp contrast to the 'conspiracy of silence' that may have become established in their home life. Finally, hospitals ideally provide patients with many opportunities to ask questions to staff and other patients about their illness, its treatment, and any unfamiliar symptoms. Without access to this form of reassurance, aches and pains can assume threatening proportions.

The idea of returning to life before cancer is an illusion; rarely can people 'take up where they left off'. Not only has the patient been changed by what they have been through, but other people have changed or moved on too. 'Everyday life' has to be constructed anew, and for many it will be radically different from life before cancer.

> Since I left hospital, I made a huge effort to be cheerful and positive and to put on a brave face. Nevertheless, sometimes, as was the case this evening, the horror of what happened to me just overwhelmed me, without any warning at all.

There may be expectations from family and friends that people's relationships with one another will soon return to the way they were before cancer, but this does not always follow. Many relationship difficulties and breakdowns following cancer are attributed to the disease which also causes sexual problems within couples (*see* Chapter 3). Returning to work and resuming other social roles after many months of absence can be daunting as people struggle with their lost confidence. For example, those working in emotionally draining occupations (e.g. teachers, mental health personnel, cancer professionals, etc) may discover they have lost the emotional resilience they once had, and feel unable to resume their careers. Patients may have to face the world knowing they look different, feel different, and must now cope with disabilities. In one study over 70% of breast cancer patients reported that they were treated differently after people knew they had cancer, and 52% said they were avoided as a result.[115] As many as a quarter of cancer patients may face unemployment as a result of their treatment, while the proportion facing discrimination in the workplace is higher still. In countries, such as America, where medical insurance is vital to one's healthcare, cancer patients also have more difficulty obtaining health and life insurance.[116]

Studies have indicated that hospital patients do not receive enough clinical information to prepare them for the transition home. Institutions which facilitate the transition out of hospital benefit in terms of cost-effectiveness, and patients are more satisfied.[117] Maintaining an ongoing but less frequent relationship with the hospital (such as attendance at a support or rehabilitation group) may enable patients to negotiate the transition from patient to survivor more easily. Professionally led and self-help survivor groups not only provide people with emotional support as they 'pick up the pieces of their lives' but also help to provide some aspects of the 'safety net' that is felt to be missing at the end of treatment. Finally, reassuring patients and their families that the healthcare team will continue to be a resource for them to draw upon in the future provides a sense of safety.

Healthcare implications

- Preparing patients and their families for what to expect in the months following discharge allows them to be able to predict the future with more certainty and thus feel more in control over it.

- Preparation for discharge should provide patients and their families with a clear road map of:

  - follow-up care (e.g. care at home, hospital visits expected of the patient, etc.) over the foreseeable future;

  - why and how long medication should be continued;

  - the likelihood of prolonged side-effects and what patients can do about them;

  - the availability of further medical and emotional support prior to the next outpatient appointment;

  - what telltale symptoms of recurrence patients should look out for and how and when they should react to them.

- Rehabilitation programmes can help people regain their physical and social confidence in themselves as well as ease the transition from hospital to community (*see* Chapter 5—Rehabilitation).

- Discharge is an important opportunity to reassess the impact of the treatment on the individual and their loved ones. The emotional and physical exhaustion of treatment may well have exacted its toll on the patient and family by the time patients' active treatment ends, so the potential crisis of ending is a further chance to assess people's ongoing concerns (*see* Chapter 6).

Living with uncertainty

Cancer treatments are not pleasant but at least they give patients the sense that something is being done, and while this continues there is an illusion of safety. When active treatment finally ends and the apparent safety of this contact is no longer available, the individual has to learn how to live with uncertainty. The prospect of recurrence and physical deterioration is rarely far from people's minds.[118] However, for those who survive, the passage of time eventually helps to restore a sense of safety from cancer, particularly as significant prognostic markers (e.g. 2 years, 5 years, etc.) are passed.

Follow-up contact with healthcare staff is a mixed blessing. On the one hand it offers reassurance and safety, yet on the other it poses a threat. Each follow-up visit is often preceded by weeks of apprehension and worry. In particular, waiting for test results is a form of mental torture: '*What if they find something this time? What then?*' It is essential that healthcare staff tackle this 'What then?' question. After all the heroic and exhaustive treatments they have undergone, many patients fear that if there were a recurrence of their disease no more treatment will be offered. It is therefore vital to reassure patients and their families that they will never be abandoned, and that some form of further treatment and care will always be offered, even if no longer with the aim of cure.

The possibility of recurrence can become a significant and distressing problem for the patient and their carers. Almost 90% of one sample of breast cancer patients were thinking about recurrence eight years after their initial surgery.[87] For some, the fear of recurrence only diminishes with repeated reassurances from professionals, and then only temporarily. Repeated visits to the family doctor, or phone calls to the hospital, become a way of coping with the uncertainty, albeit a miserable one. For a few, the fear leads to extensive self-checking rituals and an anxious preoccupation with the disease. Rather than re-engaging with their lives, they live from one day to the next in anticipation of their inevitable recurrence. Many of these unfortunate people find it oppressive to be alone, with little other than their own frightening thoughts to stimulate them. Worry is not exclusive to fears of recurrence (*see* Chapter 6—Anxiety, Worry, and Uncertainty).

> I am much better at waiting to hear results – I suppose that it's because they can't tell me anything that I'm not already partly prepared for now. I feel that I've confronted the worst case scenario and that I could deal with it if I had to.

Essentially, the challenge for all patients living with uncertainty is to achieve a balance between maintaining a 'sensible' level of surveillance over their bodies, and a healthy participation in stimulating meaningful activities which provide distraction from these worries.[118] What is a 'sensible' level of self-observation, however, is often difficult for patients to judge. Healthcare staff, however, are in a better position to provide clear information about what symptoms to be aware of, what symptoms are more likely to be residual side-effects from treatment, and how persistent symptoms need to be before the patient should seek medical advice. Again, reassurance that the healthcare team will always have something to offer, and goals to achieve no matter what the future holds, helps to contain many of the anxieties of patients and families.

Many other people are discharged from active treatment knowing that their cancer remains. For increasing numbers of patients, cancer is a chronic disease that must be integrated into a life that is otherwise rich and meaningful. Feelings of uncertainty remain, of course, though they usually have more to do with length of survival and what the end will be like. For those with advanced cancer, these concerns will be particularly prominent, so patients appreciate being able to discuss their fears of dying with the doctors and nurses caring for them.

Healthcare implications

- Fears of recurrence are very common among people who have finished active treatment. Rather than seeming to ignore it, it is helpful if healthcare staff acknowledge that patients normally find living with uncertainty difficult at first.

For those with more advanced cancer, worries about the future are not only about how to interpret new symptoms, but are also to do with uncertainty surrounding the entire process of dying.

- Opportunities should be given to patients to articulate their fears and concerns about the future. Some of these fears may be based on inaccurate assumptions—about the course of the disease, how possible scenarios will be managed by the medical team, and may be easily corrected.

- Patients should be educated in how to identify and respond appropriately to plaus-ible symptoms of recurrence. This will help them discriminate between a genuine cause for concern and more benign symptoms (such as residual side-effects of treatment). To the extent that this can be accurately and explicitly described, the clearer the patient will be. However, depending on the cancer, even doctors can find this a hard assessment to make. But rather than warning people that breast cancer, for example, can recur at any time it is more helpful to tell patients that their chances of relapse after a certain date are negligible.

- At the same time, patients should be warned that becoming preoccupied with their natural fears of recurrence can become a problem in itself. The best way to prevent this is to re-engage in meaningful goals and activities (e.g. contact with family, friends, work, hobbies, recreational activities, etc.) that provide healthy distraction from unproductive worrying. Excessive time on one's hands is likely to breed worrying thoughts.

- At follow-up assessment clinics patients and their loved ones are often highly anxious and vulnerable. It helps to acknowledge this anxiety and to encourage people to express their fears. Waiting for test results is highly stressful and has been described as a form of 'mental torture', so ensure that results for any follow-up investigations are delivered as soon as possible.

- Many patients worry that if their cancer returns, or their symptoms become unmanageable, they will be abandoned by the healthcare team. Reassurance that the healthcare team will always have something to offer the patient helps to contain many of the anxieties that people feel when they face an uncertain future.

References

1. Sikora K, Thomas H. (1989). *Fight cancer: how to prevent it and how to fight it.* London: BBC Books.
2. Sontag S. (1991). *Illness as metaphor.* London: Penguin. (First published in 1978).
3. *The Book of Job: The Bible, Old Testament.*
4. Holland JC. (1998). Societal views of cancer and the emergence of psycho-oncology. In: JC Holland (ed.), *Psycho-oncology*, Oxford: Oxford University Press.
5. Open University's U205 Course Team (1985). *Experiencing and explaining disease.* Milton Keynes: Open University Press.
6. Burish TG, Meyerowtiz BE, Carey MP, and Morrow GR. (1987). The stressful effects of cancer in adults. In: A Baum and JE Singer (ed.), *Handbook of psychology and health*, Vol.5, New York: Erlbaum.

7. Sheldon F. (2003). Social impact of advanced metastatic cancer. In: M Lloyd-Williams (ed.), *Psychosocial issues in palliative care*, Oxford: Oxford University Press.

8. Blackwell N. (1998). Cultural issues in indigenous Australian peoples. In: D Doyle, GWC Hanks, and N MacDonald (ed.), *Oxford textbook of palliative medicine*, Oxford: Oxford University Press.

9. Good M, Munakata T, Kobayashi Y, Mattingly C, and Good BY. (1994). Oncology and narrative time. *Social Science and Medicine* **38**:855–62.

10. Kashiwagi T. (1998). Palliative care in Japan. In: D Doyle, GWC Hanks, and N MacDonald (ed.), *Oxford textbook of palliative medicine*, Oxford: Oxford University Press.

11. Olweny CLM. (1998). Cultural issues in sub-Saharan Africa. In: D Doyle, GWC Hanks, N MacDonald (ed.), *Oxford textbook of palliative medicine*, Oxford: Oxford University Press.

12. Mansfield CJ, Mitchell J, and King DE. (2002). The doctor as God's mechanic? Beliefs in the Southeastern United States. *Social Science and Medicine* **54**:399–409.

13. Lam WW and Fielding R. (2003). The evolving experience of illness for Chinese women with breast cancer: a qualitative study. *Psycho-Oncology* **12**:127–40.

14. Cella DF, Mahon SM, and Donovan MI. (1990). Cancer recurrence as a traumatic event. *Behavioral Medicine* **13**:15–22.

15. Armstrong L. (2001). *It's not about the bike – my journey back to life*. London: Yellow Jersey Press.

16. Smith MY, Redd WH, Peyser C, and Vogl D. (1999). Post-traumatic stress disorder in cancer: a review. *Psycho-Oncology* **8**:521–537.

17. Gregory R. (ed.) (1987). *Oxford companion to the mind*. Oxford: Oxford University Press.

18. Moos RH. (1986). *Coping with life crisis: an integrated approach*. New York: Plenum Press.

19. Bowlby J. (1979). *The making and breaking of affectional bonds*. London: Tavistock Publications.

20. Shou KC and Hewison J. (1999). *Experiencing cancer: quality if life in treatment*. Buckingham, UK: Open University Press.

21. Salander P and Windahl G. (1999). Does 'denial' really cover our everyday experiences in clinical oncology? A critical review from a psychoanalytic perspective on the use of 'denial'. *British Journal of Medical Psychology* **72**:267–79.

22. Weisman AD. (1979). *Coping with cancer*. New York: McGraw-Hill.

23. Altschuler J. (1997). *Working with chronic illness*. Basingstoke, UK: Macmillan.

24. Thomas C. (2001). *What are the psychosocial needs of cancer patients and their main carers? A study of user experience of cancer services with particular reference to psychosocial need*. Lancaster: Institute for Health Research, Lancaster University.

25. Heider F. (1959). *The psychology of interpersonal relations*. New York: Wiley.

26. Taylor SE. (1983). Adjustment to threatening events: a theory of cognitive adaptation. *American Psychologist* **38**:1161–73.

27. Lowery J, Jacobsen BS, and DuCette J. (1993). Causal attribution, control, and adjustment to breast cancer. *Journal of Psychosocial Oncology* **10**:37–53.

28. Sikora K and Smedley H. (1988). *Cancer*. London: Heinemann Medical Books.

29. Fox BH. (1998). Psychosocial factors in cancer incidence and prognosis. In: J Holland (ed.), *Psycho-oncology*, Oxford: Oxford University Press.

30. Petticrew M, Fraser JM, and Regan MF. (1999). Adverse life events and risk of breast cancer: a meta-analysis. *British Journal of Health Psychology* **4**:1–17.

31. Barraclough J. (1996). Adverse life events and the development of breast cancer. Other studies have found no association. *British Medical Journal* **312**:845.

32. Price MA, Tennant CC, Smith RC, Butow PN, Kennedy SJ, Kossoff MB, *et al.* (2000). The role of psychosocial factors in the development of breast carcinoma: Part 1. *Cancer* **91**:679–85.

33. Cella DF, Tross S, Orav EJ, Holland J, Silberfarb P, and Rafla S. (1989). Mood states of patients after the diagnosis of cancer. *Journal of Psychosocial Oncology* **7**:45–54.

34. Harcourt D, Rumsey N, and Ambler N. (1999). Same-day diagnosis of symptomatic breast problems: psychological impact and coping strategies. *Psychology, Health and Medicine* **4**:57–71.

35. Taylor SE. (1990). Health psychology: the science and the field. *American Psychologist* **45**:40–50.

36. Lindley C, McCune JS, Thomason TE, Lauder D, Sauls A, Adkins S, *et al.* (1999). Perception of chemotherapy side-effects – cancer versus noncancer patients. *Cancer practice* **7**:59–65.

37. Jones GY and Payne S. (2000). Searching for safety signals: the experience of medical surveillance amongst men with testicular teratomas. *Psycho-Oncology* **9**:385–94.

38. Lorber J. (1975). Good patients and problem patients: conformity and deviance in a general hospital. *Journal of Health and Social Behavior* **16**:213–25.

39. Taylor SE and Brown JD. (1988). Illusion and well-being: a social psychological perspective on mental health. *Psychological Bulletin*, **103**:193–210.

40. Corney R. (1991). Emotional responses in patients and doctors. In: R Corney (ed.), *Developing communication and counselling skills in medicine*, London: Routledge.

41. Ley P. (1997). Compliance among patients. In: A Baum, D Newman, J Weinman, R. West, and C. McManus (ed.), *Cambridge handbook of psychology, health and medicine*, Cambridge: Cambridge University Press.

42. Doyle D and Jeffrey D. (2000). *Palliative care in the home.* Oxford: Oxford University Press.

43. Sheard TAB. (1994). Unconventional therapies in cancer care. In: CE Lewis, C O'Sullivan, and J Barraclough (ed.), *The psychoimmunology of cancer,* Oxford: Oxford University Press.

44. Alter CL, Pelcovitz D, Axelrod A, Goldenberg B, Harris H, Meyers B, *et al.* (1996). Identification of PTSD in cancer survivors. *Psychosomatics* **37**:137–43.

45. Sreekumar C. (1997). Paper presented at the 2nd psychosocial oncology conference, Thiruvananthapuram, Kerala, India.

46. Rajagopal MR, Joranson DE, and Gilson AM. (2001). Medical use, misuse, and diversion of opioids in India. *The Lancet* **358**:139.

47. Shelby RA, Taylor KL, Kerner JF, Coleman E, and Blum D. (2002). The role of community-based and philanthropic organizations in meeting cancer patient and caregiver needs. CA: *A Cancer Journal for Clinicians* **52**:229–46.

48. Parle M, Jones B, and Maguire P. (1996). Maladaptive coping and affective disorders among cancer patients. *Psychological Medicine* **26**:735–44.

49. Harrison J, Maguire P, Ibbotson T, MacLeod R, and Hopwood P. (1994). Concerns, confiding and psychiatric disorder in newly diagnosed cancer patients: a descriptive study. *Psycho-Oncology* **3**:173–9.

50. Jones RV, Hansford J, and Fiske J. (1993). Death from cancer at home: the carers' perspective. *British Medical Journal* **306**:249–51.

51. Barker C, Pistrang N, Shapiro DA, and Shaw I. (1990). Coping and help-seeking in the U.K. adult population. *British Journal of Clinical Psychology* **29**:271–85.

52. Brown GW and Harris TO. (1978) *Social origins of depression: a study of psychiatric disorders in women.* Tavistock: London.

53. Northouse LL, Dorris G, and Charron-Moore C. (1995). Factors affecting couples' adjustment to recurrent breast cancer. *Social Science and Medicine* **42**:69–76.

54. Rodrigue JR, Behen JM, and Tumlin T. (1994). Multidimensional determinants of psychological adjustment to cancer. *Psycho-oncology* **3**:205–14.

55. Neuling SJ and Winefield HR. (1988). Social support and recovery after surgery for breast cancer: frequency and correlates of supportive behaviours by family, friends and surgeon. *Social Science and Medicine* **27**:385–92.

56. Wellisch D, Kagawa-Singer M, Reid SL, Lin Y, Nishikawa-Lee S, and Wellisch M. (1999). An exploratory study of social support: a cross-cultural comparison of Chinese-, Japanese-, and Anglo-American breast cancer patients. *Psycho-oncology* **8**: 207–19.

57. Glasdam S, Jensen AB, Madsen EL, and Rose C. (1996). Anxiety and depression in cancer patients' spouses. *Psycho-Oncology* **5**:23–9.

58. Kissane DW, Bloch S, Burns WI, McKenzies D, and Posterinos M. (1994). Psychological morbidity in the families of patients with cancer. *Psycho-oncology* **3**, 47–56.

59. Dunkel-Schetter C. (1984). Social support and cancer: findings based on patient interviews and their implications. *Journal of Social Issues* **40**:77–98.

60. Pistrang N and Barker C. (1992). Disclosure of concerns in breast cancer. *Psycho-oncology*, **1**:183–92.

61. Pistrang N and Barker C. (1995). The partner relationship in psychological response to breast cancer. *Social Science and Medicine* **40**:789–97.

62. Sabo D, Brown J, and Smith C. (1986). The male group and mastectomy: support groups and men's adjustment. *Journal of Psychosocial Oncology* **4**:19–31.

63. Radley A. (1994). *Making sense of illness: The social psychology of health and disease.* London:Sage.

64. Seligman ME. (1975). *Helplessness: on depression, development and death.* New York: WH Freeman.

65. Mellette SJ. (1985). The cancer patient at work. CA: *A Cancer Journal for Clinicians* **35**:360–73.

66. Maunsell E, Brisson C, Dubois L, Lauzier S, and Fraser A. (1999). Work problems after breast cancer: an exploratory qualitative study. *Psycho-oncology* **8**:467–73.

67. Garfield CA. (1980). Emotional aspects of death and dying. In: RG Twycross and V Ventrafridda (ed.), *The continuing care of terminal cancer patients*, Oxford: Pergamon Press.

68. Worden JW. (1986). *Grief counselling and grief therapy.* London: Tavistock Publications.

69. Weisman AD and Worden JW. (1976). The existential plight in cancer: significance of the first 100 days. *International Journal of Psychiatric Medicine* **7**:1–15.

70. Aldwin CM and Sutton KJ. (1998). A developmental perspective on posttraumatic growth. In: RG Tedeschi, CL Park, and LG Calhoun (ed.), *Posttraumatic growth: positive changes in the aftermath of crisis*, Mahwah, NJ: Lawrence Erlbaum Associates.

71. Nunn K. (1996). Personal hopefulness: a conceptual review of the relevance of the perceived future to psychiatry. *British Journal of Medical Psychology* **69**:227–45.

72. Tennen H and Affleck G. (1998). Personality and transformation. In: RG Tedeschi, CL Park, and LG Calhoun (ed.), *Posttraumatic growth: positive changes in the aftermath of crisis*, Mahwah, NJ: Lawrence Erlbaum Associates.

73. Frank-Stromberg M, Wright PS, Segalla M, and Diekmann J. (1984). Psychological impact of the "cancer" diagnosis. *Oncology Nursing Forum* **11**:16–22.

74. Tedeschi RG, Park CL, and Calhoun LG. (ed.)(1998). *Posttraumatic growth: positive changes in the aftermath of crisis*, Mahwah, NJ: Lawrence Erlbaum Associates.

75. Moos RH and Schaefer JA. (1984). The crisis of physical illness: an overview and conceptual approach. In: R Moos (ed.), *Coping with physical illness: new perspectives*, Vol. 2, New York: Plenum Press.

76. Nerenz DR and Leventhal H. (1983). Self-regulation theory in chronic illness. In: TG Burish and LA Bradley (ed.), *Coping with chronic disease: research and applications*, London: Academic Press.

77. Gill S and Gilbar O. (2001). Hopelessness among cancer patients. *Journal of Psychosocial Oncology* **19**:21–33.

78. Dew AM, Bromet EJ, and Penkower L. (1992). Mental health effects of job loss in women. *Psychological Medicine*, **22**, 751–64.

79. MacLeod AK, Tata P, Evans K, Tyrer P, Schmidt U, Davidson K, *et al.* (1998). Recovery of positive future thinking within a high-risk parasuicide group: Results from a pilot randomized controlled trial. *British Journal of Clinical Psychology* **37**:371–9.

80. Carver CS, Pozo C, Harris SD, Noriega V, Scheier MF, Robinson DS, *et al.* (1993) How coping mediates the effects of optimism on distress: a study of women with early stage breast cancer. *Journal of Personality and Social Psychology* **65**:375–90.

81. Norem JK and Cantor N. (1986). Defensive pessimism: harnessing anxiety as motivation. *Journal of Personality and Social Psychology* **51**:1208–17.

82. Brennan J. (2001). Adjustment to cancer – coping or personal transition? *Psycho-oncology* **10**:1–18.

83. Beck AT. (1967). *Depression: clinical, experimental, and theoretical aspects.* New York: Harper and Row.

84. Greenstein M and Breitbart W. (2000). Cancer and the experience of meaning: a group psychotherapy program for people with cancer. *American Journal of Psychotherapy* **54**:486–500.

85. Csikszentmihalyi M and Csikszentmihalyi IS. (1988). *Optimal experience: psychological studies of flow in consciousness.* Cambridge: Cambridge University Press.

86. Frank AW. (1992). The pedagogy of suffering: moral dimensions of psychological therapy and research with the ill. *Theory and Psychology* **2**:467–85.

87. Polinsky ML. (1994). Functional status of long-term breast cancer survivors: demonstrating chronicity. *Health and Social Work* **19**:165–73.

88. White CA. (2000). Body image dimensions and cancer: a heuristic cognitive behavioural model. *Psycho-oncology* **9**: 183–93.

89. White CA and Unwin JC. (1998). Post-operative adjustment to surgery resulting in the formation of a stoma: the importance of stoma-related cognitions. *British Journal of Health Psychology* **3**:85–93.

90. Passik SD, Newman ML, Brennan M, and Tunkel R. (1995). Predictors of psychological distress, sexual disfunction and physical functioning among women with upper extremity lymphoedema related to breast cancer. *Psycho-oncology* **4**:255–63.

91. Kugaya A, Akechi T, Okamura H, Mikami I, and Uchitomo Y. (1999). Correlates of depressed mood in ambulatory head and neck cancer patients. *Psycho-oncology* **8**:494–99

92. Breitbart W, Chochinov HM, and Passik S. (1998). Psychiatric aspects of palliative care. In: D Doyle, GWC Hanks, and N MacDonald (ed.), *Oxford textbook of palliative medicine,* 2nd edn, Oxford: Oxford University Press.

93. Maguire P. (1992). Improving the recognition and treatment of affective disorders in cancer patients. *Recent Advances in Clinical Psychiatry* **7**:15–30.

94. Ward SE, Goldberg N, Miller-McCauley V, Mueller C, Nolan A, Pawlik-Plank D, *et al.* (1993). Patient-related barriers to management of cancer pain. *Pain* **52**:319–24.

95. Hopwood P. (1993). The assessment of body image in cancer patients. *European Journal of Cancer,* **29A**:276–81.

96. Taylor EJ, Outlaw FH, Bernardo TR, and Roy A. (1999). Spiritual conflicts associated with praying about cancer. *Psycho-oncology* **8**:386–94.

97. Gallup G. (1995). *The gallup poll: public opinion 1995.* Wilmington DE: Schoolarly resources. Cited in Mytko JJ and Knight SJ. (1999). Body, mind and spirit: towards the integration of religiosity and spirituality in cancer quality of life research. *Psycho-oncology* **8**:439–50.

98. Feher S and Maly R. (1999). Coping with breast cancer in later life: the role of religious faith. *Psycho-oncology* **8**:408–16.

99. Maltby J, Lewis CA, and Day L. (1999). Religious orientation and psychological well-being: the role of the frequency of personal prayer. *British Journal of Health Psychology* **4**:363–78.

100. Cole B and Pargament K. (1999). Re-creating your life: a spiritual/psychotherapeutic intervention for people diagnosed with cancer. *Psycho-oncology* **8**:395–407.

101. Moadel A, Morgan C, Fatone A, Grennan J, Carter J, Laruffa G, *et al.* (1999). Seeking meaning and hope: self-reported spiritual and existential needs among an ethnically-diverse cancer patient population. *Psycho-oncology* **8**:378–85.

102. Cordova MJ, Cunningham LL, Carlson CR, and Andrykowski MA. (2000). Posttraumatic growth following breast cancer: a controlled comparison study. *Health Psychology* **20**:176–85.

103. Miller MW and Nygren C. (1978). Living with cancer – coping behaviors. *Cancer Nursing* 297–302.

104. Cella DF and Tross ST. (1986). Psychological adjustment to survival from Hodgkin's disease. *Journal of Consulting and Clinical Psychology* **54**:616–22.

105. Andrykowski MA, Brady MJ, and Hunt JW. (1993). Positive psychosocial adjustment in potential bone marrow transplant recipients: cancer as a psychosocial transition. *Psycho-oncology* **2**:261–76.

106. Kennedy BJ, Tellegen A, Kennedy S, and Havernick N. (1976). Psychological response of patients cured of advanced cancer. *Cancer* **38**:2184–91.

107. Gritz ER, Wellisch DK, Siau J, and Wang H. (1990). Long-term effects of testicular cancer on marital relationships. *Psychosomatics* **31**:301–12.

108. Curbow B, Somerfield MR, Baker F, Wingard JR, and Legro MW. (1993). Personal changes, dispositional optimism, and psychological adjustment to bone marrow transplantation. *Journal of Behavioral Medicine* **16**:423–43.

109. Dunkel-Schetter C, Feinstein L, Taylor SE, and Falke RL. (1992). Patterns of coping with cancer. *Health Psychol* **11**:79–87.

110. Koenig HG, Bearon LB, Hover M, and Trasis JL. (1991) Religious perspectives of doctors, nurses, patients and families. *Journal of Pastoral Care* **45**:254–67.

111. King DE and Bushwick B. (1994) Beliefs and attitudes of hospital inpatients about faith healing and prayer. *Journal of Family Practice* **39**:349–52.

112. Cunningham A, Stephen J, Phillips C, and Watson K. (2001). Psychospiritual therapy. In: J Barraclough (ed.), *Integrated cancer care: holistic, complementary and creative approaches.* Oxford: Oxford University Press.

113. Kissane DW, Bloch S, Miach P, Smith GC, Seddon A, and Keks N. (1997). Cognitive-existential group therapy for patients with primary breast cancer—techniques and themes. *Psycho-oncology* **6**:25–33.

114. Arnold EM. (1999). The cessation of cancer treatment as a crisis. *Social Work in Health Care* **29**:21–38.

115. Peters-Golden H. (1982) Breast cancer: varied perceptions of social support in the illness experience. *Social Science and Medicine* **16**:483–91.

116. Kornblith AB. (1998). Psychosocial adaptation of cancer survivors. In: J Holland (ed.), *Psycho-oncology*, Oxford: Oxford University Press.

117. Seaborn D, Lorenz A, Gunn W, Gawinski B, and Mauksch L. (1996). *Models of collaboration: a guide for mental health professionals working with health care professionals.* New York: Basic Books.

118. Somerfield MR, Stefanek ME, Smith TJ, and Padberg JJ. (1999). A systems model for adaptation to somatic distress among cancer survivors. *Psycho-oncology* **8**:334–43.

Chapter 3

Other people

What is social support and why is it important? 92
    What kind of social support do people with cancer need? 93
    What is emotional support? 94
    The social context of social support 95
    Helpful and unhelpful reactions to cancer 96
Family context 98
    Family turmoil. 99
    Family roles, relationships, and communication 100
    Families and the healthcare team 102
    Supporting families 103
    What and when to tell children 106
    People on their own. 110
    Older people 111
Partner relationships 113
    Partner relationships and communication 114
    Gender differences in partner support 120
    Gay and lesbian couples 124
    Communication advice for couples 126
    Sexual problems. 127
Caring. 134
    The stress of caring 135
    Assessing distress among carers 137
    Supporting carers. 137
References 139

> I am writing this because I know I might need to read it again when perhaps one day I might be standing at the gate at the end of my life … I want to read how it all began and how strong I felt then with everyone I love holding me together.

In the face of any crisis, it is often the people we know who exert the greatest influence over how we get through it. In fact, it would be no exaggeration to say that every person's experience of cancer is decisively shaped by the people they know: their family, friends, colleagues, and acquaintances, as well as the people they come to know, such as healthcare staff and other patients. There are also, of course, broader social and economic conditions which affect how people interpret and respond to their illness and these are explored in Chapter 4. But this chapter looks at the contribution of people closest to the patient, what is academically referred to as *social support*. Social support is critical to how people manage their particular cancer and adjust to its implications.

The crisis of cancer is obviously shared by families, partners, friends, and carers. It will be these people who will be most involved in supporting and caring for the patient during their treatment so it is essential that healthcare staff understand how cancer impacts on these most important people in the patient's life. Many of these people will wish to maintain close contact with the healthcare team, so from the outset patients must be able to define who is their 'family' and who they wish to be given information. And relatives and friends need to know how to access information about their loved one, and to feel comfortable about doing so.

When a significant experience like cancer occurs, we not only look to other people for our physical safety (i.e. the medical team), we also look to other people (family and friends) to understand, corroborate, and emotionally concur with our perceptions and feelings about what is happening. We need our loved ones to reassure us that they will always be there for us, and that they will continue to love and value us. These key relationships, or 'attachments', help cushion us from the immense stress that the threat of cancer poses, enabling us to feel more robust in the face of it. As described below, this is the reason why social support is so powerful in protecting people from the effects of stressful events; simply put, it facilitates coping and adjustment.

The difficulty, however, is that partners, families, and other carers are themselves having to cope with all the changes brought about by the illness, and they too are having to adjust to the knowledge that someone they care about has a life-threatening illness. As we will see in this chapter, not only are patients, partners, and families frequently highly distressed, their relationships with one another are often put under great strain.

What is social support and why is it important?

Social support is one of the most widely studied and commonly cited concepts within the medical and social sciences, a fact that testifies to the importance of other people in our relationship to the world. Without the glue of family and other social relationships no knowledge or culture would be created, and without the development in childhood of an awareness of other people's feelings and intentions few people would survive long. In very general terms, social support simply refers to the help that people give one another. One way of studying social support has been to compare people with many friends and relationships with those who are more socially isolated. Not surprisingly, it has been found that people with many relationships live longer and have better physical and mental health than those without such 'social ties'.[1] According to this view, the individual's social network enmeshes them in a web of relationships that helps sustain them through good times as well as bad.

The other main way of researching social support has been to work out what type of social support is helpful in what sort of situation.[2] There are several forms of social support but the three most important types of support seem to be *practical* help, *informational* help, and *emotional* help. To take a simple example, moving house is a stressful experience for most people. The support given by a friend might involve their practical assistance shifting furniture, providing information about where to find a good removals company, or simply being there to talk to about how exhausting it all is. In practice, a friend might provide all three forms of help or, equally, they may not be able to help at all, though any form of help in this situation might be quite welcome. On the other hand, if a fire broke out in your home, you might appreciate practical support (i.e. help putting it out) rather more than emotional support, however well intentioned. So, according to this second view, social support acts as a kind of psychological 'shock absorber' between the individual and the stress they happen to be facing, *provided* there is a sensible match between the type of stress involved and the type of social support provided.[3]

What kind of social support do people with cancer need?

People's foremost need is to survive, so they obviously look to the healthcare team for this form of practical support. They also need information about their illness and the treatment being offered to them, so that they can predict and feel a sense of control over what is happening to them. Again, the most reliable source of this will be their medical team. Finally, they also need emotional support to help them integrate the many changes they are undergoing and consider the uncertainties that lie ahead. Emotional support is especially important in cases where the individual believes they have little control over the stress itself.[3] Cancer is a prime example of such a situation.

While the emotional support of healthcare staff is essential, it is to partners, family, and friends that people immediately turn when confronted by the stress of cancer. Interview studies, which have asked people with cancer what forms of support were particularly useful, found that over 80% regarded emotional support as the most helpful, 41% mentioned informational support (if provided by healthcare staff), and only 6% rated practical assistance as being important (their medical treatment was not included).[4] Some of the most *un*helpful behaviours concerned family or friends giving the patient information and advice. Other studies have confirmed that people with cancer require plentiful emotional support but frequently complain that what they receive is insufficient.[5, 6] Moreover there is evidence that the presence of emotional support from doctors during 'bad news' consultations is associated with less depression and fewer symptoms of post-traumatic stress[7] (*see* Chapter 6—Eliciting Concerns). In short, it is clear from copious research that those who are emotionally well supported experience less psychological distress (e.g. feelings of anxiety and depression) than those who are not well supported.[6, 8–10]

What is emotional support?

> Spoke to several people and felt very good about myself. Am really appreciating the good friends that I've got – my attitude to friendship will never be the same again.

In Chapter 2 we highlighted some of the many ways in which cancer and its treatment can impact on the individual. Although it can sometimes have ultimately positive effects, cancer often undermines and threatens people's roles in life, how they see themselves and their bodies, their relationships with others, their confidence in themselves, and their sense of purpose and meaning. Yet there is good evidence that emotional support can help protect or buffer people from many of these negative effects.

There is still debate as to how emotional support does this but a plausible explanation goes something like this. Emotional support involves having people in one's life to confide in and feel valued by. It seems to entail two main components: empathy and validation. The idea of empathy is not difficult for most people to grasp but it is far more difficult to define. Empathy involves one person trying to understand what it must feel like to be another person, but it also involves being able to convey this understanding back, without making a value judgement about what has been said. In other words, the person in distress feels that their words and feelings have been both understood and acknowledged. Remarkably, this simple exchange can lead people to feel they have shared something of the burden of their distress, which then feels lighter ('a problem shared is a problem halved'). Empathy, of course, does not always have to involve words; sitting in silence with someone ('being there'), or simply physically embracing the other person can be hugely empathic.

Emotional 'validation' largely comes from feeling reassured through the use of words. The very act of trying to put diffuse thoughts and feelings into words gives them shape and form which often makes events feel more controllable, predictable, and therefore more manageable.[11]

> When you are in your thoughts your mind can go all over the place and I sometimes have the most frightening thoughts about the future. But when I talk about it in words, logic kicks in and it feels easier to handle.

The process of telling the story of what has happened helps to integrate it into one's ongoing 'life narrative' (which, as we saw in Chapter 1, is an important aspect of a person's mental maps). While empathy encourages people to articulate their thoughts and feelings, validation works by confirming helpful perceptions and querying unhelpful ones. For example, if someone is feeling distressed because they believe they have become a burden on their family, the person providing support can help by acknowledging these feelings and perhaps questioning the assumptions upon which they are based. More directly, validation can involve reminders to the patient that they are still valued and loved (sometimes referred to as *esteem support*), and will not be abandoned.

> The thing I felt most curative, while still in the ward, was love. Friends and letters and family brought it and it was drug-like. I dont mean hippy love, I mean care, kindness, being made to feel that I mattered to everybody, and feeling the shock of that.

Much of what people talk about has to do with comparing their version of events with the perception of others. Having one's perceptions validated confers a sense of safety. As ethologist Robert Hinde, has written:

> It is in our nature (for obvious adaptive reasons) to try to achieve a feeling of security and coherence, of being in control, and we can achieve that the more readily if our psychological world is compatible with those of others. We attempt to validate our view of the world by comparing it with those of others.[12]
>
> (Hinde 1998, p. 176)

So, in summary, social support is an essential resource for people negotiating the many stresses of cancer. Emotional support is particularly important because it provides a safe environment in which people can release, share, and clarify their feelings and thoughts.[13] Expressing thoughts and emotions has been shown to reduce the physiological arousal associated with stress.[14] It helps people consider the problems they face and the options available to them, and it provides reassurance to people when making decisions. Finally, using words to explore the meaning of stressful events enables people to integrate them with their core assumptions about the world, so that the events become part of the individual's ongoing life narrative.

But, as already mentioned, there is a complicating factor. Although partners, families, and friends are the most important source of support in people's lives, they can also be a source of stress, particularly at times of crisis. Those providing support are facing enormous changes in their lives and they too are frightened and unsure. Just as the patient is compelled by events to reexamine many of their assumptions and expectations, so too loved ones are often examining theirs. Not surprisingly, relationships change and often become more complicated and strained just at the time when they are needed most.

The social context of social support

The way in which support is expressed and received varies from person to person, family to family, and culture to culture. There are cultural expectations regarding caring and the expression of emotion,[15] and culturally defined gender roles within families. These are not static expectations but continually shift and evolve in response to factors such as economic climate, social mobility, education, technology, and communication.

Every society contains norms, ideals, and myths about what constitutes a 'couple' or a 'family', and how members within these groups should behave towards one another. These expectations include how people should respond to a loved one facing an adversity like serious illness. Such beliefs and expectations are uniquely drawn from the society and culture which has surrounded people throughout their lives and which shapes their individual and collective experiences. For example, in England, new couples tend to be expected to form their own separate household. Consequently, unlike many other cultures, having more than two generations in the same household has been historically relatively rare.[16] In some parts of the West, moreover, families are probably more varied in composition than ever before: couples and parents are not always heterosexual, and there may be any number of 'parents' in a family. In working with couples and families, healthcare professionals therefore need to be sensitive to the cultural expectations, beliefs, and pressures surrounding every one of us, and to respect any differences that do emerge.

Healthcare in the West has also been changing over the past few decades. As more people survive serious disease and live longer, families are being expected to shoulder more of the burden of care. Patients have shorter hospital stays, but they leave 'quicker and sicker'.[17, 18] It is ironic that, as medical technology improves, there are more ill people in the community being cared for by their families. However, as the proportion of older and ill people in the community continues to increase, there are growing numbers of people living on their own,[19] and less traditional family stability or an extended family structure to support people being cared for at home. Consequently there is greater reliance on nursing homes and other forms of institutional care.

Cultural background also influences what families expect of themselves. The extended family is valued by most cultures but, for example, middle-class White Americans are thought to place less value on strong family ties than do African, Asian, or Latino-Americans, and are therefore probably less able to benefit from family support.[20] A person's gender and age is also likely to affect the availability of support.[21] During adolescence, for example, family support tends to increase for girls and decrease for boys. Adult women generally have larger social networks than men and more access to emotional support, and this becomes more pronounced with age; at the same time, the older people are, the smaller their range of social support tends to be. (*see* Gender Differences; also Older People.)

Helpful and unhelpful reactions to cancer

> No one, but no one said a word to me about my situation – it was as though it were a complete non-event, of no importance. I felt very hurt at this, and slipped out and cried all the way home. Later understanding came and I realised that it was probably because no one knew what to say. What do you say to someone who has just been announced to have cancer?

Not everyone reacts supportively when they hear someone is ill. In fact, there is considerable clinical and research evidence that people with cancer are frequently disappointed with the quality and level of support that they do receive. Friends fail to contact the patient, neighbours avoid the family, and even relatives sometimes react with such false optimism that the family can feel their plight is being ignored or trivialized. In many instances, of course, it is simply the social awkwardness of not knowing what to say that causes people to avoid the patient and the family. People are usually concerned, but do not wish to upset the patient by saying the wrong thing and making the situation worse. Social awkwardness (i.e. fear of embarrassment, humiliation, and shame) is a force that should not be underestimated, and is not only a British affliction. But alongside this, people with cancer also sometimes experience social rejection based on fear. The sheer presence of someone with cancer can be a reminder to other people of their mortality, or it may provoke other latent fears (e.g. that cancer is contagious).

While friends and relatives are often keen to help, they may be unclear in their offers. It obviously helps if offers of support are specific. 'Would you like to meet for a chat?' or 'Can I drive you to your treatment?' 'I've got some time on Thursday afternoon; let me know what you would like me to do?' These are questions more likely to elicit a response than 'Let me know if there's anything I can do to help' which is too ambiguous—the patient does not know how to interpret it, so both they and the potential supporter are left waiting for the other person to contact them.

> People say you find out in these situations who your real friends are but I don't think you quite do that. You find out how people deal with these situations. Their friendship may be great but their fear of impotence in the face of illness may be greater ... I mean, it isn't what people do, it's the attention they apply in trying to do the right thing for you. That they are trying on your behalf to manage whatever their own fears are.

Research suggests that the most unhelpful reactions from friends involve *withdrawal* or *avoidance*, while the most unhelpful reactions from those closer to the patient (e.g. partners and close family members) involve *minimizing* the seriousness of the situation, *forced cheerfulness,* or *criticizing* the way the patient is handling their cancer.[4] Helpful behaviours include emotional support from close relatives and friends. Like professionals, other patients are valued for both the information and the emotional support they can provide.[22]

> People around me want me to be positive because it reassures them. What is happening to me is not only threatening for me, but for everybody that knows me. It reminds us that one day we will have to face death. Why are we so reluctant to think about it and to try to come to terms with this fact?

Probably the most insidious and unhelpful response from other people is the pop psychology idea that to survive cancer one must rely upon 'positive thinking'. While, of course, it is important to focus on the positive aspects of any situation, it is both unrealistic and unhelpful to expect anyone to maintain the mental straight-jacketing that positive thinking seems to require. As the diarist above suggests, it is likely that people who insist on positive thinking either feel uncomfortable handling other people's emotional distress, or wish to avoid their own distress (e.g. a man who is afraid of losing his wife upon whom he depends). The main problem with positive thinking is that it expects people to censor rather than express whatever they are really feeling and thinking, and this does little to aid adjustment.

Finally, many people with cancer are simply reluctant to cause distress to their loved ones:

> In the course of the conversations I had with other patients in hospital, it came out that we all tend to keep our 'bad patches' to ourselves. I wonder why? Is it because we fear that in showing our vulnerability, we would most certainly upset our loved ones and, therefore, make it all the more difficult?

Family context

To understand how cancer impacts on families, it helps to understand something about families. Like partners, families can either be an enormous source of support, or an additional source of distress. Healthcare professionals who are sensitive to these issues can provide more sensitive care, though rarely does this require the intervention of a specialist.

From the moment we are born we turn to our families or carers for support; we quickly learn that our carers are there to provide us with the safety, nurturing, and guidance that we need. Throughout childhood and beyond we depend upon our families for understanding and reassurance when we are in trouble. Such 'attachments' help to ensure our survival.[23] Knowledge builds upon previous knowledge so that a person's earliest experiences (which usually involve their biological family) are likely to be particularly important in shaping the expectations they hold about relationships in general. With the child's developing awareness of other people's perspectives and experiences (their 'theory of mind', *see* Chapter 1) comes the opportunity for deeper, more empathic relationships.

It is from the secure base of the family that we feel the confidence to explore the world beyond it. As we emerge out of childhood, partners and friends come to assume more importance as sources of social support, particularly emotional support. Close personal relationships, such as partners and family members continue to be an important source of emotional support to people throughout life; they are the secure base to which we return at times of crisis or uncertainty. As already described, emotional support is particularly effective as a psychological shock absorber in situations, like cancer, which are frightening, ambiguous, and apparently uncontrollable. But although a supportive family may help cushion the shock of cancer on the individual, the family itself will also reverberate from its impact. Like the individual with cancer, the family is a living open system and must adapt itself to the new situation of having an ill member. Not surprisingly, those families that are able to maintain a sense of coherence in the face of illness tend to be more resilient and maintain a high family quality of life.[24]

Families vary in size, structure, and complexity.[25] They vary in the beliefs they hold and the way members communicate with one another. They vary in the age of their members, the shared history of their relationships with one another, and their shared experience of stressful events. Every family has its own history or 'family narrative'.

They vary in their resilience and ability to adapt to change, and they vary from the extremes of being highly rigid to being highly chaotic. They vary according to how closed or open, how cohesive or differentiated, and how strict or liberal they are. In short, families are complex systems that can differ from one another in a large number of ways.

As Tolstoy famously asserted, 'all happy families resemble one another, each unhappy family is unhappy in its own way.'[26] There is certainly no 'normal family', nor is there a family without some tensions or difficulties. It is therefore essential that problems within families are not instantly regarded as 'pathological' (or the family seen as 'dysfunctional') but, rather, understood in context, in terms of what the problem may be expressing about the family as a whole, or the function the problem serves within the family system.[18] For example, in families where one of the parents is ill, a child who becomes fractious and angry may be expressing their own distress at the situation, but equally their anger may indicate that the child's developmental needs are being neglected, or that information is not being fully shared within the family.

Family turmoil

When cancer affects one of its members for the first time, the family faces a situation with which it has never had to cope before. Even when there has been previous disease in the family, the new illness must be confronted afresh, albeit with expectations coloured by previous experiences. Individual members must adapt their *roles* within the family to fit in with new requirements imposed by the illness; for example, adolescent children may be required to help with the cooking when one of their parents is ill and the other parent is visiting the hospital. The *structure* of the family may have to alter temporarily; a grandparent may have to stay with the family to help look after the children of a single parent. Members of the family may also find themselves *communicating* with one another in a different way; for example, after learning he has cancer, a father may want to become more emotionally involved with his children. In short, each family member's mental maps of the world must adjust to the implications of the patient's illness.

> A lot of good has come out of all this: the family are much closer, W [husband] & I are on the way to a stronger relationship, the kids are mature and caring, I've learnt to really appreciate the value of real friends and I've met some wonderful people who I hope I will never forget.

Many of the challenges faced by families parallel those faced by the individual. The trajectory of a family is shaped by its evolving history and guided towards the future by shared values and goals.[27] Each member will have their own views and expectations about illness and how to respond to it. Family members are expected, by themselves and by others, to care for their sick member at a time when they are often feeling shocked and terrified. For a while the family may become more 'permeable' as extra support is drawn in: healthcare professionals, extended family, friends, and religious organizations.[18] As the crisis subsides or intensifies, the family's relationship to this 'outside world' will vary, but many family members will experience prolonged distress.[28]

The primary task of the family with cancer, therefore, is to be able to respond flexibly to the changing needs imposed by the illness and the treatment, while maintaining its integrity as a family and its other functions. As with personal crisis, family turmoil is not always ultimately negative; some families have reported that cancer has led to more time for family activities[29] and brought the members closer.[30] For some, however, it revives unresolved problems from the family's history. In any event, the family must not become frozen in the past, functioning as if nothing has happened, nor paralysed by the illness such that children's developmental needs are ignored.

> So easily, family needs can come second to the needs of the illness ... We need to help families hold on to their competence, and integrate their experience of illness in a way that retains some identity unrelated to illness[18]

(Altschuler 1997, p. 47).

Family roles, relationships, and communication

In studies of family communication, patients who show the lowest distress also report the best patient–family communication. Good family communication is associated with frequent opportunities for patients to discuss the illness and its consequences, and for the family to be a strong source of emotional support.[31] It seems that where open communication is maintained and people are free to express themselves, families are more effective in supporting the patient and managing the changes that cancer involves.[32–34]

However, the threat of cancer may be so unspeakably dangerous to the security of family members that open communication within the family system becomes tense and uncertain. Consequently, relationships between family members become strained and challenged. The demands on families vary according to the stage of the disease and the developmental needs of family members. The immediate concern of the family is with the threat of death and how this would impact on each member personally, as well as other members of the family. The enormity of this threat, however, can be too frightening to talk about, especially with loved ones who would be most affected. A 'conspiracy of silence' may hang over the family, as members either withhold information from one another, or react to it by minimizing or trivializing the threat facing them all. Thus, at a time when family members need each other most, they can suddenly find themselves inhibited from talking with one another, not knowing what it is safe or potentially damaging to discuss.

> I'm feeling so miserable now. I've had a little cry. I want to talk to Mum but I know I'll just cry. I can't talk to anyone 'cos I'll cry. I'll just have to cry on my own. I just wish it were over. I'm already tired of being brave.

During the initial phase of treatment, the family becomes centred around the demands imposed by the treatment calendar (i.e. hospital appointments). This phase requires considerable domestic upheaval and the reorganization of family roles and responsibilities. Social activities are reduced, employment and household activities altered, child care responsibilities have to be rearranged, and transport to and from the hospital must be organized. At the same time, previously laid individual and family plans may have to be postponed or abandoned, with resulting disappointment. Members of the family may be required to leave work to support the patient, with obvious consequences for the family's financial security.

While the patient and their partner, if there is one, are usually the first to learn about the threat of cancer, one cannot assume that this information will then reach other members of the family. People with cancer frequently minimize the seriousness of their situation so as to shield other members from being distressed or themselves becoming 'a burden'. Parents understandably want to filter the news that they pass on to their children. Even adult children are sometimes 'protected' by their parents from ongoing news of the illness; indeed, when they feel they have inadequate information their anger is sometimes directed towards healthcare staff.[35] Some parents with cancer suffer intense worry about the fate of their children if they were to die, yet may find it difficult to discuss such fears lest others regard them as having 'given up'.

> I have always been the strong helper but now I have to accept help and show vulnerability with friends and family. I am aware that this would be really frightening for them (or so I imagine, maybe I'm being over protective) so I keep up the strong front.

There are many ways in which relationships within the family must adjust to the demands of cancer and its treatment. Family members' desire to protect one another from distress can lead to emotional distance between them though, conversely, a particularly intense relationship between the ill person and a family member (usually their main carer) can lead other members to feel excluded and isolated.[18] The relationship between a parent and their adolescent child may be transformed when the child is required to help the parent with intimate aspects of their care, such as bathing and toileting. The new restrictions and responsibilities imposed on family members can lead to resentment, blame, and guilt, unless these feelings are openly discussed and addressed. Some children may feel they are shouldering an unfair proportion of the burden of care compared with their siblings. Young adults with cancer, having recently left home and enjoying their autonomy, may be forced to resume a more dependent relationship with their parents. Men who are required to take over more childcare responsibilities may welcome the opportunity to spend more time with their children. But, while a father is being challenged by his new role, his partner may feel that her normal role has been taken away from her.

> I have distracted myself from D. [son] during all this time. Why did I do that? I love him, so much. He needs me. Have I hurt him because I have not been me? What the hell was I doing? Trying to protect him so that when I die it will not be so hard? This hurt right now is way beyond me.

Sometimes family members, including the patient, emotionally withdraw in order to begin the process of separation that will inevitably occur at the moment of death.

Such premature withdrawal is almost always misguided and can be challenged by asking the person concerned whether they have considered the wishes of the rest of the family (e.g. '*Are you sure they want you to withdraw? What do you think they are wanting from you right now? Would you be happy for them to withdraw if it were they that were ill?*')

It is essential that the patient is not relegated to a role in the family which is solely defined by their illness. The challenge for the family system is being able to respond and adapt to the needs of the illness and its treatment, while maintaining the integrity of its relationships. For example, an ill parent may need the emotional and practical support from others in the family, but they can still maintain their role as a parent who *provides* support. To maintain an adaptive family system requires open channels of communication so that differences and conflicts can be aired and resolved, and the needs of each member can be understood by the others.

Any of these problems may be magnified in single parent and lower income families.[25] These families are frequently already dealing with major stresses with little support. A single parent may turn to their child for someone to talk to, or practical support, when no one else is available. The child, in turn, may be more reluctant to burden their sole parent with their own needs yet may worry about being orphaned if they were to lose their sole parent. Also, the financial strains of lower income families can lead older children to drop out of school and seek work.

Families and the healthcare team

Holding regular meetings with families, especially early in the treatment, not only helps to establish shared goals and expectations (a 'road map'), it can help identify difficulties they may be having. Equally important, it is an opportunity to provide the family with guidance on what care is expected of them – this information is widely appreciated by family members, who frequently feel helpless yet want to be active in their support. Interestingly, adult children of cancer patients are sometimes angry and demanding, perhaps driven by their helplessness to advocate actively on behalf of their parents, or possibly because of their anticipatory grief.[36]

One focus group study that questioned patients and providers about optimal doctor–family communication asked how best to integrate family members into the process of healthcare.[37] Families certainly wanted to be seen as a resource for the rest of the healthcare team. Both healthcare providers and patient groups regarded families as a useful 'extra set of ears' in recalling relevant information for both the patients and the medical staff. (In fact, when a family member is present, doctors have been observed to provide more information but less emotional support.[38]) They were seen as a source of comfort and emotional support, as well as a help for patients making critical decisions about their treatment.

Patients may wish to have a member of their family present in consultations with their doctors and this should always be facilitated whenever possible. However, while family-centred care may be the ideal, it is important to note that in a huge UK national survey of 65 000 cancer patients conducted in 2000, 14% stated that they did *not* want family and friends to be involved in decisions about care and treatment and a further 6% reported that they had no family or friends to be involved.[39] Therefore the patient's wishes regarding family involvement must always be ascertained first.

In the focus-group study, healthcare staff reported finding families difficult to work with when information was being deliberately concealed from one family member by another. The staff suggested the following strategies:[37]

- ask the patient in advance how much information they want the rest of the family to know;
- communicate with patients and families together as much as possible;
- ensure that the same information is given to both patient and family;
- make it clear that the patient cannot be treated if the family do not allow them to know about their illness;
- remind the family that the patient is the team's first priority;
- ask the family how they would feel if information was withheld from them.

Supporting families

To summarize, families are complex systems that vary from one another along many dimensions. The structure, cohesiveness, and communication within families can differ according to many cultural factors, so it is essential to respect the uniqueness of *every* family and the way they are attempting to manage the threat of the illness. It is generally unhelpful to think in terms of 'normal' families or to imagine that there exist families without conflict or difficulties.

Families can be a vital source of emotional and practical support to people with cancer. However, family members are often highly distressed and in need of support themselves. The family is a living system of relationships and, as such, must adapt to the changing demands of cancer, while continuing to see to the developmental needs of all its members. This is achieved through open communication between members of the family so that differences and problems can be understood and resolved. However, family members are often inhibited about expressing their own feelings because of a desire to protect themselves or others from further distress, and this can be interpreted by others as withdrawal at the very time when support is needed. Consequently, a number of difficulties can develop in families as they struggle to manage the illness and its treatment.

- It is essential that the patient defines which people constitute their 'family' and who they wish to support them. It will be these people who will be most involved in caring for the patient and maintaining contact with the healthcare team.
- The healthcare team assumes major importance to families as a source of information and support. What professionals say to family members is often later scrutinized

and dissected. Healthcare staff can do much to reassure families by listening to and 'containing' their fears and concerns. The family needs detailed ongoing information so that it can adjust to the current situation and prepare itself for the future.[40]

- Contacts between healthcare staff and family members are typically very limited, yet family members want to be treated as integral members of the healthcare team, with information to give as well as receive.[41] Because families and doctors are rarely in the hospital at the same time, the responsibility for initiating contact often rests with family members who are reluctant to bother busy doctors and nurses[17] Family members are often intimidated by healthcare professionals, especially if they are faced with several staff members at once or different staff on each visit, but they will appreciate contact particularly if it is initiated by staff.

- Professionals should aim to maintain contact with family members in a planned and systematic manner; families need to know when and where they will have contacts with the healthcare team. The use of a key worker, such as a specific nurse acting as an ongoing information access point for the family, can be helpful. Some authors have advocated the use of a family conference so that clinicians can clarify the family's understanding of the illness and identify any concerns or problems. In this way, the professional can serve as a model of open communication by sharing information and helping to resolve problems[35] Seeing a family together enables each person to express their fears with one another and for the professional to normalize their worries.[42] If family members and healthcare staff are 'in tune' with one another there will be shared expectations and fewer misunderstandings.[37]

- Families should be encouraged to draw in as much support as they feel can deal with. Too much support can destabilize and undermine families, but it is helpful to dispel the myth that all families *should* be able to cope without external support. Extended family, friends, religious organizations, health and social care agencies, and voluntary organizations can all have a role in supporting the family.

- Lower-income families often face considerable financial and practical burdens as a result of the illness, though they may be reluctant to voice their concerns for fear of losing dignity and respect in the eyes of professional staff. Thus, easy access to information about social welfare should be made available to *all* families, whether or not they are likely to require it.

- Like patients, families often wish to be actively involved during the treatment. '*Doing something*' helps to avoid the unpleasant sense of helplessness and passivity that patients and families too often feel. Healthcare staff can help by suggesting ways that the family can support the patient (e.g. encouraging the patient to talk about whatever they wish to discuss, helping with their practical needs, being encouraging, demonstrating their love, aiding their rehabilitation).

- It should not be assumed that information will automatically be transmitted through the patient to and from their partner, if there is one. Although the final decision must rest with the patient, they may find it helpful to discuss what information is shared with whom in the family. *Have you managed to tell people in the family about your illness? How much do they understand?* People with cancer sometimes find it helpful to obtain guidance on how other people handle such delicate issues (e.g. *see* What and When to Tell Children). In general, people with cancer should be encouraged to be as open as possible with other members of the family so that misunderstandings can be minimized from the start.

- Discharge planning should include family members so as to dispel any anxieties they may have around caring for the patient at home. Teaching family members as part of a rehabilitation programme, or asking families to attend a session where they will obtain information and learn practical caring skills, can leave families feeling both more involved and more competent in facing what often feels like an uncertain future.

- Professional staff should routinely assess how the patient feels about their level of family support. Such an assessment can start by acknowledging the many different ways families cope with the diagnosis of cancer, thus attempting to normalize whatever response the patient may have already received from their family, for example:

Families seem to have all sorts of ways of reacting to cancer, some helpful, some perhaps not so helpful. After all, this is a situation none of you have had to face before.

- How do you feel your family has been managing since you've been ill?
- Are you worried about any particular person in the family?
- Do you feel you are all managing to talk to one another openly about the situation and any difficulties that crop up?
- Do you feel your role in the family has changed?
- How do you feel the children are getting on?'

- In meeting with the family, it may be useful to review the following issues:
  - Has the patient, because of their illness, been moved to the periphery of the family? To what extent are they able to maintain their normal roles and relationships?
  - Are the patient's needs being recognized and attended to by other family members?
  - Does the family have access to support from other people and agencies?
  - Are there pre-existing family issues that have re-emerged since the illness began?
  - If there are two parents, how is their relationship faring? Are they able to communicate effectively about the family?
  - Are the developmental needs of all family members being addressed?

- Certain features of family functioning may give cause for concern and should be used as a cue for referral to a specialist, such as a family therapist or social worker, after discussion with the patient. Staff should be concerned where ... [40]
  - the family seems unable to provide adequate care or support to the patient;
  - the patient is not complying with treatment without their family's agreement;

- the family's behaviour disrupts the work of the unit (e.g. the family upsets other patients, is excessively angry, etc.);
- there is conflict between the family and professional staff;
- there are signs of extreme anxiety or depression in a family member;
- a family member has severe physical complaints;
- there is clear conflict between the patient and the family.

What and when to tell children

One of the most distressing tasks for any parent (or other relative) with cancer is having to tell their children that they have a life-threatening illness. It is even more distressing when children must be told to prepare themselves for the death of their parent. Given the enormity of the news they have to convey, many parents worry about damaging their children by saying the wrong thing, at the wrong time, and in the wrong way. This is particularly the case for single parents who may have no one to talk these issues through with. Parents often imagine that unless they 'get it right', their children will be emotionally scarred for the rest of their lives. So parents often turn to professionals for guidance on how best to talk to their children.

First, it is important to state that parents know their children better than any 'expert' could. Therefore parents' judgements about what is the right thing to do for their children should be supported and encouraged, and the 'advice' below should never be used to undermine this basic premise. By helping parents to reflect on what they instinctively feel is right, healthcare staff can enable them to feel more confident about their judgements. Of course, if there are two parents, these discussions should involve both of them together to ensure that children hear a consistent message.

The second thing to say is that children are developing all the time. Consequently their understanding (i.e. their mental maps of the world) is also constantly changing. Therefore, information that may be appropriate at one time may no longer be sufficient at another. Like adults, children require sufficient time to absorb information and it is essential therefore to ensure that they have easy access to further information and are able to ask further questions whenever they wish.

Children are quick to pick up that something is amiss. If they are deprived of information about what is happening children are likely to generate their own ideas; in other words, they will fantasize and worry. If they later discover they have been misled, it may be difficult to regain their trust. Young children may worry that the parent's illness is their fault, especially if they are sent away to be looked after by another relative. They quickly become aware of changes in the way their parents are caring for them and often long for their previous level of contact with a parent. Some children even worry that they will be entirely abandoned.

The evidence suggests that fully informing children about a terminal illness reduces their anxiety and helps them deal with it better.[43] However, in the case of cancers with a longer-term prognosis, it is less clear whether a full exploration of future possible scenarios may do more harm than good. Children's need for 'the truth' must be balanced by their need to know they are loved, safe, and will not be abandoned. So, while it is important to tell children honestly that the parent has cancer, it is equally vital to reassure them (without making promises) that, where there is a reasonable prognosis, the parent fully expects to overcome the illness and continue to be there for them. In the absence of any firm prospect of death (i.e. a short prognosis) there is little point in children needlessly worrying about their parents and their future security; if there is a turn for the worse, there is almost always enough time to prepare the child for the parent's death. Of course, in such an event, children must be given sufficient warning of their parent's imminent death so they can prepare for the loss, though even doctors usually find it difficult to anticipate accurately when someone will die.

Practical guidance

- If a parent asks healthcare staff for advice about talking with their children, professionals should reassure and support the parent in their role and not leave them feeling undermined and deskilled. The parent's knowledge of the child and their feelings about what is the right thing to say should always be respected.

- It can be helpful to establish what and why parents want to tell their children about the illness. There are many good reasons for telling children about cancer but it is helpful if the parents can articulate these for themselves. This discussion may then guide their thinking in terms of what they subsequently tell their children. Parents understandably worry about upsetting their children and getting upset themselves. It can help parents to rehearse what it is they want to say to their children, as well as anticipate what their children are like to say and do in response. Reassure parents that it is not harmful to get upset in front of their children. If there is more than one parent, encourage them to be consistent with one another in talking to their children.

- It is useful if the parent starts by asking the child what they understand about what has been happening. The parent can then correct any misunderstandings as well as gently bring the child up-to-date with the current situation.

- The way in which information is conveyed to children must be appropriate to the age of the child. A very young child's beliefs about illness may be quite limited, while an older child may already have picked up some powerful associations of what cancer 'means'. Younger children will tend to worry about the safety of the family, their own security, and whether or not they are to blame for the illness. They should be very clearly reassured about this. Older children are more likely to be concerned about the impact of the illness on their own lives. Adolescent children often feel conflict between wanting to support the ill parent and wanting to continue to develop their independent life away from the family (consequently feeling guilty when they are not at home). They may also have concerns about their own risk of developing cancer, especially in cancers where there is a known genetic risk and, indeed, may begin to view the future course of their own lives differently.[44]

- Parents should be guided by the child's reactions. Make the illness manageable for the child by not presenting it as a tragedy. Break the news a little at a time. The attention span of young children is short, so long-winded answers are likely to miss their mark. Smaller chunks of information are preferable. The child should be given ample time to react and say what they feel. If a child withdraws, it may be a sign that they have had enough for the moment. The parent should suggest that they return to the conversation when the child feels ready to know more.

- Parents should use simple unambiguous language so as to avoid misunderstanding. For example, saying that one may have to 'lose' a breast can be confusing to a young child who is accustomed to losing things all the time. Either demonstrate using your body, or use suitable media according to the child's developmental stage: e.g. perhaps toys or pictures with a very young child to demonstrate the loss of a breast.

- Parents should be encouraged to use the term 'cancer' because, by using it, the word becomes less emotionally charged. If the child is in school, explain a few of the basic facts about cancer so that, if they later hear the word used on the playground, they will be better equipped to separate fact from fiction. For example, parents should make it clear that cancer is not contagious, that there are many different types of cancer, and that not everyone dies from it, that everyone is unique, etc.

- While being open and honest with one's child is essential, it is important to balance this with the child's other needs. Children do not need to be told about every follow-up test that their parent undergoes or the fact that a blood test indicates a slight elevation in liver enzymes. It may be more sensible to discuss the state of the disease with the children only when there is something definite to report that has significant implications for the child.[45]

- Pointing out that the medical team has plans, that there is treatment to be had, or that, in the case of incurable disease, there is still time to be had with the dying parent, allows the child to retain a sense of safety and hope. The child should always be reassured that, no matter what happens, their need for security and love will be met. In particular, children who face the loss of their only parent need reassurance that they will continue to be cared for, so it is essential that these practical issues have been thoroughly explored and guardians identified.

- It is important that parents warn the children about the side-effects of treatment: hair loss, nausea, fatigue. Children may worry that these are signs that the parent is becoming more ill rather than being treated. Parents should explain that, while the parent is undergoing treatment, things around the home may be different, and that people in the family may be a bit more emotional than usual. The child should be warned that they may feel a bit left out because the parent needs more attention and care than normal.

- Parents should ask the child if they have any questions of their own. When a child asks a direct question it should be answered rather than evaded. If one is unsure about an answer it is better to say 'I don't know but I'll try to find out' than to guess or lie. Avoiding difficult questions merely fuels the child's fears. The most anxious children are likely to be those who feel unable to discuss their parent's illness with them.[46]

• Children should be reassured that they will be kept informed and can ask further questions whenever they have them. They should be encouraged to talk to other trusted adults if they wish. It obviously helps if other adults, such as teachers, coaches, friends, and relations continue to be involved in the child's life so they can be a source of ongoing support to them.

• Allow the child to use whatever defences they have. Sometimes adolescent children *appear* heartlessly uncaring which can be hurtful to a sick parent. Other children may act out their fear and anger in some other setting such as school. Children, like adults, need time in which to make sense of the news. It can help parents to know that there are many different reactions among children and that regression (i.e. to a younger stage of development) is quite common when the child's world feels threatened.

• If a parent is going to be absent for a while (e.g. hospitalization), warn the child of this and try to preserve whatever means of communication are possible. Parents should expect that on their return home children sometimes appear rejecting and angry, while still pleased to see them. When the parent's appearance has radically changed as a result of the illness or its treatment, the child should be warned of this before seeing them (a photo can help prepare the child). Reassure children that the parent is still the same inside even if they look different as a result of their treatment.[47]

• Maintain continuity for the child. A predictable world is one where people feel in control and safe. Retain the child's focus on the normal activities of their lives rather than the parent's illness. It is essential that the child's developmental needs are not ignored or neglected, and that they continue to feel loved and secure.

• Communicate to the child that both the family and the healthcare team (as well as the child) are working together to help the ill parent. This will help the child feel part of a larger team of people on the side of the parent. Asking children to help more with domestic tasks may not always be welcomed, but some children like to be able to contribute their support.

Worrying about children

For ill parents of young children the spectre of their own death is often unthinkably distressing to bear. Regardless of how good a prognosis they may have received, parents often suffer with intrusive images of their children suffering intense grief on the day of their funeral, or other disturbing thoughts about the fate of their loved ones. Often such thoughts cause parents restless insomnia at night and intensely poignant contact with their children during the day.

As is typical of worry, individuals allow their minds to 'witness' these painful images until their distress becomes too overwhelming. They then try to distract themselves with more cheerful thoughts or busy activity. In time, however, the same images and thoughts inevitably intrude once again. It is fruitless for others to challenge these images because, certainly in the case of those with advanced cancer, they may be entirely realistic. Worry, after all, is merely a facet of the mind's very adaptive capacity to anticipate the future; it does not necessarily distort it. The answer lies in helping people to think *beyond* the 'snapshot moment' of their children's most intense grief. By imagining, and putting into words, the days, months, and years which follow their funeral, people can begin to accept that their children's suffering will pass and that they will adjust to a world in which their parent is no longer with them. This thought can be powerfully reassuring to parents whose primary concern will be for the welfare of their children. As David Spiegel has noted, 'talking about the worst somehow detoxifies it'[48] (Spiegel 1990, p. 1423).

This form of intervention necessarily involves exploring the patient's worst fears and therefore often provokes intense distress in the short term. It should not be pursued lightly, and only when the patient has understood its purpose and agreed to it, and there is sufficient time and privacy (*see* Chapter 5—Worry).

People on their own

The economic wealth of the West has led to large numbers of people establishing households that are separate from their family of origin. Many of these people live alone and, indeed, many have chosen to live alone. They include single, divorced, separated, and widowed people. In fact, in Britain 17% of the adult population were living on their own in 2000 and this proportion has been increasing over the past decade.[19] Half of the people over the age of 75 live on their own.

Although there has been little academic attention paid to the needs of people with cancer who live on their own, they can present with distinct concerns. A UK national survey of 65 000 cancer patients in 2000 reported that 6% of them had no family or friends to be involved in decisions about their care and treatment.[39] It is unknown how many of these were socially isolated or were finding it difficult to access adequate support. Even among people on their own who are relatively well supported, many fear that they will become a burden on their friends or a source of distress to their families. Here is how one 35-year-old single woman, not a cancer diarist, described her wish for a partner:

> It would be having that person in the house so that when you are feeling low at that instant they are there … You might want them to give you a hug. The worst time is just when you are going to bed – then the thoughts start again and there's no one there to talk to.

People who wish to have a partner may feel that the vestiges of their cancer preclude this possibility, either because of disability or disfigurement, or because of a loss of function (e.g. fertility). This, and a loss of confidence, obviously carry the risk of self-fulfilling prophecy if they lead individuals to avoid social opportunities to meet new people. It therefore helps if people on their own can discuss their fears and apprehension about making new social contacts, their reluctance about turning to friends and family for support, as well as any difficulties they have re-integrating with their social lives.

Young people often turn to their family of origin for support yet may feel ambivalent, appreciating the support of their parents yet resenting them for their own adolescent fear that they have regressed to a child again. Many young people also have to 'grow up fast', facing their mortality at an age when their contemporaries are exploring and testing themselves within the social world. They may find it hard to re-integrate socially with friends and peers in light of the life-changing experiences they have been through. For example, there may be a tendency to dismiss their friends' concerns as trivial when compared with the life-threatening drama they have been through in which they were centre stage. Or it may simply be difficult learning not to 'play the cancer card' when, in the past, it has generated such a powerful reaction in others.

Older people

The incidence of cancer rises with age. Over half of all cancers occur in people over the age of 65, and the incidence of the most common cancers (prostate, breast, colorectal) increases significantly in people over this age. But older age is not just associated with a higher incidence of cancer. Other chronic conditions such as arthritis, hypertension, and hearing and visual impairments are also more common among older people. Progressive loss in physiological functioning in older age is also associated with reduced ability to perform 'activities of daily living' (cooking, cleaning, self-care), a weaker immune system, and reduced ability to recover from traumatic events such as falls, surgery, or acute illness.[49] So cancer among older people often occurs in the context of other illnesses.

Unlike many other cultures in the world, in which older people are revered for their life experience and wisdom, older people in some Western countries often feel they are regarded as irrelevant, redundant, or a nuisance. Older people frequently feel invisible and ignored, and they are rarely afforded the respect and dignity they receive in other cultures. The uniqueness and diversity of every individual seems to be lost in a culture obsessed with youth. This gradual social exclusion is manifest in the healthcare provided to older people in that healthcare resource allocation unduly disadvantages the older person[50] American studies show that older patients are less likely than younger people to receive aggressive forms of cancer treatment despite being as willing to choose them. They are also less likely to have alternative therapies presented to them or to be offered adjuvant therapy.[50] Furthermore, even though older people may be suffering from a number of other physical complaints (particularly arthritis), pain is under-diagnosed and under-treated, especially among patients who are female and poor.[50]

The fact that serious illness is often seen as less timely or 'appropriate' among younger people in no way lessens its impact on older individuals whose core assumptions may be similarly violated, albeit in different ways. Yet this assumption of 'timeliness' may be responsible for the fact that older people tend to under-report their symptoms compared with younger people, seeing them as 'normal' or 'inevitable'.[49]

Older people are thought to suffer more psychological problems than younger people, with rates of suicide, depression, and organic brain disease (dementia) increasing with age. Loneliness, other psychosocial sources of distress (e.g. loss of a partner), as well as social deprivation (e.g. poverty), and discrimination are commonly reported among older people with cancer. Older people often have less involvement in roles that formerly sustained their sense of control and worth in society at large.

This general picture of decline, however, should not be overstated. Older people are as diverse as any other section of the community and many people adapt positively to their advancing years, remaining actively engaged in meaningful goals until late in life. However, the supportive care and psychosocial needs of older people have been neglected features of geriatric care generally, and especially among those living in nursing homes.[51]

As people grow older in the West more of them live on their own. In Britain, this applies to 60% of women and 33% of men over the age of 75.[19] Living alone and experiencing loneliness do not necessarily mean the same thing, but people who live on their own generally experience more loneliness than those who live with someone else.[52] The decline of secure and meaningful relationships among older people not only affects their sense of loneliness but also their opportunities to manage and integrate the many frightening elements of cancer and its treatment. In one Swedish study, eight out of ten prostate cancer patients who were not living with a partner had no one to confide in, while men who did have someone to confide in reported better emotional and physical well-being.[53]

Healthcare staff should be attuned to the fact that older patients are often more needy than is apparent, and may be more reluctant than younger people to report their distress, whether it is largely a physical concern (e.g. pain), a social problem (e.g. isolation), or emotional suffering (e.g. depression). Yet all these factors can interact and influence one another so any assessment of an older person should attend to this holistic context. Where family members and other carers are available, they may be a valuable source of additional information in assessing the needs of older people,[51] provided their views do not eclipse those of the patient. This may be especially valuable where the patient has cognitive impairments such as those caused by dementia. The ability of the family to provide emotional support and practical care-giving is critical to the well-being of older people with cancer. However, the well-meaning desire of the family to provide comprehensive care must not undermine the older person's sense of autonomy or encourage a premature sense of dependency.[49]

Above all, healthcare staff must avoid the common tendency to generalize about older people and thereby neglect the wide diversity of experience and need in this growing population. For example, many older people have poor hearing but not all; rather than raise their voice, thus appearing to patronize older people, healthcare staff should first establish how well the patient can hear. Professionals commonly underestimate psychological distress among older people,[54] just as older people are more likely to present their distress as a 'medical' problem: insomnia, poor appetite, etc.[55]

Too often chronological age is used as a proxy for the individual's physical or mental status, their capacity to absorb bad news, or their wish to collaborate in planning their treatment. Older people feel pain no less acutely, and experience fear and loss just as intensely as younger people. Healthcare professionals frequently underestimate older patients' competence and potential for rehabilitation,[49] as well as their responsiveness to psychological forms of therapy.[56] Above all, it is important to take a psychosocial history of older patients. Apart from eliciting their concerns, one of the potential added advantages of taking such a history from older patients is to reveal their unique life story and, by doing so, lift them out of anonymity in the eyes of their healthcare team. Older people have had long lives and deserve due respect.

Partner relationships

It has long been recognized that confiding relationships act as a protection or buffer against depression for those facing chronic stress.[57] As discussed above, intimate relationships provide emotional support which helps people make sense of, and adjust to stressful events; this form of social support is especially important when what is happening feels beyond the individual's immediate control. Although not all confiding partnerships involve marriage, this has been the most widely studied type of relationship. Being married is consistently related to better health and a reduction in the negative emotional effects of all types of life strain,[58] though the benefits are almost always greater for men than for women.[59] One of the most important positive health effects of being married is that marriage involves people in a greater number of family ties and social networks, thus preventing social isolation.[60]

When people are distressed they are most likely to turn to their spouse or partner for support.[61] In adulthood, partners to some extent replace parents as being the 'secure base' in people's lives from which they can explore the wider world. Adult relationships provide security and safety by enabling partners to trust and depend on each other in good times and in bad. This capacity for sustained intimacy, for mutual concern, and sensitivity to another's point of view, as well as the ability to reflect on one's actions in the face of criticism, are all qualities that children learn, or fail to learn, from their families of origin.[62] For a relationship to remain alive and creative, partners must be emotionally accessible and responsive to one another, as well as comfortable with feeling somewhat dependent on the other person.[63]

However, when both members of a couple are under stress, their relationship often becomes strained. Obviously the quality of their previous relationship will have a large bearing on how the couple cope with the new threat facing them both. Cancer may not always cause problems, but it can often aggravate existing ones. If the couple have a successful history of sharing problems and confronting them together, they are likely to use this same strategy in the face of cancer. But if the couple has a history of poor communication or conflict, they may find it harder to support one another throughout the long ordeal of treatment. Their relationship to one another during the course of the illness will inevitably change, and prior expectations and assumptions about each other and their relationship will be tested.

Partner relationships and communication

> It's not been a brilliant weekend – C. has been in a foul mood and we just ended up shouting at each other. He refuses to entertain the idea of getting any help yet says he has too much to do and is falling behind with his work. He also seems to be forgetting that I'm not feeling overly wonderful.

There is a wide spectrum of ways in which people respond to the illness in their partner. Partners can be:

- supportive and caring, able to focus on the positive without denying the fears and doubts;
- involved but trying to fix the problem, with a tendency to give advice, or be overly positive ('*I won't hear you talking negatively*');
- dismissive, trivializing, or minimizing of the seriousness of the situation;
- silent and withdrawn;
- critical, needling, and undermining.

Partners can be a potent source of support throughout the cancer experience or an added source of distress for the patient. When people with cancer have a partner in whom they can confide, it can provide them with a source of emotional support and also a larger network of support than they would otherwise have. Indeed, the evidence strongly suggests that a good partner relationship, which involves emotional support, is associated with less distress among people with cancer.[6, 8, 64–66]

However, the couple relationship itself comes under enormous strain as the partners, individually and together, attempt to manage and adjust to the shifting challenges of cancer. Inevitably relationships alter when partners are required to adopt new roles and responsibilities towards one another, as one partner becomes defined as the patient and the other the carer. Previous assumptions about there being mutual support in the relationship are tested to the full and, for some people, these assumptions are disappointed, if not shattered. In one study of couples that divorced after Hodgkin's disease, nearly half attributed the cause of the divorce to the illness,[67] and marital tensions and strains have been reported to occur in 10% to 20% of couples affected by cancer.[33] Relationship conflict is particularly important because, even among healthy couples, people reporting marital dissatisfaction are 25 times more likely to be depressed than single people.[68] Thus, far from being a powerful source of support, a poor partner relationship often represents an additional source of stress for the patient.

> Little shit. Here I was, totally bald bar a bit of downy hair, still not having completed my course of chemo and he's yelling and being verbally abusive towards me. He hasn't said it, but I think he resents my 'freaky' appearance. Maybe it frightens him, a visual reminder of my condition. And just perhaps he's jealous of the attention and sympathy that other people give me.

One of the difficulties in working with couples affected by cancer is disentangling how much problems in the relationship are due to challenges triggered by the illness, and how much they are the result of pre-existing difficulties in the relationship. So, before discussing more long-term problems that couples sometimes face, we look at common responses among couples to the stress of cancer.

Partner distress

One reason many couples struggle in the face of cancer is that the patient's partner is frequently highly distressed and in need of emotional support themselves.[35, 69] Some studies have even reported partners being more distressed than the patients[70, 71] while other research indicates that women, whether patients or partners, are at higher risk of distress than their male partners.[72, 73] For one thing, the stress of caring is considerable, and can sometimes lead to resentment and hostility (*see* Caring). Partners are frequently obliged to fulfil not only their existing responsibilities but those of the ill person as well, leaving them little time to engage in activities unconnected with the illness.[66] Understandably, they may begrudge restrictions (e.g. to employment, recreational and social activities) imposed by cancer treatments or time spent caring for the patient.

Communication failures

> It wasn't a particularly good weekend – C. was getting more and more wound up as we went along and I don't know what to say or do to help [him]. Everything is just so frustrating and that's probably because reality is beginning to set in after the whirl of the last couple of weeks. We ended up rowing at bedtime but did manage to resolve it a bit afterwards. We've a long way to go yet and can't afford to be falling out too much.

Couples adapt best when they find a way to discuss the real issues facing them, their private concerns as well as their shared ones, and how they will manage the changes to their relationship.[25] Attempting to avoid hurting one another can paradoxically lead couples to feel isolated from one another.[18] Of course some partners discourage or withdraw from open communication lest they say 'the wrong thing' and make matters worse, so they become silent or spend as much time away from the patient as possible. The insistence on 'positive thinking' has a similar effect of inhibiting people from discussing openly what they may be privately thinking and feeling. Minimizing the seriousness of the illness in the belief that one should remain positive at all costs, or as a way to avoid talking about their fear and despair, is usually interpreted by the other person as insensitive and rejecting.[74]

If I'm happy, he's happy. I sometimes feel he wants me to be positive so he can be. He's always saying 'Be positive'.

Was not nice to W. – he wanted to cheer me up. I think it is easier for him if I am always bright and brave and he doesn't seem to realise that there are times when I can't/don't want to be like that – sometimes I need to be melancholy.

Mind-reading

'Mind-reading' is another common communication difficulty among couples, especially those who have known each other a long time and assume they know each other well. Trying to guess what your partner may be feeling or thinking, and responding accordingly, can lead to misunderstandings and hurt feelings. This is especially the case when both members of a couple are trying to mind-read one another. For example, a man whose wife recently had a mastectomy may try to be sensitive by assuming she would not want him to make sexual advances. While this assumption may be accurate in the early days, over time she may interpret, or mind-read, his behaviour as revulsion towards her changed body and a loss of sexual desire for her.

Dependency

As many people have observed, the first thought that cancer evokes is the possibility of death. The prospect of permanent separation through death brings to the surface many powerful feelings that partners have long harboured for each other, but not necessarily expressed. Expectations and assumptions about the partner and the relationship are brought into focus and re-examined.

Among these feelings, the most important is likely to be dependency. Many people, especially men,[75] equate adult maturity with having separated and gained independence from their family of origin. Feeling dependent on someone else therefore threatens this belief in their self-sufficiency and autonomy. When people feel uncomfortable with their own dependency and vulnerability they tend to respond defensively by withdrawing, avoiding, or becoming critical and undermining towards the person who is evoking these feelings (whether it be parents, a partner, or someone else). For example, when a woman becomes seriously ill she may understandably withhold some of the support she had previously given to her partner. Her partner may resent this loss of support and react with different degrees of hostility (critical, needling, and undermining). Not surprisingly, female patients feel poorly supported by male partners who are critical or withdrawn.[76, 77]

Security of the relationship

Where there is a lack of security in the relationship, patients may harbour fears that they will be abandoned by their partners. In fact, it is not uncommon for the patient's need for closeness with the partner to conflict with the partner's need for a degree of separateness from the 'implosive' effect of the illness on the relationship.[25]

In some instances, however, *either* partner may have to deal with the added stress of their own conflicting feelings. Some relationships may have been on the threshold of ending when one of the partners develops cancer. For example, the healthy partner may feel compelled to stay in the relationship to support the patient, while silently feeling desperate to leave it. They may feel too guilty to leave, or they may worry how it would look to others to be leaving at such a vulnerable time for the patient. In any event, they feel trapped.

Support for the partner

People are best able to support other people when they are well supported themselves. Partners often lack social support from friends and family who see the patient as the person most in need of help,[78] and this may contribute both to their own emotional vulnerability and to a diminished capacity to support the patient (*see* Caring). This may be particularly true of men who tend to have a smaller network of friends than women (*see* Gender Differences). But it can be easily overlooked that although the patient may be dealing with their illness and its treatment, they can usually continue to offer support to their partner. If cancer is posed as a *mutual* problem, rather than one that the patient faces alone, the couple will be in a better position to support one another. To do so therefore requires both partners to be able to acknowledge the needs and difficulties of the other and to be committed to keeping the channels of communication open between them.

Positive changes

> One good thing to have come out of this whole depressing business is an improvement in my relationship with W., – he changed almost instantly when he understood what I faced. I know now that he cares and that he will be with me. Something good has come of it all.

Although changes to the relationship frequently cause strain, they also offer positive opportunities for the couple to re-examine and realign the way they live together and communicate. This may involve helpful insights into the stresses faced by the other, and an opportunity to acknowledge the trust and affection that may have long been taken for granted. Many couples report that facing cancer together strengthened their relationship[79] and forged greater intimacy. Conversely, some people, rather than continue to endure a relationship that has long lost any meaning, choose to take charge of their lives and change the situation, even if this means ending the relationship.

However, whatever strains there are in the relationship in the early stages of the illness, they are likely to be more pronounced in the more advanced stages. As death becomes a more imminent prospect, the dying patient must relinquish their roles to a partner who may be overwhelmed by their own sense of impending loss.

Relationship difficulties

Unfortunately, many relationships have a history of communication difficulties that work against the ideal of mutual support and open communication. Peteet and Greenberg have identified four common relationship difficulties[80] which often warrant referral to a specialist:

Immature relationships Young couples, without much history of resolving problems between themselves, may find the crisis of cancer particularly overwhelming. Either partner may find the reactions of the other unsympathetic and disappointing (often in comparison with their parents' comfort and support). They may have little under-standing of how to support each other, and may still be more attached to their family of origin than to their partner. When people discover their partners have returned to their family of origin for support, they are likely to feel that their partner has been dis-loyal or that they have been abandoned.

Hostile dependent relationships   These relationships are characterized by poor commu-nication and an intolerance of difference. Hostile arguments are interspersed with brood-ing truces which maintain an atmosphere of irritability and a tendency for both partners to provoke one another. They often find the disruption caused by the illness intolerable and the crisis of cancer thus escalates problems in an already difficult relationship.

Abusive relationships   Healthcare staff tend to avoid the issue of domestic violence when it is reported or identified because it can seem complex and intimidating. However, it is essential to explore all forms of physical and emotional abuse in the home. When such couples are confronted by cancer their changing needs create dis-ruption to the established way of communicating and this can precipitate an escalation of abuse. Domestic violence is common and, where it occurs, the safety of the victim and the rest of the family must be paramount. Issues of confidentiality should be weighed against this priority. Where abuse is detected, hospital social workers and mental health professionals may be as helpful to the medical team as they are to the couple. Staff may have strong feelings towards the partner who is perpetrating the abuse so it is useful to clarify these feelings. Sometimes it also helps to enlist the sup-port of someone 'neutral', outside the immediate healthcare team, who can be a con-duit for ongoing communication with the abusing partner.

Detached relationships   In relationships characterized by emotional detachment and lack of intimacy, the crisis of cancer has the effect of highlighting these shortcomings. The patient may suddenly realize that their partner is not someone they can emotion-ally depend upon in a crisis. This disappointing insight deeply challenges their implicit expectation that the relationship would be mutually supportive. Sometimes this leads to a complete re-evaluation of the relationship and a decision to end it.

Rarely do problematic relationships present in the orderly way in which we have described them. In fact, most relationships probably include an element of at least some of these styles of communication at one time or another. By presenting these dysfunctional types of relationship, we are not encouraging healthcare staff to 'spot-diagnose' couples using these labels. Rather, we do encourage staff to consider the couple before them in terms of their shared history, the way in which they communicate with one another, and the extent to which they appear to be facing the crisis of cancer separately or together.

In view of the lack of mental health professionals with the requisite skills working in oncology, some authors have suggested that the patient's primary oncology physician should intervene with couples in crisis.[80] However, we would temper this view by noting that therapeutic work with couples can be complex and potentially damaging and should not be undertaken lightly. Couples sometimes require extensive long-term work and a well-meaning novice can deter couples from pursuing the kind of help they might ideally need. If a doctor or other healthcare professional wishes to intervene therapeutically with a couple's relationship, supervision from a competent and experienced specialist in this field should always be sought.

> Today I was depressed for a while in the morning and had a bit of a cry. G. [husband] came home shortly after and knew straight away that I was down, so [he] cuddled me tight. I can't get used to having no hair and it disturbs me when I touch my head or go to twiddle my hair and it's only 1 cm long.

Healthcare implications

- It is essential that healthcare staff recognize the distress of *both* the patient and the partner, rather than simply focusing on either the patient or the person who appears to be most distressed. Cancer affects the relationship between two individuals as much as it affects the two individuals separately. It is important to identify with both partners' distress.

- Emphasize what patently works in the relationship rather than focusing exclusively on the difficulties in the relationship. It can help if the couple can see that they are both in a period of transition in their lives and that it is recognized that both of them are struggling; facing the crisis together will enable them both to manage it better.

- By focusing on underlying *feelings* rather than the 'surface issue' healthcare staff can enable the couple to understand each other's positions and experiences.

- Go at a pace that does not leave the less emotionally articulate partner (often the man) behind. Expecting someone emotionally illiterate to express their feelings quickly can lead them to feel interrogated and is likely to provoke defensive hostility.

- Partners are frequently highly distressed and should therefore be encouraged to access additional support from outside the relationship. This may include help from other family members, friends, community and religious organizations, self-help groups, and support from healthcare professionals. Support from other people may reduce the 'intensity' of the patient–partner relationship.

- The healthcare team should be seen as a source of information and support to both patients and partners. Partners need easy access to accurate information about the patient's condition, treatment, and what is expected of them in terms of care. Like the rest of the family, partners usually want to have an active role in caring for the patient but are often unsure what they can do.

- Partners, like patients, often harbour considerable fears about the future. Staff can help by exploring the partner's worst fears, both alone and with the patient, in a way that both clarifies and normalizes their concerns. They should demonstrate that openly sharing concerns and fears can lead to mutual comfort and a release of pent-up tension.

• It is important to avoid any implication of blame for problems within the relationship. It helps to think of a relationship as almost a separate living organism whose life is sustained by the communication within the couple. Both partners constitute the couple and both are having to cope with the stress of the illness, albeit from different positions. When someone is depressed they are likely to overestimate their own contribution to relationship problems they may be having (e.g. feeling a burden), while someone who is angry is more likely to blame their partner.[80]

• Couples do best when they are able to confront the challenge of cancer together and maintain open, emotionally supportive communication with one another while respecting each other's needs for separateness (*see* Communication Advice for Couples). Rather than trying to imagine what their partner may be thinking and feeling, couples should be encouraged to ask their partner. Similarly, rather than expecting partners to read each other's mind, couples should be encouraged to express their concerns and needs *to* one another.

• Some couples are surprised by their sudden difficulty communicating with one another but are otherwise highly committed to their relationship. By exploring what may be shared about their experience, healthcare staff can help them move away from positions that have become polarized or extreme.[18] Rather than viewing their differences as problematic, staff can show the couple how to respect and value differences. In other words, different perspectives do not have to result in hostile conflict but can be understood and respected. Couples should be reassured that conflict can be healthy and creative provided that open communication is also felt to be safe.

• The partner relationship can be a significant source of additional stress to people with cancer, so additional support should be on hand in these instances. Some couples have pre-existing communication difficulties that may require specialist help.

Gender differences in partner support

Healthcare professionals are aware that men and women react to serious illness in ways that are usually similar but sometimes different. Professionals bring their own cultural assumptions of what is appropriate behaviour for a man or a woman and this can influence how their patients feel they are expected to behave. In this section we consider the evidence for some of these presumed gender differences and the factors behind them, but start by thinking about what we mean by a person's gender.

The term 'sex' denotes a person's biological sexual characteristics: male or female. By contrast, the term 'gender' signifies general tendencies within people (e.g. 'his feminine side') or particular behaviours (e.g. 'masculine' behaviour) that have become associated with one of the sexes within a particular society. The gender terms 'masculinity and femininity' have been described as *floating signifiers*, describing two ends of a particular social continuum. They mean different things in different social contexts.[81]

For example, male friends or relatives often hold hands in public in Arab and some Latin countries, but not in Britain where physical contact between males is rare except in sporting contexts where usual inhibitions between men are often suspended.[81]

One must be cautious when ascribing behaviour to the sexes. A person's sex may be clear but the individual will vary along the masculine–feminine continuum according to the situation they find themselves in. Therefore, although there appears to be evidence in the research literature that men and women differ in certain ways (e.g. in the way they express their feelings and respond to the needs of others), one should never assume that a particular individual conforms to the general tendencies ascribed to their sex within the population as a whole.

In facing illness, men and women are often forced to adopt roles for which they may be ill-prepared. Some of these roles may even challenge their notions of what it is to be masculine or feminine. For example, caring is associated with a traditionally female role, while acting in the public arena of work has traditionally been the preserve of men. Of course, such 'gender roles' not only vary from culture to culture, but are constantly changing and evolving over time within cultures.

In traditional families, serious illness in the wife or mother often poses the greatest risk to how the family and couple function, because women generally assume many of the practical and caring roles within the family.[25] On the other hand, the financial security of such families often depends on the father's income, so the livelihood of the entire family may be jeopardized if it is he who becomes chronically ill. The situation in many industrialized countries of the West, at least in regard to family income, has changed in recent decades with more women gaining paid work, though the domestic division of labour has remained relatively unaltered with women still assuming most of the domestic and care-giving roles and responsibilities.[82]

The social legacy of our biological identity (e.g. child-bearing) is the traditional division of labour between the sexes and the somewhat different psychologies of men and women. While women's lives have centred on the importance of nurturing and socializing children and valuing their relationships with others, men have been required to view the goal of development and adult maturity as the achievement of autonomy ('standing on your own feet') which comes with a wariness of dependence on others.[75, 83] Not surprisingly, men are characteristically less confident and familiar with the language of emotion, relationships, and care. As John Gottman has put it, 'the world of feelings is by and large outside most men's comfort zone'[84] (Gottman 1994, p. 139).

But of course, while this may often be true, it is also something of a caricature. Men and women vary along many dimensions, both within their sex and between the sexes, and research suggests that psychological similarities between the sexes greatly outweigh the differences.[85] In fact, on the basis of a review of the literature, it has been argued that knowledge of a person's sex adds little to our ability to predict how they will behave in most situations.[86]

R. [husband] comes into the spare bedroom concerned that I hadn't returned upstairs (oh yes, so worried that he only slept soundly for 6 hours). He asks what is wrong. If he doesn't know, then I'm not going to tell him (I can be so horrible at times). He guesses – wrongly, but I still refuse to communicate. He proposes to take the day off work but I tell him his priority is obviously the Management Meeting ... he has never, and will never understand the complexities of my emotions. He asks me to be more honest with him. I agree and he phones work to say that he will be in late; after he has taken me to the doctor's. The Management Meeting was cancelled.

There do, however, appear to be a few general tendencies that have a bearing on how men and women view their relationships with one another. For example, there is a modest tendency for women to use more self-disclosure than men, as well as for women to perceive closeness in intimate relationships as meaning 'being emotional and interdependent', while men are more likely to perceive closeness as 'involving sex'.[87] Research also indicates that, while men have a greater tendency than women to withhold their emotions, they feel more comfortable expressing them to women than expressing them to men.[88] As we will see, this is particularly pertinent to how couples support one another when they are confronted by cancer. But perhaps it is not so surprising that women continue to be seen as the main source of emotional support by both men and women, in view of their central position in child-rearing. One survey has found that the majority of adults in the UK have contact with their mothers at least once a week, while over 10% see them daily.[89]

These findings from studies of healthy people are generally consistent with those conducted in the cancer field, though relatively few studies have compared men and women in similar situations. First, it seems that women generally report more psychological distress than men, whether they are the patient or the partner.[73, 90, 91] But, while the psychological distress of healthy husbands makes a significant contribution to the distress of female patients, the distress of healthy wives seems to make only a minor contribution to the distress of male patients.[60] In other words, men's emotional well-being is mostly influenced by their own condition, while women's well-being is more easily influenced (than that of men) by the distress of their partner.[72]

There also may be differences in the way that men and women care for one another when one of them develops cancer. In one study, nearly 40 per cent of women with breast cancer, who initially viewed their male partners as their most important source of support, subsequently changed this view, mostly in favour of another woman.[92] Women in the study reported that communication with their partners was more difficult than with friends and relatives; consequently, despite wanting to talk more, they withheld from talking to their partners. Other studies have confirmed that women often turn to other women for support, in the belief that only another woman can give them the kind of empathy and support that they need.[93] Some research has found that men are more likely than women to be withdrawn and critical when they find themselves having to support their partners,[77] while another study of breast cancer patients and their husbands found that men often prefer to adopt a protective, reassuring, and minimizing role rather than getting too closely involved with their wives' distress.[74] By contrast, there is no published evidence that many men are unsatisfied with the support they get from their female partners.

So why are men sometimes emotionally distant, or even critical and undermining, at a time when their partners need them most? Some authors have speculated that in chronic illnesses men resent the fact that their wives' condition imposes limitations on their social, recreational, and sexual activities.[94] Others have suggested that these communication problems are more to do with men's difficulties dealing with feelings (for example, not knowing what to say for fear of making the situation worse), rather than a failure to understand their partners' concerns.[92] People obviously tend to avoid situations where they feel incompetent, socially awkward, or potentially overwhelmed, so it is likely that men's lack of confidence with the language of emotion inhibits their expression of care.

Because men are more likely than women to confide solely in the partners,[95, 96] they may resent her sudden preoccupation with her illness and her apparent withdrawal of support to him. Thus, paradoxically, a man sometimes resents his partner's need for support because, being distressed himself, he is in need of *her* support. Men are thus often in a 'gridlock of over-dependence on women'[97] (resenting women for their own feelings of dependence on them). Conversely, a woman sometimes maintains this relationship of dependence by withholding her own needs and not making burdensome demands on her partner.[18]

By contrast, when the couple is able to face the crisis of cancer together, both partners can derive much-needed support:

> D. [husband] is wonderful about everything. He is there when I need him. We said today, (and we both feel like this) that we want to be near each other all the time. Just to be in sight is ok. We feel so close all the time.

Healthcare implications

Healthcare staff approach their interactions with patients and families with their own stereotypes and assumptions about what is 'appropriate' behaviour for a man or a woman. The cultural assumptions of staff can influence what the patient believes is expected of them. Men and women do sometimes conform to the gender stereotypes that prevail within a particular culture, but often they do not. Women do not always show their feelings openly and can sometimes be poor at showing support to others. Men frequently do cry and feel despair intensely, but they may be less inclined than women to show their distress in front of other people. Men can also be extraordinarily supportive as carers, and are increasingly able to articulate a language of emotions and relationships. What is important is that healthcare staff are sensitive and responsive to every individual's unique experience, whether they are a man or a woman, a patient or a partner. Rather than adopting a fixed view of what is appropriate or expected behaviour for either sex, it is preferable to appreciate that every person may be constrained by implicit gender expectations but that no one is bound by them.

The crisis of cancer is not the optimal time to challenge gender differences in how people communicate. A man who wishes to protect his family by 'being strong' in the face of cancer should be respected for doing what he feels is right in the circumstance. Thus, offering counselling and therapy to men can sometimes be tantamount to challenging their self-image as someone who is managing the crisis, unless one is able to reassure him about the normality of his feelings. To express his feelings and 'break down' in tears might lead him to conclude that he is patently *not* coping. It may therefore be preferable for some men to retain their dignity and self-respect by seeming to be in control and silent. It is for this reason that it is sometimes harder for healthcare staff to elicit the personal concerns of men.

Healthcare staff can reassure people about the many different ways that men and women manage the stress of cancer. For example, it may be helpful for a woman to learn that her husband's withdrawal in the face of her cancer is not necessarily a rejection of her; rather, he may be feeling overwhelmed or confused by his own feelings, or simply afraid of saying something that might upset her. (*see* Communication Advice for Couples).

Gay and lesbian couples

Just as single people have rarely been studied, very little research has been conducted on the needs of gay, lesbian, and transgendered people with cancer. However, the social conditions for most lesbian women, gay men, bisexuals, and transgendered (LGBT) people remains chronically stressful. LGBT people continue to suffer persecution and discrimination in large parts of the world. Even the liberal and libertarian West has seen only slow progress in improving the social position of this part of the community.

Little is known about rates of cancer among people of diverse sexual orientations because little information about people's sexuality is collected. However, possible barriers to accessing health services by lesbians have been identified as a research priority by the US Institute of Medicine.[98] It is thought that many lesbians experience difficulty communicating with and receiving standard clinical care from doctors and healthcare systems. Preliminary data suggest that gay men and lesbians are at increased risk for certain cancers, though there is insufficient data to be able to infer whether transsexual people are at greater risk. Higher rates of cancer among gay men are partly due to higher rates of AIDS among this population and consequently the presence of AIDS-related cancers such as Kaposi's sarcoma and AIDS-related non-Hodgkin's lymphoma.

Lesbians may be at higher risk than heterosexual women for breast cancer due to higher rates of certain risk factors (e.g. obesity, alcohol consumption, nulliparity, and lower rates of breast cancer screening). Lesbians also receive less frequent gynaecological care than heterosexual women so may be at greater risk of gynaecological cancers, particularly ovarian cancer.[98] Recent research indicates that lesbian women generally have less body image concerns, receive better support from their partners than heterosexual women and are more likely to cope by expressing their anger, but are considerably less satisfied with the care received from their physicians.[99] Although this research found no differences in levels of mood or sexual activity between lesbian and heterosexual women, lesbians were less likely to view the healthcare system as supportive of their needs.

When an LGBT person develops cancer, their private or hidden sexuality sometimes becomes public for the first time, and at a time of great vulnerability.[25] Since heterosexuals are not routinely victimized for being heterosexual, it is prudent to ask LGBT patients (who offer information about their sexuality) how open they wish to be about it. Much communication in healthcare contains an implicitly heterosexist bias that can leave gay and lesbian patients and their partners uncomfortable about expressing their needs and concerns.[100] Healthcare staff who harbour homophobic attitudes may find it too threatening to engage with the LGBT patient as a whole person, with the result that they neglect their broader psychosocial needs. Gay and lesbian partners rarely have automatic legal standing as next of kin in the way that a married partner does, so healthcare staff should make every effort to ensure that the wishes of the patient are acknowledged and followed. For example, at an appropriate time it may be helpful for LGBT patients to consider writing a will that makes it clear who will inherit their estate.

Impotence resulting from surgery or radiotherapy can leave gay men, like heterosexual men, feeling mutilated, and unattractive to prospective sexual partners. But cancer and its treatment can have particular consequences for gay men. Removal of the anus or rectum in gay men practicing anal penetration requires that they find alternative sources of sexual stimulation, while incontinence can be embarrassing and inhibiting for anyone. The loss of a testicle to a gay man or a breast to a lesbian woman may seem no more devastating than the same loss in a heterosexual person, but those with same-sex partners must confront the wholeness of their partners' bodies, thus underlining their own incompleteness.[101]

The life-threatening nature of cancer leads many people to confront their mortality and re-examine some of the deeply held assumptions by which they have lived their lives (see Chapters 1 and 2). Consequently, like anyone else, LGBT people often find themselves reassessing their own behaviour and relationships. For some this can reawaken feelings of self-loathing caused by internalized social prejudice regarding their sexuality. For others, however, it can lead to a determination to be proud and open about their sexual feelings and preferences. For example, some families learn for the first time that their son is gay when he tells them he has AIDS. Bisexual men and women may finally wish to give expression to a side of their sexuality that has thus far been suppressed and hidden within their 'conventional' heterosexual relationship. A lesbian couple may wish to 'come out' on learning that one of the partners has breast cancer.

While often liberating, such revelations can be stressful for all concerned—ignorance and prejudice must be confronted and relationships may be required to change. 'Coming out' is usually daunting at the best of times; it is far harder during the stressful period following a cancer diagnosis. Sometimes a family may not be willing or able to accept the gay or lesbian partner, or the individual's transsexuality. In the worst situations, there is a painful conflict between family and partner over who is seen as the primary care-giver. Ultimately, the decision is the patient's, although where there is conflict, both the family and the partner should be afforded as much support by the healthcare team as they are willing to accept. Preferably they should be helped to overcome their differences in the best interests of the patient.

In the context of the multiple stresses of cancer and the sometimes tenuous support from families of origin (compared with heterosexual patients),[99] LGBT patients may benefit from joining others of similar sexual orientation in a support group. Mutual sharing of information, cohesiveness in the face of stigmatization, managing difficult symptoms, discussing difficult relationships with family members, and emotional expression and support are all potential benefits from group approaches. Preliminary evidence for the effectiveness of such a group with lesbian breast cancer patients has already been reported.[102]

Finally, it is often the subtleties of communication that reveal the attitudes that healthcare staff harbour towards gay and lesbian individuals and couples. LGBT patients often have to anticipate what level of disclosure it is safe to risk with their healthcare providers; they are likely to disclose more if they feel that the healthcare team will be sensitive to and supportive of their needs. Healthcare teams may therefore wish to reflect together on how to ensure that same-sex relationships are as respected and valued as heterosexual ones.

Communication advice for couples

> I have never felt so close, yet so distant from each other in all the time we have been together. I think we both knew we were hiding our worst fears from each other.

Cultures have different views as to appropriate respective roles of men and women. A comparative study of Chinese-American, Japanese-American, and European-American women with breast cancer found a number of qualitative differences in the perception of their husbands' support.[103] Asian-American women, for example, tended to be more self-sacrificing and less inclined to assert their needs than European-American women. Asian-Americans were also more likely to value non-verbal communication and the goal of harmony in their relationship compared with European-Americans who rated direct verbal communication with the goal of intimacy as being more important. Therefore the following advice may have particular relevance for couples in 'Western' countries that strive for social and interpersonal equality between men and women.

1. People are less likely to develop problems like depression and anxiety if the couple manage to face the stress of cancer together.

2. Let each other know what you are feeling but do not interrogate your partner, nor expect them to know immediately what you or they are feeling. This may take time, especially for men, so be patient.

3. Do not assume you know what your partner is feeling or thinking. This is mind-reading. Be open with one another about what you feel and think.

4. Do not interrupt your partner when they are speaking or you may miss the main point of what they wanted to say (see Point 3).

5. Try to be supportive, not critical of your partner. Remember that it is a stressful time for both of you.

6. Being overly positive, giving advice and finding solutions is not always what is needed; try instead to find out whatever your partner would find it helpful to talk about.

7. Do not worry too much about saying the wrong thing; it is more important to try to understand and 'stay with' whatever your partner is feeling.

8. Do not withdraw from your partner; this is a time when you both need one another.

9. Try to listen more than to talk. Try to accept that what your partner is saying is their point of view, so acknowledge it first and only then respond to it openly, calmly, and honestly.

10. Find someone else you can talk to on a regular basis. Diversify your sources of support; do not depend entirely on your partner for your support but share and discuss your feelings with other adults too.[104]

Sexual problems

The taboo of talking about sex is only equalled by that of talking about death, so it is not surprising that many healthcare workers find it difficult to talk about sex with their patients. Yet sexual problems can occur as a result of cancer of any kind and are thought to be common.[105] Roughly 30% of women have been found to end their treatment with some form of sexual dysfunction.[106]

As in any other area of human behaviour, sexuality is characterized by its diversity. A person's sexuality is uniquely their own. It is influenced by beliefs and expectations that have been shaped by their social background and personal experiences. People even vary according to what they regard as their sexuality; some define sexual satisfaction in terms of frequency of intercourse, while others see it in terms of intimacy with others or their own feelings of attractiveness. People vary in terms of who and what they find sexually exciting, and how much importance they place on their sexuality. Everyone may have the potential to be sexual, but it is not only nuns and priests who choose not to be sexually active. Sexuality is an important part of some people's overall identity while for others it assumes less importance.

It is essential that healthcare staff do not make assumptions about a person's sexuality on the basis of superficial characteristics such as their age, sexual orientation, or whether the individual happens to have a partner. Older people are often sexually active and masturbation, which frequently begins in infancy, is a common and normal feature of a person's sexuality throughout life.[107]

Cancer can affect a person's sexuality in many ways. High levels of fear, and particularly fears about dying, can alter people's attitudes to both their sexuality and their intimacy. Either partner may want more or less of either, leading people to feel rejected and hurt at a time when the other person is most needed. Furthermore, feeling ill or suffering pain, whether due to the illness or the effects of treatment, is likely to decrease a person's interest in sex. Muscle weakness, bone metastases or difficulty in breathing, can make it physically challenging to engage in strenuous sexual activity. In short, sexual couples often find themselves having to relearn how to have a mutually satisfying sexual relationship after one of them has been ill.

Sexual problems in people with cancer can be caused by any combination of physical damage, treatment side-effects, and psychological causes:

Physical damage

Physical damage to the sexual response can be directly caused by cancer itself. For example, central nervous system tumours can cause men to have difficulty obtaining an erection, as can invasive tumours in the pelvic region. But much more often it is caused by surgical attempts to remove the cancer.

A number of surgical interventions can result in permanent damage to parts of the body which are involved in the sexual response. Pelvic surgery can cause sexual problems in both men and women. In men, nerve damage as a result of surgery or damage to pelvic blood vesicles (e.g. radical prostatectomy, orchidectomy, and penectomy) can lead to impotence or sometimes a difficulty in controlling and delaying his orgasm. In women, surgery to the pelvic region (e.g. hysterectomy, oopherectomy, or vulvectomy) is often associated with loss of sexual desire, and painful intercourse.[108] The regular use of vaginal moisturizers, and the use of vaginal lubricants during penetrative sex, may be useful where there is scarring or narrowing of the vagina. Women receiving extensive surgery, such as pelvic exenteration (removal of the bladder, vagina, uterus, ovaries, and rectum), should always be offered additional support in recovering psychologically. Surgical removal of the ovaries results in the sudden loss of ovarian testosterone, which leads to a loss of libido and ability to achieve an orgasm (*see* Chemotherapy), as well as decreased oestrogen levels (*see* The Menopause).

Of course, surgery also has many indirect effects on the sexual response when it results in mutilation of the body. For example, a mastectomy can be a major loss, robbing the woman of an important aspect of her sexuality. Although women may fear that their partner will no longer find them sexually attractive, the great majority of partners do not lose sexual interest, provided the couple previously enjoyed mutual sexual attraction.[109] Similarly, radical surgery to the head or neck can cause disfigurements and disabilities that can profoundly undermine the individual's perception of themselves as a sexual being.

Among women, colorectal surgery involving a colostomy does not directly interfere with fertility, pregnancy, or childbearing, but intercourse can be painful while the surgical wound is healing.[110] Surgery for colorectal cancer can sometimes cause sterility and impotence in men if the parasympathetic nerves, prostate glands, seminal vesicles, or ejaculatory ducts are damaged. The presence of a stoma following colostomy or ileal conduit (in bladder cancer) not only leads to changes in body image in both male and female patients but also presents a challenge to how the couple manage this intrusion into their sexual relationship. It can be helpful to explore various methods of concealing the stoma under nightshirts and camisoles.[111]

Treatment side-effects

Radiotherapy There are a number of side-effects of radiotherapy, especially when given to pelvic and abdominal areas, which can have an impact on sexuality. These include fatigue, nausea, diarrhoea, frequent urination, and skin reactions. Radiation to the vagina can cause painful intercourse and loss of sexual pleasure as a result of a decrease in vaginal lubrication, as well as vaginal narrowing and shortening, while radiotherapy to the ovaries will cause sterility depending on the age of the patient and the dose given. Women receiving pelvic radiation should always be provided with a vaginal dilator, whether or not they have a partner.[108] Pelvic and abdominal radiation in men can lead to temporary or even permanent impotence, probably as a result of fibrosis of pelvic vesicles and damage to pelvic nerves.[112]

Chemotherapy and hormone therapy Certain types of chemotherapy, especially alkylating agents, as well as adriamycin, can affect sexual or reproductive functions (*see* Table 3.1), causing loss of libido, sterility, and impotence in men, and loss of libido, sterility, vaginal atrophy and dryness, and painful intercourse in women. In both sexes, testosterone (androgen) is the hormone largely responsible for the individual's feelings of sexual desire or libido. In addition, in women, oestrogen is important for physiological aspects of sexual excitement, such as vaginal lubrication. People without adequate levels of testosterone either cannot achieve an orgasm at all or, if they can, the pleasure of it is severely diminished. Unless contraindicated, testosterone replacement can be helpful in restoring sexual desire and the ability to achieve an orgasm, though this form of treatment has been often neglected.[109]

A number of hormone manipulation therapies are currently used in cancer care. For example, hormone therapy for metastatic prostate cancer aims to reduce the presence of androgens and consequently results in impotence and the loss of sexual desire in about 80% of men[113] (*see* Chapter 5—Prostate Cancer). In women, the ovaries are responsible for the secretion of both oestrogen and testosterone, both of which are vital to normal sexual functioning. Thus, hormone treatments such as anti-oestrogens

Table 3.1 Chemotherapy agents which affect sexuality or fertility

Agent	Complication
Alkylating agents	
Busulfan Chlorambucil Cyclophosphamide Melphalan Nitrogen mustard	Amenorrhoea, oligospermia (reduced concentration of sperm), azoospermia (absence of sperm), decreased libido, ovarian dysfunction, erectile dysfunction
Antimetabolites	
Cytosine arabinoside 5-fluorouacil Methotrexate	As for alkylating agents
Antitumour antibiotics	
Doxorubicin Plicamycin Dactinomycin	As for alkylating agents
Plant products	
Vincristine	Retrograde ejaculation, erectile dysfunction
Vinblastine	Decreased libido, ovarian dysfunction, erectile dysfunction
Miscellaneous agents	
Procarbazine	As for alkylating agents
Androgens	Masculinization (in women)
Antiandrogens	Gynaecomastia, impotence
Oestrogens	Gynaecomastia, acne
Antioestrogens	Irregular menses
Progestins Antiglutethimide	Menstrual abnormalities, changes in libido
Corticosteroids	Masculinization (in women)
Interferons	Irregular menses, acne, transient impotence, amenorrhoea

Groenwals SL, Goodman M, Hansen Frogge M, Henke Yarbro C. (1997). *Cancer nursing principles and practice*, 4th edn. Sudbury, Mass.: Jones and Bartlett Publishers.

(tamoxifen) and corticosteroids can cause a number of sexual problems through masculinizing women and inducing a premature menopause (*see* The Menopause). Tamoxifen has been reported by some women to cause loss of libido and loss of orgasm, although as yet the effects of tamoxifen on sexual desire are relatively unexplored[114] and it is claimed that only 3% of women discontinue the drug as a result of side-effects[109]. Soreness, drying, and shrinking of the vagina, which is reported by some women taking tamoxifen, are symptoms of oestrogen deficiency which, if not detected early, can lead to vaginal atrophy which can be severe and irreversible.[109]

The Menopause The menopause technically refers to the last menstrual period, though it is generally used to denote a process that has completed when the woman has had no menstrual periods for a full year.[115] Roughly half of the testosterone (responsible for libido) in premenopausal women is made by the ovaries, while the other half is manufactured by the adrenal gland. After a normal menopause the ovaries go on secreting some testosterone for many years which, together with the testosterone produced by the adrenal gland, maintains reasonable levels of libido and orgasm in most women.[109]

Whether caused by surgery (oopherectomy—removal of the ovaries), oblation of the ovaries (by radiotherapy), or anti-oestrogen hormone therapy (e.g. tamoxifen), premature menopause can be psychologically devastating. Frequently the woman concerned must face the consequences and implications of her menopause with little warning or preparation. She not only loses the normal cycles and rhythms of female life, but she has also lost her fertility. The loss of fertility can be a significant loss for any woman since it represents the end of a physical capability that may have formed an important part of her sense of herself and her future. Without it she may feel redundant and of less value.

With this loss comes the onset of hot flushes, changes to the skin and hair, vaginal dryness, and mood changes associated with the loss of oestrogen. Hot flushes are the most commonly reported menopausal symptom triggered by low oestrogen levels, but they are poorly understood. They can be so severe, however, as to cause intense night sweats that interfere with sleep and necessitate a change in bed linen.[115] Other symptoms associated with decreased oestrogen include heightened tension and anxiety, decreased libido, mood swings, depression, headaches, and palpitations.[115] But once again, expectations can be important. A prospective study of healthy menopausal women found that women who associated the menopause with physical and emotional problems were more like to report depressed mood when they themselves were going through the menopause.[116]

All women facing a premature menopause or decreased oestrogen levels should be given sufficient preparation, support and information for what is to follow. The psychological and physical effects of the menopause are not all inevitable and many symptoms can be alleviated. Follow-up by a gynaecologist who is familiar with both the endocrinal side-effects of cancer treatment as well as the safety of hormone replacement therapies in cancer care should be a routine part of rehabilitative care.

Psychological causes

Hair loss, weight gain, mutilating surgery, intense fatigue, having to cope with catheters or colostomies, and fearing the possibility of one's death can be devastating to a person's sense of themselves as a sexual object. In view of the number of ways that cancer and its treatment can affect the body, it is little wonder that shame, embarrassment, and a fear of hurting one's sexual partner, where there is one, lead people to feel inhibited talking about the way cancer has affected their sexuality. Furthermore, sexual problems may be particularly hard to discuss among people from cultures where sex is not openly discussed. Consequently, healthcare staff must be particularly sensitive to the fact that talking about gynaecological, urological, and gastrointestinal problems is acutely embarrassing for some of their patients, especially when they are not of the same sex as the clinician.

In the end, it is communication between partners that is required to re-establish a sexual relationship. Without trust and intimacy in their relationship, any couple can easily become sexually inhibited and withdrawn. Patterns of sexual avoidance often become established when partners anticipate rejection and fail to voice their fears. Not surprisingly, the ability to communicate effectively about the sexual relationship will depend decisively on the couple's previous communication history (*see* Partner Relationships and Communication). For example, patients often report that they enjoy being touched by their partners but are not necessarily interested in this contact being or becoming sexual; without open communication, this situation can easily lead to both partners feeling misunderstood and hurt. Adjusting to a change in the relationship, whether sexual or not, requires patience, openness, and sensitivity on both sides, and not surprisingly many couples find this hard to sustain.

People without sexual partners may not be under pressure to satisfy another person sexually, but they face the prospect of having to discuss the permanent effects of their cancer and its treatment with any future partner. In getting to know a prospective partner, they may wonder at what point they should mention the fact that they are infertile, or have had a mastectomy or an orchidectomy. Early, so as to avoid later rejection? Or later, once a more trusting relationship has developed, with the risk of a more painful loss if one is then rejected?

Where there is a partner, the couple will need to relearn patiently how to give each other sexual pleasure and gratification. As a result of pain, disability or practical necessity (e.g. a colostomy bag) couples may have to alter their previous sexual practices or learn new positions and techniques. It may take longer to achieve sexual satisfaction, and sex may have lost its former spontaneity. If problems require professional help, it will be useful to explore the couple's pre-existing sexual relationship and any difficulties that predated the cancer, as well as latent problems within the couple relationship.[109] Sexual satisfaction is also difficult to achieve in the presence of anxiety or clinical depression. One of the clinical signs of depression is loss of libido so the extent and causes of depression should always be assessed in the presence of sexual difficulties.

Above all, couples will need to communicate their needs to one another as openly and honestly as they can; this can represent a significant challenge in couples who are unused to discussing sex or for whom it is culturally embarrassing. Fears of failure and pressures to satisfy one's partner are common in sexual relationships, especially after an interval without sex, and people tend to avoid such situations of anxiety and uncertainty. Sometimes, when a person feels they can no longer be sexually aroused by their partner, couples may need to redefine their relationship in ways that compensate for the loss of the sexual component; for example, by emphasizing other aspects of mutual intimacy and nurturance.[25]

The longer any of these problems are avoided, however, the more anxiety-provoking they are likely to become and the more rejected and hurt the couple are likely to feel by one another. It is therefore essential that healthcare professionals, while showing sensitivity to cultural differences regarding modesty etc., are as open as possible about what couples should expect as a result of the cancer and its treatment (i.e. potential sexual problems), be prepared to explore what the couple wish to aim for in their sexual relationship, and encourage them to communicate in helpful ways (i.e. with openness, honesty, and patience).

Help with sexual problems

- Information which helps people to form realistic expectations about their sexuality during and following treatment is likely to help reduce anxiety and prevent unnecessary problems. In particular, potential damage to a person's sexuality should be thoroughly and openly discussed prior to the commencement of treatment. In particular, potential damage to nerves, blood vesicles, and the production of hormones involved in the sexual response should be clearly explained. Written information should support these discussions, not replace them.

- Professionals who are embarrassed when talking about sexuality should probably not do so. If healthcare workers show they are not embarrassed but feel comfortable with the subject of sex, the person they are speaking to is more likely to relax too.

- It is important to consider the cultural appropriateness of the contact when discussing sexuality. For example, in many cultures a male patient may not feel comfortable talking about his sexual difficulties with a woman; or vice versa.

- It is essential not to make assumptions about a person's sexuality on the basis of surface characteristics such as age, gender, or disability.

- Simple guidance can reassure people about what it is reasonable to achieve in their sexual lives, and in what time frame. For example, one piece of simple guidance might be that masturbation removes the performance anxiety associated with sex and is often a helpful starting point for people resuming sexual activity. Other good advice is to encourage couples to proceed slowly, without any expectations of themselves or their partner. By starting with non-sexual cuddling and proceeding slowly, in gradual steps, each partner can retain a sense of control and safety as they relearn how to give one another pleasure.

- As with other psychosocial concerns, patients do not generally volunteer information about their sexual difficulties unless the subject is introduced by a healthcare professional. Indeed, they may anticipate considerable shame by doing so. For example, while women are increasingly learning that the sexually transmitted human papilloma virus is a major cause of cervical cancer, they may fear that they will be perceived as having been sexually promiscuous by others if they are diagnosed with this form of cancer.[108]

- If either patient or partner asks for help with their sexual relationship, healthcare staff should show that they take the issues seriously and that the person's concerns are normal and understandable. Professionals may be able to help their patients rehearse what they would like to discuss with their partner since the single most important factor in resolving sexual difficulties is open, honest communication.

- Couples need to recreate a sexually satisfying relationship by learning what is best for whom, and when this contact is welcome and when it is not. They need a trusting intimacy in which to share their fears and concerns with one another, and discover new ways of sexually satisfying one another. If there are pre-existing sexual or communication problems in the relationship, referral to a specialist in psychosexual problems may be warranted (for couples who wish to have such help).

- Vaginal dryness, atrophy, and shrinkage are more easily prevented than cured and should be treated with moisturizing creams (e.g. Replens). Where there is painful intercourse, or following pelvic radiation, the use of vaginal dilators to relax the pelvic muscles is recommended, as well as the use of vaginal lubricants during intercourse [108]. Where there is androgen deficiency the use of non-virilizing doses of testosterone can be effective in restoring libido and the ability to orgasm.

- A useful guide as to whether a man's impotence is caused by physical damage or psychological factors is to ask him whether he has erections at night. Most men have spontaneous erections as part of the sleep cycle. If a man is not experiencing nocturnal erections and is unable to obtain an erection through masturbation, it is more likely that there is a physical basis to his impotence. Specialist assessment, however, is essential.

Caring

In most chronic illnesses, the majority of people's care occurs in their community and is largely provided by 'informal carers', predominantly partners or family members, rather than professionals. Therefore it is essential that healthcare staff do what they can to support the patient's carers so as to enable them to sustain this vital role over sometimes protracted periods of time.

Over the past few decades there has been increasing attention paid to the needs of people who care for those with physical or mental disabilities and illnesses. This interest in the needs of carers is most likely due to the widespread shift in policy towards care in the community.[117] Indeed, as cancer has increasingly become a chronic illness in the West, there has been a corresponding tendency for cancer patients to be cared for at home, mostly by family members and particularly spouses, where there is one. In the last year of life 90% of patients spend the majority of their time at home. The capacity of carers to sustain and support patients is therefore critical.

Women have historically born the brunt of care-giving in society, and continue to do so. Epidemiological studies suggest that about 70% of carers among older people are women[118] (who include partners, daughters, daughters-in-law, and sisters), though this gender difference is less evident among older couples where there is a more even balance of care between men and women.[119] One explanation for this gender difference is that the more restricted employment opportunities for women has historically led to less 'cost' to the family in women giving up work to look after a relative. However, as female employment in the West has increased relative to male, those traditionally providing care and support may now be in the labour force.[16] Another explanation is to do with filial obligation, although this does not explain why it is women, as opposed to men, who so often provide the bulk of care in a family.[118] An alternative view is that caring is considered 'women's work' and that this gender role is socially reinforced; a failure to engage in care may simply be more threatening to a woman's self-esteem, due to social expectations, resulting in more feelings of guilt than it would in a man.[75]

Although there has been a preoccupation in the research of recent years to focus on the burden of caring, it is important to balance this with the recognition that caring can also be a source of satisfaction and meaning to those providing it.[117] Care-giving works both ways, and the patient's responsiveness to the carer may play a decisive role. Studies indicate that 80% of carers find some elements of care-giving satisfying.[117] If the carer has a good relationship with the patient, derives meaning from their role, and feels they are able to make a difference, they are more likely to derive satisfaction from being a carer.

Similarly, the carer's expectations of their role, and thus their satisfaction with it, are shaped by their own individual context: prevailing cultural expectations, their past and present experiences of caring, the history of their relationship with the patient, and the amount of support available to them. For example, adult children who provide intimate physical care (washing, toileting, etc.) for their mother or father may find the role-reversal as distressing as it is for their parents, yet at the same time they may derive satisfaction from being able to reciprocate the care they once received. In short, every caring situation is unique and evolving.

The stress of caring

Unlike healthcare staff who are paid to care while they are at work, 'informal carers' are required to sustain practical and emotional support to the patient over extended periods of time, often with little or no support for themselves. For them caring is part of the fabric of their everyday lives;[120] the needs of the patient become paramount and their own distress is frequently muted. In fact, most people who care for others do not define themselves as 'carers' at all, perhaps because the term implies a high level of dependency that is inappropriate in many instances (e.g. where people have been recently diagnosed and are in reasonable health).[121] Their care is born out of a mutual history of concern and love for the patient, but nonetheless a relationship that may imply an obligation to care.[122]

One of the key tasks for carers is to provide support that does not undermine the patient's identity, dignity, sense of control, and independence.[117,121] The problem is that the carer's own needs can become lost in this pursuit. There is a tendency for carers, especially close family members, to hold unrealistic expectations of their roles as caregivers. They may assume they *should* face the burden of care-giving competently and on their own, and may even regard shared responsibility for care, or respite from it, to be a shameful sign of weakness and failure.[123] Alternatively, they may be more than willing to care but not physically or emotionally capable of it, or they may be fearful of the responsibility involved.

Although there is evidence of high levels of distress among carers,[35] there is little to suggest that the stress of caring is related to the amount of care given[117] or the nature of the care-giving situation.[124] The type of care involved may be a better predictor of burden on the caregiver than the total number of tasks or the time taken in caregiving. Personal tasks (such as feeding, washing, toileting, and dressing the patient) are considered more burdensome, particularly if they restrict the freedom of the caregiver,[94] than non-personal tasks (such as doing the shopping), while emotional support is considered one of the most stressful aspects of the role.[125]

It is the relationship between carer and patient that is probably the most important determinant of how stressed a carer becomes. Although little is known about changing patterns of care-giving in relation to the course of cancer[125] this is clearly a central question in a disease that is increasingly becoming defined as chronic. It seems likely that the emotional distress of patients can gradually erode the capacity of carers to provide emotional support, through what has been termed a 'contagion of distress',[126] although more research on this question is required. Stress is more likely where the patient is constantly demanding, negative, and grumbling, gives no positive feedback to the carer, resists the need for help, or expects more than the carer can provide.[117]

Care-giving is always a dynamic and evolving relationship which changes in response to many factors: the patient's condition, the personal resources of the carer, the nature of their relationship, conflict with or support from other family members and the wider community, financial resources, healthcare support, quality of housing, etc. The caring relationship and situation are rarely static for long, yet are often a chronic source of stress for the carer who, like the patient, has to face many uncertainties. Carers must endure both the exhausting demands of physical care, as well as the emotional drain of supporting a loved one through a long, often progressive illness. Both the patient and the carer must negotiate and integrate the many changes and challenges involved in cancer. Both need the opportunity to talk about their experiences, express their feelings and thoughts, and have them acknowledged, yet typically it is only the patient who is identified as suffering.

Finally, there appear to be differences between men and women in the distress associated with care-giving in cancer. One study of patients with prostate cancer found that their wives demonstrated significantly higher levels of distress than the patients themselves.[71] A study of care-giving in advanced cancer found that women expressed a greater need to stand by their ill husbands and reported more care-giving demands than did men in the equivalent role,[127] while other work suggests that women who feel they are doing a poor job at caring suffer the greatest distress.[128]. Other studies have found that wives shoulder a greater housework burden that men and a disproportionate share of responsibility for organizing the family and providing emotional nurturance to others, regardless of whether they are patients or carers.[129, 130]

Assessing distress among carers

Healthcare staff need to remember that carers are likely to understate their own needs in favour of those of the person they are caring for. Yet it is commonly this very preoccupation with the patient's needs that leads carers to feel unsupported and alone in their role. The carer may feel guilty and undeserving of such attention although, for some, the relief of finally talking about their own distress can involve a tearful release of pent-up feeling. It may help to consider the following potential components of stress that have been derived from a factor analysis of a number of carer distress scales[124]:

Relationship:	Does the relationship depress the carer?
	Is the relationship strained?
	Does the carer feel resentful towards the patient?
	Does the relationship give the carer pleasure?
Emotional burden:	Does the carer feel frustrated, nervous, helpless, or overwhelmed in their role?
Social impact:	Does the carer take less part in organized social activities?
	Do they see less of their family and friends?
Patient demands	Does the carer feel the patient tries to manipulate them?
	Do they feel the patient makes more demands than necessary?
Personal cost	Does the carer feel their personal life has suffered?
	Do they feel their own health has suffered?
	Do they feel that the patient has only the carer to depend on?
Financial strain	Does the carer worry about their finances?

Supporting carers

• Try to engage family members or other loved ones in a discussion about their potential role as carers. Refrain from merely seeing carers as appendages to the patient who can be used as an extra healthcare resource. Rather than assume they are prepared to take on this role, explore it with them. Like patients, carers have an ethical right to be as fully informed as possible. They should be told what caring for the patient at home is likely to involve, the probable course of the disease, and the sources of support that will be available to them.

- Assess not only a person's willingness to care but also their physical and emotional ability to care.

- Spend time with the patient and carer considering whether home care is practically viable. What additional resources would be required for caring to take place at home? This may involve physical aids, equipment, redesigning the way the home is used, and financial support. A home assessment by a specialist, such as an occupational therapist, may be required.

- Provide carers with adequate levels of information, especially about medication and its side-effects, treatment plans, and the likely course of the disease (a 'road map').[121] Involve carers in discharge planning so that the care plan is suited to the unique care-giving situation,[131] and keep them informed about any changes that may affect this situation. Again, to ease communication, it is helpful if a member of the healthcare team is identified as the key worker for the family.

- Provide carers with training and information about the tasks expected of them, and offer them back-up telephone support if required. Carers are often anxious about the responsibility they are taking on, especially at the start of a period of home care.

- Positive relationships between carers and patients are more likely to develop if carers feel they are valued and appreciated and their skills acknowledged.[117] Enable carers to 'tell their story' so as to be able to identify positive elements in their role as carers. Remember that women in particular may be carrying the stress of additional domestic and caring responsibilities.

- Recognize and acknowledge carers as an important resource to the patient's healthcare. They often have expert knowledge about the patient's symptoms, response to treatment, preferences, and the way they manage at home.[117] However, they may be reticent about speaking in the healthcare setting if they feel they are interfering in the doctor–patient relationship.[121]

- Provide carers and patients with a list of professionals they are likely to encounter so that they understand their respective roles.

- Encourage carers to galvanize the support of other family members and friends so that they can share both the physical and the emotional strain of caring. Point out that other people are often willing to help if they are given concrete examples of tasks that would be helpful. 'Let me know if there's anything I can do' may sound like an empty gesture but, equally, it may be a genuine offer of support. By suggesting a choice of a few things that the person could actually do to help, the carer enables them to be supportive in a practical fashion.

- When patients are in hospital, ensure carers have easy access to the patient, according to the patient's wishes, but be clear about institutional restrictions too. Staying overnight on the ward may be appropriate when a patient is critically ill or dying, but it can also be obstructive to nursing staff and other patients at other times.

- Assess the emotional state of the carer as often as possible, while remembering that many carers stifle their own needs in favour of those of the patient. Where possible, encourage the carer to consider the possibility of respite care which, although it is no panacea, may provide them with a much-needed break.

- Loss of the caring role when the patient dies (or is hospitalized or cared for in an institution) is a major transition for which the carer may require additional support. If the care has been prolonged, a bereaved carer may have complicated ambivalent feelings of sadness and relief, and also anxiety about a future without their caring role. Those who are socially isolated may especially need professional support in the form of bereavement counselling.

- The emotional strain of helplessly watching a loved one deteriorate is a profound form of suffering. Whenever possible, make time to listen to the carer's experiences. They are, of course, more likely to talk about the patient rather themselves and embed their own concerns in the patient's story,[122] but helping them to voice their own, often suppressed, needs and concerns is highly supportive and therapeutic.

References

1. Wallston BS, Alagna SW, DeVellis BM, and DeVellis RF. (1983). Social support and physical health. *Health Psychology* **2**:367–91.
2. Cohen S and Wills TA. (1985). Stress, social support and the buffering hypothesis. *Psychological Bulletin* **98**:310–57.
3. Cutrona CE and Russell DW. (1990). Type of social support and specific stress: toward a theory of optimal matching. In: BR Sarason, IG Sarason, and GR Pierce (ed.), *Social support: an interactional view*, New York: Wiley.
4. Dunkel-Schetter C. (1984). Social support and cancer: findings based on patient interviews and their implications. *Journal of Social Issues* **40**:77–98.
5. Neuling SJ and Winefield HR. (1988). Social support and recovery after surgery for breast cancer: frequency and correlates of supportive behaviours by family, friends and surgeon. *Social Science and Medicine* **27**:385–92.
6. Helgeson VS and Cohen S. (1996). Social support and adjustment to cancer. *Health Psychology* **15**: 135–48.
7. Mager WM and Andrykowski MA. (2002). Communication in the cancer 'bad news' consultation: patient perceptions and psychological adjustment. *Psycho-Oncology* **11**:35–46.
8. Northouse LL (1988). Social support in patients' and husbands' adjustment to breast cancer. *Nursing Research* **37**:91–5.
9. Northouse LL, Dorris G, and Charron-Moore C. (1995). Factors affecting couples' adjustment to recurrent breast cancer. *Social Science and Medicine* **42**:69–76.
10. Rodrigue JR, Behen JM, and Tumlin T. (1994). Multidimensional determinants of psychological adjustment to cancer. *Psycho-Oncology* **3**:205–14.

11. Brennan J. (2001). Adjustment to cancer – coping or personal transition? *Psycho-Oncology* **10**:1–18.

12. Hinde RA. (1998). Mind and artefact: a dialectical perspective. In: C Renfrew and C Scarre (ed.), *Cognition and material culture: the archaeology of symbolic storage*, Cambridge: McDonald Institute for Archaeological Research.

13. Rafferty JP. (1985). The psychosocial adjustment problems of the cancer patient. In: DJ Higby (ed.), *The cancer patient and supportive care*, Boston: Martinus Nijhoff Publishers.

14. Mendolia M and Kleck RE. (1993). Effects of talking about a stressful event on arousal: does what we talk about make a difference? *Journal of Personality and Social Psychology* **64**:283–92.

15. Wellenkamp J. (1995). Cultural similarities and differences regarding emotional disclosure: some examples from Indonesia and the Pacific. In JW Pennebaker (ed.), *Emotion, disclosure and health*, Washington, DC: American Psychological Society.

16. Richards M. (1995). Family relations. *The Psychologist* **8**:70–2.

17. Northouse LL. (1988). Family issues in cancer care. *Advances in Psychosomatic Medicine* **18**:82–101.

18. Altschuler J. (1997). *Working with chronic illness: a family approach*. London: Macmillan.

19. Office for National Statistics (2002). *Living in Britain – results from the 2000/01 general household survey*. London: The Stationery Office.

20. Meyerowitz BE, Richardson J, Hudson S, and Leedham B. (1998). Ethnicity and cancer outcomes. *Psychological Bulletin* **123**:47–70.

21. Vaux A. (1985). Variations in social support associated with gender, ethnicity, and age. *Journal of Social Issues* **41**:89–110.

22. Dakof GA and Taylor SE. (1990). Victims' perceptions of social support: what is helpful from whom? *Journal of Personality and Social Psychology* **58**:80–9.

23. Bowlby J. (1988). *A secure base: clinical applications of attachment theory*. London: Routledge.

24. Anderson KH. (1998). The relationship between family sense of coherence and family quality of life after illness diagnosis. In: HI McCubbin, EA Thompson, AI Thompson, and JE Fromer. (ed.), *Stress, coping, and health in families: sense of coherence and resiliency*, London: Sage Publication.

25. Rolland JS. (1994). *Families, illness and disability: an integrative model*. New York: Basic Books.

26. Tolstoy L. *Anna Karenina*, 1873–7. (Translated by L. and A. Maude) London: Everyman's Library

27. Weihs K and Reiss D. (1996). Family reorganization in response to cancer: a developmental pespective. In: L Baider, CL Cooper, and A Kaplan De-Nour (ed.), *Cancer and the family*, Chichester: John Wiley.

28. Ell K, Nishimoto R, Mantell J, and Hamovitch M. (1988). Longitudinal analysis of psychological adaptation among family members of patients with cancer. *Journal of Psychosomatic Research* **32**:429–38.

29. Lewis FM, Ellison ES, and Woods NF. (1985). The impact of breast cancer on the family. *Seminars in Oncology Nursing* **1**:206–13.

30. Cooper ET. (1984). A pilot study on the effects of the diagnosis of lung cancer on family relationships. *Cancer Nursing* **7**:301–8.

31. Gotcher JM. (1992). Interpersonal communication and psychosocial adjustment. *Journal of Psychosocial Oncology* **10**:21–39.

32. Vess JD, Moreland JR, and Schwebel AJ. (1985). An empirical assessment of the effects of cancer on family role functioning. *Journal of Psychosocial Oncology* **3**:1–16.

33. Keller M, Henrich G, Sellschopp A, and Beutel M. (1996). Between distress and support: spouses of cancer patients. In: L Baider, CL Cooper, and A Kaplan De-Nour (ed.), *Cancer and the family*, Chichester: John Wiley.

34. Spiegel D, Bloom JR, and Gottheil E. (1983). Family environment as a predictor of adjustment to metastatic breast carcinoma. *Journal of Psychosocial Oncology* **1**:33–44.

35. Kissane DW, Bloch S, Burns WI, McKenzies D, and Posterino M. (1994). Psychological morbidity in the families of patients with cancer. *Psycho-Oncology* **3**:47–56.

36. Kissane DW and Bloch S. (2002). *Family focused grief therapy: a model of family-centred care during palliative care and bereavement.* Buckingham, UK: Open University Press.

37. Speice J, Harkness J, Laneri H, Frankel R, Roter D, Kornblith AB, *et al.* (2000). Involving family members in cancer care: focus group considerations of patients and oncological providers. *Psycho-Oncology* **9**:101–12.

38. Labrecque MS, Blanchard CG, Ruckdeschel JC, and Blanchard EB. (1991). The impact of family presence on the physician-cancer patient interaction. *Social Science and Medicine* **11**: 1253–61.

39. Airey C, Becher H, Erens B, and Fuller E. (2002). *Cancer National Overview 1999/2000.* London: UK Department of Health.

40. Lederberg MS. (1998). The family of the cancer patient. In: J Holland (ed.), *Psycho-oncology*, Oxford: Oxford University Press.

41. Baxandall S and Reddy P. (1993). *The courage to care: the impact of cancer on the family.* Melbourne: David Lovell Publishing.

42. Black D and Wood D. (1989). Family therapy and life threatening illness in children or parents. *Palliative Medicine* **3**:113–8.

43. Rosenheim E and Reicher R. (1985). Informing children about a parent's terminal illness. *Journal of Child Psychology and Psychiatry and Allied Disciplines* **26**:995–8.

44. Wellisch DK, Gritz ER, Schain W, Wang H-J, and Siau J. (1992). Psychological functioning of daughters of breast cancer patients. Part II: characterizing the distressed daughter of the breast cancer patient. *Psychosomatics* **33**:171–9.

45. Harpham WS. (1994). *After cancer: a guide to your new life.* New York: WW Norton and Co.

46. Nelson E, Sloper P, Charlton A, and While D. (1994). Children who have a parent with cancer: a pilot study. *Journal of Cancer Education* **9**:30–6.

47. Stokes J and Crossley D. (2001). *As big as it gets: supporting a child when someone in their family is seriously ill.* Gloucester, UK: Winston's Wish Publications.

48. Spiegel D. (1990). Facilitating emotional coping during treatment. *Cancer* **66**:1422–6.

49. Hansson RO and Carpenter BN. (1994). *Relationships in old age.* London: The Guilford Press.

50. Roy DJ and MacDonald N. (1998). Ethical issues in palliative care. In: D Doyle, GWC Hanks, and N MacDonald (ed.), *Oxford textbook of palliative medicine,* 2nd edn. Oxford: Oxford University Press.

51. Ferrell BR and Ferrell B. (1998). The older patient. In: J Holland (ed.), *Psycho-oncology*, Oxford: Oxford University Press.

52. Holmén K and Furukawa H. (2002). Loneliness, health and social network among elderly people – a follow-up study. *Archives of Gerontology and Geriatrics* **35**:261–74.

53. Helgason ÁR, Dickman PW, Adolfsson J, and Steineck G. (2001). Emotional isolation: prevalence and the effect on well-being among 50–80-year-old prostate cancer patients. *Scandanavian Journal of Urology and Nephrology* **35**:97–101.

54. Small GW. (1991). Recognition and treatment of depression in the elderly. The clinician's challenge: strategies for treatment of depression in the 1990's. *Journal of Clinical Psychiatry* **52** (Suppl):11–22.

55. Addonizio G and Alexopoulos GS. (1993). Affective disorders in the elderly. *International Journal of Geriatric Psychiatry* **8**:41–7.

56. Woods RT. (1999). *Psychological problems of ageing: assessment, treatment and care.* Chichester, UK: John Wiley & Sons, Ltd.

57. Brown GW and Harris TO. (1978). *Social origins of depression: a study of psychiatric disorders in women*. London: Tavistock.

58. Jackson PB. (1992). Specifying the buffering hypothesis: support, strain and depression. *Social Psychology Quarterly* **55**:363–78.

59. House JS and Kahn RL. (1985). Measures and concepts of social support. In: S Cohen and SL Syme (ed.), *Social support and health*, London: Academic Press.

60. Baider L, Kaufman B, Peretz T, Manor O, Ever-Hadani P, and Kaplan De-Nour A. (1996). Mutuality of fate: adaptation and psychological distress in cancer patients and their partners. In: L Baider, CL Cooper, and A Kaplan De-Nour (ed.), *Cancer and the family*, Chichester: John Wiley.

61. Barker C, Pistrang N, Shapiro DA, and Shaw I. (1990). Coping and help-seeking in the U.K. adult population. *British Journal of Clinical Psychology* **29**:271–85.

62. Clulow C. (1996). Preventing marriage breakdown: towards a new paradigm. *Sexual and Marital Therapy* **11**:343–51.

63. Morgan M and Ruszczynski S. (1998). Psychotherapy with couples: in search of the creative couple. Paper presented at the 50th Anniversary Conference of the Tavistock Marital Studies Institute, 2nd–3rd July 1998.

64. Shag CA, Ganz PA, Polinsky ML, Fred C, Hirji K, and Peterson L. (1993). Characteristics of women at risk for psychosocial distress in the year after breast cancer. *Journal of Clinical Oncology* **11**:783–93.

65. Roberts C, Cox C, Shannon V, and Wells, N. (1994). A closer look at social support as a moderator of stress in breast cancer. *Health and Social Work* **19**:157–64.

66. Fuller S and Swenson CH. (1992). Marital quality and quality of life among cancer patients and their spouses. *Journal of Psychosocial Oncology* **10**:41–56.

67. Fobair P, Hoppe RT, Bloom J, Cox R, Varghese A, and Spiegel D. (1986). Psychosocial problems among survivors of Hodgkin's disease. *Journal of Clinical Oncology* **4**:805–14.

68. Schulz KH, Schulz H, Schulz O, and von Kerekjarto M. (1996). Family structure and psychosocial stress in families of cancer patients. In: LL Baider, CL Cooper, A Kaplan De-Nour (ed.), *Cancer and the family*, Chichester, UK: John Wiley.

69. Glasdam S, Jensen AB, Madsen EL, and Rose C. (1996). Anxiety and depression in cancer patients' spouses. *Psycho-Oncology* **5**:23–9.

70. Keitel M, Zevon M, Rounds J, Petielli N, and Kousis C. (1990). Spouse adjustment to cancer surgery: stress and coping responses. *Journal of Surgical Oncology* **43**:148–53.

71. Kornblith AB, Herr HW, Ofman US, Scher HI, and Holland JC. (1994). Quality of life of patients with prostate cancer and their spouses. *Cancer* **73**:2791–802.

72. Hagedoorn M, Buunk BP, Kuijer RG, Wobbes T, and Sanderman R. (2000). Couples dealing with cancer: role and gender differences regarding psychological distress and quality of life. *Psycho-Oncology* **9**:232–42.

73. Manne S. (1998). Cancer in the marital context: a review of the literature. *Cancer Investigation* **16**:188–202.

74. Sabo D, Brown J, and Smith C. (1986). The male group and mastectomy: support groups and men's adjustment. *Journal of Psychosocial Oncology* **4**:19–31.

75. Gilligan C. (1982). *In a different voice: psychological theory and women's development*. Cambridge, MA: Harvard University Press.

76. Pistrang N and Barker C. (1995). The partner relationship in psychological response to breast cancer. *Social Science and Medicine* **40**:789–97.

77. Manne SL, Taylor KL, Dougherty J, and Kemeny N. (1997). Supportive and negative responses in the partner relationship: their association with psychological adjustment among individuals with cancer. *Journal of Behavioral Medicine* **20**:101–25.

78. Northouse LL, Templin T, Mood D, and Oberst M. (1998). Couples' adjustment to breast cancer and benign breast disease: a longitudinal analysis. *Psycho-Oncology* **7**:37–48.

79. Gritz ER, Wellisch DK, Siau J, and Wang H. (1990). Long-term effects of testicular cancer on marital relationships. *Psychosomatics* **31**:301–12.

80. Peteet J and Greenberg B. (1995). Marital crises in oncology patients. *General Hospital Psychiatry* **17**:201–7.

81. Moynihan C. (1998). Theories in health care and research: theories of masculinity. *British Medical Journal* **317**:1072–5.

82. Canary DJ and Emmers-Sommer TM. (1997). *Sex and gender differences in personal relationships*. New York: The Guildford Press.

83. Dinnerstein D. (1976). *The rocking of the cradle: the ruling of the world*. New York: Harper and Row.

84. Gottman J. (1994). *Why marriages succeed or fail*. New York: Simon & Schuster.

85. Hyde JS and Plant EA. (1995). Magnitude of psychological gender differences: another side to the story. *American Psychologist* **50**:159–61.

86. Aries E. (1996). *Men and women in interaction: reconsidering the differences*. New York: Oxford University Press.

87. Canary DJ and Emmers-Sommer TM. (1997). *Sex and gender differences in personal relationships*. New York: The Guildford Press.

88. Aukett R, Ritchie JI, and Mill K. (1988). Gender differences in friendship patterns. *Sex Roles* **19**:57–66. Cited in Canary DJ and Emmers-Sommer TM. (1997). *Sex and gender differences in personal relationships*, New York: The Guildford Press.

89. Finch J and Mason J. (1993). *Negotiating family responsibilities*. London: Routledge. Cited in Richards M. (1995). Family relations. *The Psychologist* **8**:70–2.

90. Baider L. (1995). Psychological intervention with couples after mastectomy. *Supportive Care in Cancer* **3**:239–43.

91. Northouse L, Mood D, Templin T, Mellon S, and George T. (2000). Couples' pattern of adjustment to colon cancer. *Social Science and Medicine* **50**:271–84.

92. Pistrang N and Barker C. (1992). Disclosure of concerns in breast cancer. *Psycho-Oncology* **1**:183–92.

93. Omne-Pontén M, Holmberg L, Sjödén PO, and Bergström R. (1995). The married couple's assessment of the experience of early breast cancer – a longitudinal interview study. *Psycho-Oncology* **4**:183–90.

94. Manne SL and Zautra AJ. (1989). Spouse criticism and support: their association with coping and psychological adjustment among women with rheumatoid arthritis. *Journal of Personality and Social Psychology* **56**:608–17.

95. Northouse LL, Jeffs M, Cracchiolo-Caraway A, Lampman L, and Dorris G. (1995). Emotional distress reported by women and their husbands prior to a breast biopsy. *Nursing Research* **44**:196–201.

96. Harrison J, Maguire P, and Pitceathly C. (1995). Confiding in crisis: gender differences in pattern of confiding among cancer patients. *Social Science and Medicine* **9**:1255–60.

97. Rampage C. (1995). Gendered aspects of marital therapy. In: N Jacobson and A Gurman (ed.), *Clinical handbook of couple therapy*, New York: The Guildford Press.

98. Gay and Lesbian Medical Association and LGBT health experts (2001). *Healthy people 2010 companion document for lesbian, gay, bisexual, and transgender (LGBT) health*. San Francisco, CA: Gay and Lesbian Medical Association.

99. Fobair P, O'Hanlon K, Koopman C, Classen C, Dimiceli S, Drooker N, *et al.* (2001). Comparison of lesbian and heterosexual women's response to newly diagnosed breast cancer. *Psycho-Oncology* **10**:40–51.

100. Matthews AK. (1998). Lesbians and cancer support: clinical issues for cancer patients. *Health Care for Women International* **19**:193–203.

101. GaysCan – Personal communication.

102. Fobair P, Koopman C, Dimiceli S, O'Hanlan K, Butler LD, Classen C, *et al.* (2002). Psychosocial intervention for lesbians with primary breast cancer. *Psycho-Oncology* **11**:427–38.

103. Kagawa-Singer M and Wellisch DK. (2003). Breast cancer patients' perceptions of their husbands' support in a cross-cultural context. *Psycho-Oncology* **12**:24–37.

104. Hoskins CN, Baker S, Budin W, Ekstrom D, Maislin G, Sherman D, *et al.* (1996). Adjustment among husbands of women with breast cancer. *Journal of Psychosocial Oncology* **14**:41–69.

105. Kornblith AB. (1998). Psychosocial adaptation of cancer survivors. In: J Holland (ed.), *Psycho-oncology*, Oxford: Oxford University Press.

106. Anderson B, Anderson B, and deProsse C. (1989). Controlled prospective longitudinal study of women with cancer: I Sexual functioning outcomes. *Journal of Consulting and Clinical Psychology* **75**:683–91.

107. Riley AJ. (1997). Sexual behaviour. In: A Baum, D Newman, J Weinman, R West, and C McManus (ed.), *Cambridge handbook of psychology, health and medicine*, Cambridge: Cambridge University Press.

108. Auchincloss SS and McCartney CF. (1998). Gynecologic cancer. In: J Holland. (ed.), *Psycho-oncology*, Oxford: Oxford University Press.

109. Kaplan HS. (1992). A neglected issue: the sexual side-effects of current treatments for breast cancer. *Journal of Sex and Marital Therapy* **18**:3–19.

110. Mantell J. (1982). Sexuality and cancer. In: J Cohen, JW Cullen, and LR Martin (ed.), *Psychosocial aspects of cancer*, New York: Raven Press.

111. Burton M, Watson M. (1998). *Counselling People with cancer.* Chichester: Wiley and Sons.

112. Goldstein I, Feldman MI, Deckers PJ, Babayan RK, and Vrane RJ. (1984). Radiation-associated impotence: a clinical study of its mechanism. *Journal of the American Medical Association* **251**:903–10.

113. Schover LR. (1993). Sexual rehabilitation after treatment for prostate cancer. *Cancer* (supplement) **71**:1024–30.

114. Schover LR. (1998). Sexual dysfunction. In: J Holland (ed.), *Psycho-oncology*, Oxford: Oxford University Press.

115. Muscari E, Aikin JL, and Good BC. (1999). Premature menopause after cancer treatment. *Cancer Practice* **7**:114–21.

116. Hunter MS. (1992). The women's health questionnaire: a measure of mid-aged women's perceptions of their emotional and physical health. *Psychology and Health* **7**:45–54.

117. Nolan M. (2001). Positive aspects of caring. In: S Payne and C Ellis-Hill (ed.), *Chronic and terminal illness: new perspectives on caring and carers*, Oxford: Oxford University Press.

118. Orbell S. (1996). Informal care in social context: a social psychological analysis of participation, impact and intervention in care of the elderly. *Psychology and Health* **11**:155–78.

119. Payne S and Ellis-Hill C. (2001). Being a carer. In: S Payne and C Ellis-Hill (ed.), *Chronic and terminal illness: new perspectives on caring and carers*, Oxford: Oxford University Press.

120. Rose K. (2001). A longitudinal study of carers providing palliative care. In: S Payne and C Ellis-Hill (ed.), *Chronic and terminal illness: new perspectives on caring and carers*, Oxford: Oxford University Press.

121. Morris SM and Thomas C. (2001). The carer's place in the cancer situation: where does the carer stand in the medical setting? *European Journal of Cancer Care* **10**:87–95.

122. Smith P. (2001). Who is a carer? Experiences of family caregivers in palliative care. In: S Payne and C Ellis-Hill (ed.), *Chronic and terminal illness: new perspectives on caring and carers*, Oxford: Oxford University Press.

123. Rolland JS. (1994). Working with illness: clinicians' personal and interface issues. *Family Systems Medicine* **12**:149–69.

124. Cousins R, Davies AD, Turnbull CJ, and Playfer JR. (2002). Assessing caregiving distress: a conceptual analysis and brief scale. *British Journal of Clinical Psychology* **41**:387–403.

125. Nijboer C, Templaar R, Sanderman R, Triemstra M, Spruijt RJ, and Van den Bos GA. (1998). Cancer and caregiving: the impact on the caregiver's health. *Psycho-Oncology* **7**:3–13.

126. Bolger N, Foster M, Vinokur AD, and Ng R. (1996). Close relationships and adjustment to a life crisis: the case of breast cancer. *Journal of Personality and Social Psychology* **70**:283–94.

127. Stetz K. (1987). Caregiving demands during advanced cancer. *Cancer Nursing* **10**:260–68.

128. Hagedoorn M, Sanderman R, Buunk BP, and Wobbes T. (2002). Failing in spousal caregiving: the 'identity-relevant stress' hypothesis to explain sex differences in caregiver distress. *British Journal of Health Psychology* **7**:481–94.

129. Baider, L. (1995). Psychological intervention with couples after mastectomy. *Supportive Care in Cancer* **3**:239–43.

130. Baider L, Koch U, Esacson R, and Kaplan De-Nour A. (1998). Prospective study of cancer patients and their spouses: the weakness of marital strength. *Psycho-Oncology* **7**:49–56.

131. Ellis-Hill C and Payne S. (2001). The future: interventions and conceptual issues. In: S Payne and C Ellis-Hill (ed.), *Chronic and terminal illness: new perspectives on caring and carers*. Oxford: Oxford University Press.

Chapter 4

Social context

Background and introduction 148
Social class. 152
   Introduction 152
   Social class, language, and health beliefs 153
   Social class and unemployment. 155
   Social class and practicalities 156
   Social class, service providers, and support. 156
   Summary 157
Gender 158
   Introduction 158
   Gender and pain 159
   Gender and emotions 160
   Gender and support. 161
   Younger men 161
   Older men 162
   Gender and cancer information 164
   Gender and sexuality. 165
   Gender and infertility 167
   Gender and body image, disability, impairment, and stigma 169
   Summary 172
Homeless people 172
   Introduction. 172
Defining 'homelessness' 173
   Homelessness and health 173
   Homelessness and cancer 174
   Homelessness: psychosocial factors 175
   Homelessness and support 176
   Summary 177
Ethnicity. 178
   Introduction 178
Defining 'race', 'culture', and 'ethnicity' 178
   Race. 178
   Culture 179
   Ethnicity 179
   Ethnicity and essentialism 179
   Ethnicity and social class 180
   Ethnicity: West versus East 180
   Ethnicity, religion, and death 181

Ethnicity and diet 184
Racism and ethnicity 185
Ethnicity and giving support: communication, advocacy, and interpreters 189
An interpreter 190
An advocate 191
Summary 193
Refugees and asylum seekers 194
Introduction 194
Defining 'refugees' and 'asylum seekers' 194
Asylum seekers, refugees, and health 194
Asylum seekers, refugees, and mental health 195
Asylum seekers and refugees: registration and information 196
Asylum seekers, refugees, and discrimination 196
Asylum seekers and support 197
Treatment for psychological problems 197
Summary 198
Conclusion 198
References 199

Background and introduction

In this chapter we want to use a sociological approach to aspects of cancer care and focus on what the 'social' may mean in that context. By 'social' we allude to the personal and biographical context of a person, and to the conceptual issues that underpin the ways we 'see' and care for people with the disease. For example, we seldom approach our work by looking at the ways in which wider socio-economic and political forces impinge on provision of care and the ways in which we, the service providers, may be influencing the ways that people with cancer respond. Instead, we have tended to focus on the individual; on finding the 'fault' of 'sickness' or pathology *within* the person, and it is usually women, for it is they who have in the majority, been the recipients of research.[1] Cancer 'patients' cope 'well' or 'badly', the assumption being that 'dysfunction' can be treated by *individualized* psychological support. A cancer patient will return to a 'normal' state or learn to deal with illness in the ways that medicine dictates.

This individualized approach fails to take into account that distress or 'coping' can only be fully understood in the context of its experience.[1–3] Some people who, despite trying to deal with their cancer in positive, proactive ways such as seeking information or generating a 'fighting spirit,' sometimes in a quest to survive[4] simply cannot use these so-called appropriate 'coping mechanisms.' While there is no valid evidence that 'coping skills' such as, 'fighting spirit' and denial prolong survival time[5, 6] people who use them may feel in control and we would applaud such an opportunity.[7] Our worry is that people who take on this responsibility and relapse or cannot muster a positive attitude, may feel that they have failed themselves, their families, and friends. This onus to 'cope' puts a burden on individuals to 'beat' their own disease in an area of medicine where 'cure' remains a relatively rare commodity.[8] It also imputes blame. This is despite the publicly acknowledged fact that cancer treatment is often abysmally slow in its deliverance.[9] An inability to 'fight' may have nothing to do with *the person* but is likely to rely on 'social context' not to mention physical status that may in itself have many 'social' connotations.[10, 11]

'Social context' includes, the ways in which we view our bodies, age, marital relationships or friendship, employment status, sexuality, and education. However we are not so much interested in, for example, 'age' *per se* but the *meanings* it brings to an experience and the ways in which the shifting aspects of time and place will affect the ways younger or older people will view their 'social context'. Moreover, 'time and place' embrace wider parameters than those that obviously delineate the person as an individual. These wider parameters include the ways that sick people and the institution of medicine itself, engage with each other. In turn, this 'engagement' will relate to the socio-economic and political status of a society.[12, 13] The wider parameters of 'context' are important for they are, in effect, the 'cradle' in which we live; how, *in part*, our health beliefs and needs are shaped, how we access care and importantly, how it is delivered. We are of course speaking about healthcare in Western society and the cultural assumptions underlying them, particularly the UK and the USA. Even these two nations have differing ways of delivering healthcare that will orchestrate the ways in which we access needs and will in part dictate the ways in which illness affects people's responses.[13] Although a detailed exploration into these areas are beyond the remit of this book, it is worth looking at a few examples of how policy can affect cancer care, bearing in mind that ideas never emerge in a vacuum. Rather, they are 'born' (sometimes reborn, sometimes reformulated) and can only flourish if the context is conducive to its growth.

Consider the ways in which the pervasive conceptual issue of 'self-responsibility'; of coping with cancer and even extending life by adopting the 'fighting spirit' and a positive outlook, appear to be wholly individualized phenomena. If we look closely however, they may also be linked to wider political forces.[14, 15] Although 'self-responsibility' is a Victorian concept, it reinstated itself and took hold in the late 1970s and 1980s in the UK and the USA, and was heavily influenced by the 'New Right' of the 1980s where the responsibility of individuals for their own and their family's well-being was stressed.[14–16] Not coincidentally, and at the same time, stringent cuts were made in healthcare services in an effort to undercut the undesirability of a 'dependency' culture when monies were scarce and where medical science was not making the impact that had been promised.[15, 17]

Medicine then, absolved itself:[18] health as the responsibility of the individual became separated from the responsibility of the state and public services.[19] Ironically, this ethos of self-responsibility may be perceived as disastrous for a capitalist economy but exists alongside marketed goods such as stress reducing medications and even counselling (sometimes to promote a 'fighting spirit') as a means of attaining 'well-being'.[19] But as we have indicated, these 'solutions' are individualized, void of a social context, both of the person who is receiving treatment, and the part that the medical personnel play in the care of the patient.[3] This is an illustration of how one political initiative helps to manipulate the ways by which we approach disease and how it may be affecting patient's experience, despite little evidence of its' validity.[5, 6] It starts to indicate the ways in which political forces may have an impact on health beliefs and health delivery.

While the concept of 'self-responsibility' shapes the way we approach many aspects of cancer care, whether in the orthodox world of hospital medicine or in the ethos of complementary and alternative practices, we cannot explain it without thinking about another very important conceptual issue, namely the question of *power*.[12] In our work as cancer carers, we seldom, if ever, consider the potency and relevancy of this concept as we go about our work. While a debate goes on about the decline of medicine's autonomy and dominance in recent years,[20] we believe that pressures for change in medicine may both undermine *and* enhance professional powers.[20] We also believe that when theories develop which are specialized as is the case in orthodox Western medicine, a gap appears between those with specialist knowledge and the lay person, leading to a power relation between clinician and patient (and between disciplines such as medical clinicians and nurses).[12] The patient (or nurse) is subservient to the 'other' by dint of the fact that they are not considered to be 'the expert'.[17] However, other factors may also impact on power relations and they may include gender, age, social class, and/or ethnicity.[13]

We think that the ramifications of power should never be underestimated despite the advent of a 'patient-centred ethos'[20, 21] that promotes and encourages people to recognize and pursue their rights. We do not discount the debate about the ways in which people are constantly questioning not only their own lives but the authority of others in the fragmented worlds in which we now live.[18] People feel a sense of freedom to act in a quest to consume which, arguably, provides a means to a 'new empowerment' for patients.[19] Indeed there have been shifts in practice in the last decade that have seemingly enhanced patient autonomy. 'Informed decision making' is one such conceptual tool through which the patient is given centre stage. Another is the way in which the concept of 'good communication' has become an important topic of research, albeit seldom critically assessed. 'Communication' continues to be perceived as a one-way process, the clinician taking the lead role as they are taught 'good' communication skills. We know however, through work that has been documented outside the cancer field, that 'communication' is a complex and dynamic process and not a didactic one. It relies heavily on context and includes the notion of 'agency': patients are known to have their own agenda[22] notwithstanding the power relationship that is inherent between doctor and patient.

Despite these shifts, we do not think that the notion of the 'empowered consumer' necessarily lives up to its promise in the context of medicine.[20] Take for example the way that litigation against medical malpractice has risen sharply within health services with negative consequences for patients.[23] Doctors who fear being sued may not always act in the patient's best interests.[23] We know too, that the plaintiff rarely wins their case and that medical complaints are often given lip service or evaded altogether.[24] Moreover, people who are unable to converse in English, *especially* the elderly and women, do not always know the ways to proceed in order to register their dissatisfaction.[7]

Power is found in the ways that the state can undermine health services that for all intents and purposes, were conceived to give equal access to care. Patients who have to 'wait months for radiotherapy and scans'[9] are not only likely to become distressed as a result, but hardly represent an army of successful consumers. These are just a few examples of the ways that patient 'empowerment' is a spurious concept and requires critical thought, especially when speaking about 'a patient-centred ethos'.

The often subtle (and sometimes not so subtle) ways in which we use power will inevitably have an impact on the ways in which we judge situations or people, how we act and what and whom our agendas actually stand for. This requires a reflexive attitude. How do we constitute our working worlds? In whose interests do we set about our given tasks? How do we, managers, researchers, clinicians, nurses, porters, cooks, and all other members of the hospital staff influence the experience of people with cancer? Thinking about the ways in which we go about our practice is so easily whitewashed in the name of 'objectivity': a strong belief that we are without prejudice; that we have the interests of patients at heart at all times and at all levels of our working lives. A stringent 'gaze' at what we do and how we do it, may conjure a very different picture of practice.

The examples of power and self-responsibility that we have given are conceptual entities but they already begin to suggest that people's ways of 'coping' do not rely on 'personality'; that people 'adjust' or not in a social context, be it personal and/or political. Examples of 'the social' are grounded in the ways in which hospitals are structured and the 'rules' by which they operate. These 'rules' maybe impacting on patient care and the ways people react when facing an illness.[25] This can be illustrated at an everyday level; in the ways, for example, that we communicate with each other and with the people we care for.

'Communication' is a wide term and does not only include the ways in which doctors and nurses talk to their patients or vice versa or how health professionals speak to each other. It is also about the kind and quality of support we give to patients when, for example, people are facing anxious periods waiting for test results—a time when people feel a sense of abandonment and confusion. [7, 25] Bad communication includes the ways we judge people and stereotype them; the ways in which we use non-verbal body language such as yawning or fidgeting during a consultation, leaving a person in a room for long periods without explanation or just the ways in which we might sit when attending to a person with cancer.[7] Even the clothes we as professionals wear, the food that is served to sick people in hospital, and the architectural surroundings of medical institutions are forms of communication and will make an impact on the person who is ill.

In our clinical work we have noticed the ways in which distress is often linked to the inability of hospitals to fulfil certain criteria of care and this may have little to do with medical input *per se*. 'Good' communication includes clear signposting, access to information, and the ways in which it is given to people. It includes continuity of care such as the writing of notes that enable subsequent professionals to know and understand the physical and psychosocial status of a patient.[7, 25] Anxiety is provoked through a general lack of co-ordination between services and the way that patients are often passed from one medical discipline to another as if their bodies were divided into small parts with no sense of a 'whole'. When notes are lost, letters of referral 'go missing' and appointments are muddled, largely as a result of understaffing (and underfunding), people lose trust and confidence when they are especially needed.[25] These issues apply to all patients and are of major importance in fostering the adjustment process of someone who is sick, be they men or women, upper or lower social class, with black or white ethnicity.

> Then I went to yet another department to have blood given to me and there was an awful lot of 'argy bargy' about my notes. They couldn't be found. Where were they? Who was I? What was my disease status? Why was I there? All these things made me feel that I was a nobody.

> (60-year-old woman with ovarian cancer)

Bearing all these caveats in mind, we have focused below, using empirical work, on how a concept of the 'social' applies itself to people who are marginalized in cancer care and who may find it difficult to respond in ways that we as service providers, have hitherto, assumed to be 'right'. We want to look at the ways in which concepts such as social class, gender, homelessness, ethnicity, being an asylum seeker, or refugee may impact on the ways in which people may adjust to cancer and the ways in which we ourselves may be impeding that adjustment. We think that these domains are seldom scrutinized as being 'a problem' in their own right. When social constraints (or enablers) become 'background noise' or hidden altogether as they often are, we tend to individualize and pathologize the person. As we have suggested above, this can create a burden and most importantly, engenders inequalities in care.

We want to accentuate that the domains that we have chosen are not discreet; there will be many overlaps in people's responses. For example, gender *and* ethnicity may interact with social class and homelessness.[26] Age may interact with all these categories, as may a state of unemployment. Older African Caribbean men may have differing health beliefs and needs from younger ones, but may be similar to those with white ethnicity who are the same age. Health professionals may well perceive and treat older and younger women and men in differing ways according to how they perceive the sexes, 'age', the stereotypes that they bring to 'young' and 'virile' bodies, and 'old' and 'withered' ones.[27] It will depend on how their perceptions change according to social class and ethnicity. *We think it is imperative that we keep these possible interactions in mind at all times.*

Social class

Introduction

There appears to be an enduring association between socio-economic inequality, morbidity, and mortality in Western countries and this association is stark despite the differing and often confusing definitions and meanings that abide in relation to the concept of 'class'.[28] Not withstanding this confusion, there is well-documented evidence that a 'health divide' remains, *usually* in favour of upper social classes.

When men of 20–64 years and women between 20 and 59 years were studied, higher mortality rates in lower social class women with cervical and lung cancer were found, and higher rates were found amongst men in lower social class groups in relation to lung disease.[29] Conversely, the standardized mortality rates were marginally higher for upper class men and women in relation to melanoma (cancer of the skin) and breast cancer.[29] This suggests that lifestyle behaviours may help to explain these differences along with other factors such as the health beliefs and needs of people in differing socio-economic classes that may influence illness behaviour; the ways in which people access health services, the availability of the latter[19] and the ways in which health services relate to people who present with symptoms.[30] For example, middle class people are often given longer consultations during which they ask the doctor more questions and discuss more problems than their working class counterparts.[30]

Social class, language, and health beliefs

Often barriers in access to mainstream health and social care services are exacerbated by problems of language and poorly provided service information. Although this is a social class issue it is also one of ethnicity. However, barriers to access and use of services goes beyond language difficulties amongst ethnic minority groups. While not *all* individuals from minority ethnic groups are disadvantaged in every instance of health,[26] the impact of socio-economic disadvantage and discrimination on the health and well being of minority ethnic groups is very evident. Manual workers of ethnic groups show a 60% greater chance of reporting fair or poor health than those in non-manual occupations. The reporting of 'fair' or 'poor' health are independently linked to 'perceived racial discrimination', 'expressed racial harassment', and socio-economic disadvantage'.[31]

While all accounts of people's beliefs of health and illness are embedded in the wider social context[2] including social class status and the ways that healthcare is organized, there remains a danger in the way that we as social analysts may be imposing a 'smooth conceptual order on experience that may be craggy and ever changing'.[32] People's responses are seldom 'fixed'; accounts will change with time and in place and according to the 'context' of the person. Not every person has a clear conception of health, and nor is keeping healthy a main priority for everyone.[33] Furthermore, while we can be informed by people's health beliefs we have to bear in mind that they may also legitimate the person's status as an 'ordinary' and 'blameless' citizen.[33] With these caveats in mind, men and women were asked to talk about the ways in which they perceived the causes of cancer.[2] Middle class respondents were more likely to use a variety of relatively 'mentalistic' accounts when compared to manual classes. These include 'stress', 'anxiety or worry', being in 'poor psychological condition' and 'not expressing feelings'. In contrast, working class respondents use 'physicalistic' accounts to explain cancer onset, naming 'dust', 'pollution', too much alcohol', 'smoking', being 'overweight', and being in the vicinity of 'poisonous chemicals' as possible triggers to the disease.

Middle class respondents have been found to make more frequent positive mention of 'therapy' and talking, 'fighting it (cancer) psychologically', having 'support from family and friends', 'belief in treatment', 'adopting a positive attitude', and 'seeking information about cancer'. Working class respondents are likely to be fatalistic, believing that 'no help or advice' aids recovery, which in itself is a matter of 'luck'. Their solution is to put themselves into the hands of doctors and drugs.[2] This has been demonstrated in studies that show that people in lower socio-economic groups tend to present themselves relatively less frequently to psychological and psychiatric services in general[2] and psychological intervention studies for cancer in particular.[4]

The focus on language raises questions about the ways in which cancer patients may relate to health personnel and vice versa and this in turn may have social class ramifications; while no more 'intelligent', middle class people are reported to speak a 'different vocabulary' to their lower social class counterparts (as we have seen above).[34] Taken at its face value the former may appear to have knowledge that 'matches' that of the 'expert'. In reality this may not be the case. Middle class male participants who were highly educated and who had been asked what they knew about genetic cancer, presented their knowledge in 'sophisticated' ways but the content was no more accurate than the accounts by men in lower social class categories.[35] 'Accurate knowledge' depended on the accessibility and relevancy of information and a perception of the ways in which it had been presented. Even more importantly, certain knowledge was simply deemed irrelevant to a person's lifestyle and this impacted on the ways that it was assimilated and how men responded in the context of cancer genetics.

This highlights the importance of remembering how people may present themselves in clinical settings in ways that do not necessarily mirror the reality of their lives. It also illuminates the ways in which people's accounts may rely on the social aspects of their experiences. Research has shown that a group of working class families in East End of London,[36] put on their 'best face' when talking to the 'expert' by repeating what they believed to be commonly accepted views on health. This usually had moral undertones that were linked to a class ethos of work. Respondents claimed a duty to work hard and to remain well. These 'public accounts' were used to make the speaker acceptable in the eyes of a stranger who is thought to be knowledgeable and 'in charge'. When the same respondents grew to trust and accept the interviewer, they revealed their 'private accounts' but only in the context of illness and always alongside other aspects of their biographies including their age, their employment position, their place as a man or a woman in everyday life, and their past experience of healthcare.

These findings have wide connotations and even wider repercussions. They illustrate the importance of attending to the concept of *power* between 'experts' and patients. They also illustrate the importance of *trust* and the ways in which we, as health personnel, 'allow' people to express themselves; the importance of attending to how we *listen* to the differing ways in which people tell their stories and the benefits to everyone concerned of placing them in their own social contexts whatever social class they feel they belong to.

The concepts of power, trust, and listening have implications for how people from different sectors of society may make use of health services. People with cancer who are undermined by the 'strangeness' of hospital life in all its manifestations, may become distressed or even turn away from treatments if not attended to in a way that 'fits' their needs in the context of their everyday lives including their social class.

Social class and unemployment

Material circumstances may be jeopardized as a result of being ill, and this applies to both men and women.[37] We know for example, that a fear of unemployment or actual redundancy may affect a sense of identity and this may apply to both men *and* women. Studies have shown that a man's sense of masculinity is punctured as a result of unemployment and this may interact with class issues and/or age.[38] Younger men with testicular cancer are known to fear unemployment,[38] regardless of class status. However, when young men in manual classes become unemployed, they are likely to become distressed (*ibid*) in a situation that may already be exacerbated by social class status.

The ways that diagnosis and treatment may be undermining the roles a person plays both in and outside the hospital have been found to be important aspects of a cancer experience. It may help to acknowledge the ways in which job status may be affecting the sense of self. Gender theorists have focused on men's particular need to play out their lives in the public arena of work but we have no doubt that this may apply to some women too. It sometimes helps to suggest that the consultant in charge of the person who is ill, writes a letter to their employer, explaining the condition and the prospect of re-entry into the work environment. This has been especially useful for younger testicular cancer patients in lower social class groups who have every chance of leading a 'normal' life after strenuous treatments are endured, but who are particularly vulnerable as they take on piece meal manual jobs. It is important to remember, however, that consent is obtained from the person who is ill, before any correspondence takes place between the clinician and others.

> I work on a building site and my cancer meant I had to stop. It's hard enough when you are working, but my family suffered as much as I did … they had to go without.
>
> (30-year-old man with two children)

> When my boss got a letter from the doctor, it changed everything… suddenly he seemed to understand that I couldn't do a full day's work … that I got so weary so quickly. He paced my work and said that 'doctor's orders were doctor's orders!'
>
> (30-year-old single office worker)

> I had no money, no job, no manhood … who am I anymore?
>
> (26-year-old lorry driver)

Social class and practicalities

Other problems related to class status may impinge on the ways people deal with ill-ness.[39] It is important to take into account the interconnected aspects of uncertainties surrounding cancer[40] and this applies to all people with the disease. Complications of health status such as ambiguous symptoms, unclear diagnosis or prognosis, lack of infor-mation on treatment options can all create uncertainty about 'the social' aspects of a per-son's life including the financial well-being of the person who is sick. Financial resources will impact on the ways people recuperate: taking a holiday may help to restore energy: a dearth of housing space and amenities may not. Lower socio-economic groups are often located in areas that have higher noise levels, atmospheric pollution, and less availability of services such as shops and transport. The design and maintenance of housing can bring higher levels of damp, condensation, insect and rodent infestation, the risk of fire, crime, and vandalism. Where people are living in groups, housing can be especially dangerous. Often families have to share bathrooms, toilets, and kitchens.[41] These are important but obvious barriers to adjustment and/or recovery. Other more hidden barriers to adjust-ment involve for example, hospital parking fees that may seem insignificant to hospital managers but can be perceived as exorbitant in the face of waiting for hospital tests or the long hours of vigilance that are needed (and advocated) when family members are criti-cally ill. Conversely, families without cars may have to travel large distances on expensive public transport despite awkward and long working hours. At the same time hospitals themselves restrict entry beyond 'visiting time' and are often perceived as unwelcoming to latecomers in situations that are already fraught with apprehension and uncertainty. This applies to all social class groups but may be especially difficult for people who have fewer financial resources and who have difficulty in articulating their needs.

Social class, service providers, and support

We should not forget that the values of the service provider may be having an impact on patient care and this may rely on the social class of both the parties. (It may also relate to age, gender relations, and ethnicity.) As we have said, doctors are known to spend less time with working class patients.[30] This immediately, lends itself to the concept of 'inequality' but this does not only apply to consultation time. We know, for example, that in many cases health personnel including doctors and nurses perceive high social class and 'high insight verbal ability' as a precursor to the probability of selection for psychotherapy.[2] Notwithstanding the possibility that psychological interventions of any kind may not be relevant to the values and lifestyles of some peo-ple *regardless* of class, it may also be the case that people are denied access to services. While African Caribbeans are over-represented among patients who are 'compulsorily detained' they are also under-represented among those who use 'talking therapies'[42] but it is not clear as to why this is the case. 'Counselling' is a Western concept and may not 'fit' with certain cultural mores, but it may also be due to lack of resources and well-worn prejudices held about class, ethnic status, and a psychological intervention.

As Gallangher (1980) and Blair (1993)[2, 43] have argued, the psychotherapeutic community would do well to consider class experience and to revise their therapeutic techniques to accommodate class difference. This assumes of course, that an intervention of 'counselling' will iron out problems in all populations. We have little evidence that this is the case, however. (*see* under Ethnicity, Refugees and Asylum seekers). Without due attention from researchers and practitioners as to what social class (and or ethnicity) *means* to a person, the question will remain unanswered. It is worth reiterating that these ambiguities require careful thought and above all, the capacity to *listen* to people's needs in the context from which they come.

'Support' or 'counselling' includes many differing ways of delivering it. However, whichever way this is given, it will always rest itself on the concept of 'containment', a way of 'holding' the person's grief, sadness, or joy. 'Support' may mean 'counselling' on a one to one or group basis, including psychodynamic, Rogerian[44] or cognitive techniques,[45] help with relaxation or aromatherapy, or a need for more comprehensive information, including help with benefits and form filling. It is important to remember that some people are unable to read or write.[46] However, people from all social classes are known to find it particularly difficult to fill in complicated forms and many people are unaware of their rights to benefits.[47] Often people with cancer regard this type of 'support' as one of the most important aspects of their recovery.

> I didn't know about the benefits until long after I started to worry about money, and I didn't have much to start with, even less not working and being paid half. And then I had to get help with the questionnaire ... what they expect ill people to do is nobody's business!
>
> (41-year-old manual worker with a family)

Hospital personnel can do little to change the material circumstances of patients. However, we think that the study of social class and the meanings held within that term, are important on many levels. It may help us to plan needs and discharge in ways that might be conducive to positive outcomes, while also helping us to understand our own responses when caring for the people with cancer.

Summary

- People may differ from one another in terms of beliefs and needs both within classes and between them but these differences may be linked to other factors such as gender, age, and ethnicity.

- People who are members of lower socio-economic groups *seem* to have differing beliefs and needs compared to those in upper social class groups including those of health professionals. They may also have different ways of expressing them in differing contexts.

- People in economically deprived groups often live in difficult circumstances and may not have the financial resources to meet their needs. Particular care should be given to these patients when planning discharge from hospital.

- When people live in difficult circumstances, they may find it difficult to live up to certain well established (but invalid) ways of coping with cancer.
- The attitudes and assumptions of health personnel may impinge on patient care.

Gender

Introduction

Investigations into gender differences in health and illness behaviour (including prevention and utilization of health services) are fraught with methodological and conceptual problems.[48] However, health survey data has consistently indicated an excess of 'morbidity' (symptoms and ill health) among females compared to males,[48] an excess in utilization of services amongst women,[48] and an excess of mortality in males compared to females.[49]

We often make the mistake of turning to biological sex to explain these differences between men and women but seldom do we look to similarities that exist between them.[27] When we fail to consider the ambiguities that abound in terms of sexuality (some men often dress as women even without a sex change, some women wish to look and be like men, some men and women have literally taken on the 'gender' of the opposite sex and with satisfying results) we fall short of fruitful answers to explain behaviour. We then tend to turn to the social 'role' obligations to which men and women are assigned and the acquired risks linked to these roles such as stress and lifestyles. For example, men are thought to be less biologically 'durable' than women,[48] while being socialized to take the bread winning role and to face greater risks and more stress in their everyday working lives.[50] It is assumed that men have learned to be inexpressive, stoical, and 'work orientated'. Their refusal to admit weakness is said to create a barrier to an engagement with medicine[51] leading to earlier death.[52] Women are thought to be responsible for health matters as a result of their sex, specific and social status as mothers[53] and in turn, are depicted as being expressive, compliant, emotionally labile, and are thought to suffer more symptoms because of their reproductive destiny. This apparently leads them to seek medical advice more frequently than men do.

Both approaches lead us into an essentialist trap (i.e. we are 'born' with certain characteristics that relate to biological sex and we are therefore 'given' social roles). Stereotypes regarding men and women are deeply ingrained in the Western psyche. 'Inexpressive', irresponsible men and 'emotional', talkative women become 'the norm'. When these assumptions take hold, they only help to direct our attention away from structural issues that may underlie the quality of healthcare and the possible ways in which *we* as health workers, impute stereotypes onto people with cancer, their relatives, and friends. This creates and maintains untold harm not least in the ways in which inequality of care is upheld.

Here, we want to accentuate the differences *and* similarities amongst men and women with cancer.[1] No difference exists in relation to, for example, the number of days lost at work as a consequence of illness; whether people ignore, take care of themselves, seek medical care as a result of symptoms, or in the ways that different types of medication are taken by men and women.[48] Significant differences between males and females in relation to utilization of medical services such as psychological support appear to be consistent however.[48] Men are more likely to under-utilize. No obvious explanations are documented in relation to this except for the so-called irresponsibility of men towards their mental states,[50] their inability to disclose their feelings, and a dislike of 'counselling' in the name of 'masculine' ideals.[54] As we have already indicated, a 'feminine' woman's propensity to emotionality and interdependence will apparently lead her to seek help.

We think that there is no such concept as 'masculinity' or 'femininity.' Instead we want to introduce the concept of 'masculinities' and 'femininities' that are not exclusive to the biological sex of a person.[55] Men and women are no longer recognized for what they *are*, but what they *do* or achieve in 'gender relations' with other people[1] and in specific historical and political contexts. By 'gender relations' we mean the interactions that we engage in with, for example, friends and relations, medical personnel *and* institutions (including hospitals and the ethos that they promote). For example, a man may put on the stiff upper lip while talking to the clinician who is embedded in 'masculine' ideals of competitiveness, stoicism, and objectivity[27] (*see* under Gender and Emotions). However the same man may hold his teddy bear and cry in the night-time seclusion of his hospital bed.[27] *Both* ways of being are possible but usually one remains hidden as men strive to retain masculine ideals by putting on a 'brave face'.

By viewing men and women in stereotypical ways we can see how the concepts of power and conflict may impinge on care.[1, 55, 56] For example, some 'healthy' young men with testicular cancer may seem reluctant to present their symptoms to doctors. This is usually explained in terms of men's irresponsible attitude towards their bodies. It may also rely on a lack of available information regarding the disease or a previous medical encounter in which he has been made to feel ridiculed by the physician and/or ignored altogether. This in itself may be due to the real probability that his complaint was not life threatening but it may also be difficult to 'see' through a young man's seeming good health and virility.[27] This example of 'gender relations' (the way that the doctor has assumed something that has depended on the fact that he, 'the expert' is dealing with a virile young man) highlights power structures that cause conflict leading to late diagnoses and even death.

Gender and pain

The ways in which we tend to stereotype men's and women's responses and behaviour is evident in for example, the ways that we expect people to respond to symptoms such as pain. There is a belief that women have a superior endurance in their ability to cope with the latter and this relies on her biological make up and on cultural themes of roles and socialization such as giving birth and mothering.[57] In contrast, male socialization is seen to discourage men from being allowed to express pain (physical or emotional) for fear that they will be considered vulnerable (*ibid*). But as Bendelow (1993) suggests, these gendered assumptions may be 'double edged'.[57] The expectations that we hold may lead to ignoring pain and even inflicting it and these expectations are expressed in terms of ethnicity, class, age, and even sexuality. For example, men who are young, white, middle class, and heterosexual are thought to take more time to admit to being in any type of pain or to seek treatment. However (eventual) disclosure is taken more seriously by everybody, and is more likely to lead to medical action[58] while women's pain is likely to be attributed to psychogenic origins.[59] It is within the work of 'pain' that the 'social' is particularly evident. Few would argue with Bendelow (1993) when she says that pain is a 'medical(ized)' phenomenon, but it is also an 'everyday experience linking the subjective sense of self to the perceived "objective" reality of the world and other people'.[57, 58]

Gender and emotions

As we have indicated, the ways in which we, as health workers, 'see' people according to their sex is mirrored in the ways that we gender emotions other than the expression of pain. The relatively little work that has been carried out on men with cancer[1] (that is in itself a gendered response by researchers!) suggests that they react to illness in similar ways to women but this will depend on the social relations that people engage in. Men as well as women may feel lonely, sad, and emotional as they go through a cancer experience, but their feelings are seldom 'allowed' to become overt in hospital settings where health practitioners themselves take on the mantle of stoicism, competitiveness, and emotional inexpressiveness and impute them onto their practice;[27, 38] where women are *expected* to express their feelings[4] and men are not.[27, 57] How often have you heard it said and with awe that 'he took the bad news stoically' or 'what a wimp he is, he can't stop crying' or 'she hasn't come to terms with her illness because she hasn't expressed her grief'? While these responses are based on assumptions held by many professionals working with people with cancer, it has been noted that some young men may wish to remain 'silent' and withhold emotions as a means of gaining strength when facing a life-threatening disease. This suggestion runs against the tide of thought that espouses the concept of 'opening up' and can be particularly difficult for the families and friends of men who are ill as the latter 'turn their faces to the wall'. Sometimes this is quite literally the case and next of kin are left feeling helpless in the wake of seeming rejection. When this happens it may be helpful to explain this phenomenon. When illness or injury transform what men may have perceived as 'healthy' to 'the body of the lesser man',[60] young men seem to want to cocoon themselves in a mantle of stereotypical masculine ideals.[27] This does not mean that they are innately 'inexpressive'[1, 27, 38] nor that emotional support of one kind or another will not be asked for. We know for example, that when men are given a safe and empathic environment to express their needs and feelings they may do so but on their own terms and in their own time.[27]

I asked for some sort of counselling four years after I had finished treatment. At the time (of diagnosis and treatment) I was like a shutter pulled down. I didn't want sympathy, but nor did I want intolerance or dismissal … just to go it alone.

(34-year-old testicular cancer patient)

Likewise, some women may wish to go through a cancer experience without expressing emotion and denying their disease (or at least not *overtly* expressing emotion, some, or all of the time). This so-called reluctance to disclose feelings needs to be respected in *both* men and women. We believe that these responses are not 'dysfunctional' but simply 'comfortable' ways of adjusting to illness at particular times and in specific places with specific people. For these reasons they may change hour by hour, or day by day.

Gender and support

In this section we want to focus on men and support since there is little documentation of the ways in which they accept or reject help. Women are shown to accept support and express more needs than men[47] but this finding may be as much to do with the expectations we have of men and women as any truthful response. Interestingly, there are few studies that report on the effect of psychological treatment on men, despite its known efficacy on women.[61] In cancer care there is an assumption that people require formal support when they are demonstrating high scores on psychological questionnaires. However, we know that some men do welcome an invitation for support and this does not necessarily rely on high levels of severity of anxiety and/or depression.[54] Indeed need is found to relate to late stage disease and aggressive treatments.[54] However we would advocate caution. Counselling may not always benefit people in certain groups in the ways that we might expect.

Younger men

Young testicular cancer patients who were randomized to a cognitive behavioural intervention were more likely to be anxious one year post 'treatment' than those men in the control group and those men who elected not to be randomized and received standard care.[54] This may have been due to therapist effect or the fact that treated men were enabled to talk about their distress through counselling. However, we believe that when young men with cancer accept an offer of formal support, their sense of masculinity may be punctured. For these reasons we believe that a *routine* invitation to a psychological intervention is counterproductive in this group of cancer patient.

We suggest that a young man is told that a psychological support service is provided or accessible, early in the cancer experience and leave it to him to seek it out in his own time. We have found that referrals are often made without consulting the person in question. When this happens it can have wide repercussions. Just as a doctor or nurse would (we hope) explain and ask permission to carry out a medical procedure, so to, must someone be asked if they would appreciate the help of a trained counsellor. A person can feel very undermined when confronted with 'a shrink', which is how it is perceived in many cases.

If care is given by hospital staff in ways that are reflexive and sensitive to psychosocial nuances, including the recognition of mood change, we think that the need for a formal counselling may not be required in the majority of cases. Too often, 'counselling' is offered as an antidote to the perceived helplessness of medical personnel and because it is a fashionable tool with which to 'handle' cancer distress. It is as if 'a counsellor' will simply wipe out distress, rather like cutting out a tumour with a knife. But nothing is as simple as it may seem. Anxiety may be experienced as a motivating factor by some people, giving meaning to the experience of cancer. At the same time a sense of isolation and general distress can be caused by the impersonal ethos of hospitals and the ways in which we care for people in terms of, for example, gender relations and social class. Bad communication skills and a lack of relevant information may be the reasons for a person's 'morbidity' and not cancer *per se*.

> I woke up (from my operation) to find her (a counsellor) by my bed. She wasn't even pretty, but wanted to 'grieve' with me ... I told her where to get off! ... I'd had enough of people asking me to have my head examined ... I just wanted to get on with it ...

> (25-year-old single, male photographer)

When a young man is in need of support, and has agreed to accept it, it may help to 'normalize' his needs by telling him that others have requested 'counselling' and some have benefited from talking. But as with all patients, it is a mistake to take a patronizing approach. Young (and old) men and women may accept an intervention against their will, fearing that their treatment will be in jeopardy if they do not comply. When there seems to be little to offer in the face of rejection, we have noticed that one of the ways in which many men may control uncertainty and psychic pain is by focusing on 'work', be it paid employment[27, 38] or some other kind of activity such as building a wall, putting up shelves, or painting a picture. The masculine self seems to be preserved through work.[38] The latter maintains a sense of coherence in the face of loss and change when undergoing a life-threatening illness.[62] It is important to remember, however, that different classes of men (and women) may have differing responses, according to the social relations that he is embroiled in, both in and outside of the hospital setting. However we have found in our clinical work that this need in men to 'work' cuts across social class and age. Older men who have retired, also perceive 'work' as a way of gaining purpose and or pleasure. A game of golf is as significant in terms of mastery as a day at the office.

> All we could think about was our work, everyone on the ward talked about it ... would our jobs be held open? Should we tell our bosses? Would we ever get a job again? I couldn't wait to get on with it.

> (35-year-old male plumber with three children)

Older men

As we have already indicated, the age of cancer patients is a particularly important factor to take into consideration and this is the case in terms of gender. We have already looked at the ways in which younger men may react to their disease. While there is less evidence concerning older men who are ill, we know that prostate cancer patients and their carers are distressed [63, 64] but are seldom offered support[64, 65] despite their known need for it.[64] 'Support' does not necessarily mean a 'counselling' intervention but may include a perceived need for information such as brochures about services and benefits and a series of talks by health personnel regarding the medical and social aspects of prostate cancer.[64] The absence of these types of support may be due to the unavailability of services due to a lack of resources. It may also be a result of our 'blindness' in the face of older people, believing them to be 'bolstered' by age, established family networks, and stoicism relating to men in general.

Men's needs, however, require that we do not categorize them in any way. Older South Asian and white men with advanced cancer resented being 'pushed into attending support groups or day centres' as they were constant reminders of illness.[66] However, those who had attended were very satisfied with the way people provided mutual emotional support and the special bond and understanding that was created.[66] This is an example of how people's experiences differ, how men (and women) of all ethnic backgrounds including the white majority may resent the ways in which we assume that a given treatment will be 'a good thing' and how after all, some who have experienced such an intervention may find it beneficial.

We have noted how many young men with testicular cancer have a need to maintain a sense of control. As they are young and virile, the concept of control might 'fit' nicely with the representation of youth. However 'control' may also be an issue in some older men and women. All come to hospital with a life behind them and many have been in important positions at work, controlling large sums of money, and/or people or by simply living a life, keeping families fed and warm in the best way they can. Cancer can denote a loss of control and this may be the case for older people too.[62] Roles may have had to be relinquished. A person who for example, was once in charge of a multinational company may have had to resort to spoon feeding when facing a life-threatening disease. Others may have exerted their control on family members and find themselves in subservient positions through illness. The more 'in control' a person has been in life, the more they may require support in all aspects of his cancer experience. At the same time the more reluctant they may be to request it, fearing that it may further undermine a sense of self. On the other hand, there is a suggestion that sick men who have lost the control they once had in their public and private lives, may play out that control in the context of home with close relatives who are looking after them (usually women) as attention is demanded that can be overwhelming.[62] This is not to say that women too, may be controlling, but we believe that the politics of gender may play its part in this context.

Interestingly, while we have found that older men's needs are not always met in a hospital setting, work has shown that health visitors give older men with advanced cancer more of their time than they give to sick women, believing that the latter have inbuilt support networks and that men are alone and in need of help.[67] This may be true in many cases but it reinforces the argument that we 'gender' the ways in which we provide support. This inevitably leads to unequal services and less than optimal care and again, highlights the ways in which 'problems' do not necessarily lie within the person but may be linked to the ways in which medical professionals and the structure of hospitals rest their case on well-known and ubiquitous assumptions.

These are only a few examples of how gender and age interact; how older men may require support despite the fact that we do not always attend to their needs,[64, 65] and how younger ones (and older ones too) may wish to take on stereotypical responses when they are ill. These examples suggest that we might be surprised if only we *asked and listened* to the people to whom we are providing a service. People in hospital, whatever their gender, social class, their ethnicity, or age may have needs that we know little about or ignore as we impute stereotypes, assuming that people have certain requirements and not others, but nevertheless in ways that can lead to dangerous outcomes.

> I have been made to feel like an old man through having cancer … but I still have a sex life and I travel and play golf. I need to be active partly to take my mind off things, but I also, like everyone else, want to have my needs attended to … like knowing what I am in for, reassurance that I will not be sent home too early to fend for myself … and other kinds of information that will make my life better.
>
> (65-year-old single, retired man)

Gender and cancer information

Information giving is the current panacea in cancer care,[68] the belief being that without it people will be unable to fulfil expected health behaviours and will suffer negative psychological outcomes. However we think that to take a 'blanket' approach to information giving is to negate the complexity of this important health issue. We have already alluded to the ways in which men require relevant information but do not perceive it to be accessible despite the fact that they are often depicted as being irresponsible towards their bodies. For example, men wanted to know their genetic risk for cancer at the time of a marriage or birth, but it was unavailable. They perceived information to be available in doctor's surgeries, but did not find time to access it because of work commitments to subsidize families.[35] We have also referred to the ways that women seem to be proactive in matters of health and disease including information seeking. The research that has taken ambiguity into consideration has shown that *both* men and women may want transparency, require hope, and wish to avoid 'unsafe information' all or part of the time.[7, 69, 70] Moreover, because of the paucity of research that has been carried out on men with cancer compared to women[1] it is difficult to know how men might respond in this and other contexts. And while women are apparently more willing to take part in research than men[47] we believe that this rests on the assumptions we, health personnel, make about men and women preventing us from approaching male participants.[1]

Information giving does not only become problematic in the context of gender but is a problem of ethnicity too. While, for example, there is a belief amongst professionals that 'Asian' families follow a model of 'closed awareness' in that they do not disclose the diagnosis and prognosis to their sick relative, research that includes people from differing cultural backgrounds including white ethnic groups, reveals a subtle tension between the varying needs for information and the giving of it regardless of ethnicity.[7] It is easy to imagine how difficult it might be for a clinician to suggest certain very aggressive treatments when the diagnosis of cancer has not been made transparent or when further information is not asked for. Non-transparency may be dangerous in the sense that people may not understand the importance of drug taking that 'fits' with medical protocols. In these circumstances we think that very careful and sensitive 'counselling' with the sick person may often be a solution. However it must be borne in mind that people, whether they are men or women or of differing ethnic backgrounds and ages, have a right *not* to know details of their illness. The differing styles of information receiving are not necessarily indications of psychological dysfunction such as denial or anxiety, but are likely to reflect diversity in ways of adjusting to illness. Information may be asked for as time passes and when the sick person is ready, especially if they understand that professionals are at hand who are concerned and who have time to sit and listen to them. Family and friends who often guard the sick person's information pathways, need to have the importance of 'patient centredness' explained to them carefully. It needs to be conveyed that the patient must *at all times* take centre stage. It is important to maintain dignity in both people who are ill *and* their families/friends in a situation that requires the utmost sensitivity. (*See* Chapter 6 on Communication.)

Gender and sexuality

Our culture lays down 'norms' of sexual behaviour for each of the sexes that in itself is gendered.[10] But these 'norms' do not apply to every culture. For instance, there is much variation between societies in the degree of heterosexual activity permitted prior to marriage, outside of marriage, and even within marriage itself.[10] Extramarital sex is common in many societies[71] and significantly while 54% of societies allow men to indulge in it, only 11% say they allow it for women. In some societies homosexuality is completely forbidden and in others heterosexuality is prohibited for 260 days in a year. In New Guinea homosexuality is thought to make crops flourish and boys become strong (*ibid*). In the UK and the USA male behaviour that transgresses 'gender rules' of heterosexuality, is considered 'womanish' and effeminate.[72] Our assumptions that older people are less likely to have sexual lives, may rest on the ways in which sex and fertility are intertwined in societies such as ours where the importance of reproducing is widespread.[10]

This illustrates how sexuality is by no means, a straightforward concept. It is a mistake, for example, to assume that older men and women do not have an interest in their sexuality. Equally it is a mistake to think that younger men are devastated because of a loss of a testicle and especially in relation to their sex life. These assumptions obscure the many differing ways that people respond and play out their sexuality and the ways in which the latter may be contingent on time and place. Many younger men seem to sideline the sense of loss as a result of an orchidectomy (surgery to describe the taking away of a testicle) until such time that 'loss' has a meaning that is based on the reality of their lives. When older men and women in 'stable' relationships speak about their sexuality they may explain that despite 'sexual impairment', their relationships with partners are often richer since their cancer experience as they recount a closeness that cannot be measured.[1] When younger single men speak of their sexuality as being 'on hold' despite 'normal' sexual functioning, they often talk about negotiating the difficulties of revealing a 'stained' image in a first time sexual encounter.[1] Younger men with steady partners may not feel that their sex lives are constrained, despite an assumption made by clinicians and researchers that the sex lives of people undergoing treatments for cancer may be compromised.

While many men are not offered a prosthesis or replacement for their testicle when it has been removed, many men refuse the offer and claim that their body image is intact.[38] However like all the examples that we present throughout, this may depend on context-specific situations such as whether someone is in a 'stable' relationship and/or whether he is mindful of his body in a context where for example, he has to undress amongst other men such as a sports locker room. Men may wish to change their minds. We believe that men are offered a prosthesis (while being given all the possible side-effects of replacement) at the time of initial surgery with as much time as is possible to make decisions; if a man has refused, we advocate that it is offered again at follow-up, even years after diagnosis. This is a difficult proposition since many men may feel that the offer at long-term follow-up denotes a less than 'masculine' image in the eyes of the doctor. But careful wording such as 'How do you feel about a prosthesis for your testicle'? will leave an option open for the patient to state his needs. Indeed it is incumbent on health professionals to speak openly about this often 'hidden' aspect of people's lives. Too often it remains a topic to be shunned because of embarrassment on the clinician's part.[38]

All these caveats apply to women too. We tend to assume that women according to their age will neatly 'slot' into gendered 'roles'. For example, it may be assumed that because she is older and without a visible partner, she does not have or wish for a sex life. Making light of situations such as brachytherapy after surgery for gynaecological cancer through sexual innuendo, may feel degrading, as may the whole process of vaginal dilation.

> The radiographer referred to the 'thing' they put into my vagina as a penis in a jokey sort of way, and wondered whether I was using my dilator, 'for after all' she said, 'you may want a one night stand or even a toy boy one day',! I was horrified and then sad that she had treated me like this.

> (58-year-old divorced woman)

When an older women goes through menopause she is regarded as someone who has reached a 'natural' event in her life and that her libido is likely to wane in an expected way. To bolster that and other symptoms, a treatment that relies on a medical model will remedy her dry vagina, hot flushes, night sweats, osteoporosis, irritability, headaches, and dizziness by administering HRT (hormone replacement therapy) managed by clinicians albeit in ways that are not necessarily uniform. Doctors appear to prescribe HRT according to the context in which consultations take place, as well as personality, training, age, sex, and experience of the clinician and the social and cultural attributes of the patient herself.[73] This illustrates the possible gendered approach many clinicians use when attending to people whether in the context of cancer[74] or not. It also negates the ways that sociocultural 'events' that coincide with a woman's hormone depletion may help to cause the symptoms she may be experiencing. These 'events' include social transitions such as retirement and children leaving home. When women are going through premature menopause because of a cancer, these other 'events' may not be present. She may be relieved by the cessation of her periods and the possibility of unwelcome pregnancies. However, she may welcome HRT to aid her libido while her sexuality has never waned. The loss of meaning in her life may be more difficult for her than further risk to her physical well-being. On the other hand, she may be more worried about her *cancer* than she is about her loss of the so-called 'femininity'. Careful information giving and the ways we elicit the *meaning* that a menopause will have on a woman's life will help her to make her own decisions in ways that are most beneficial to herself and the life she leads.

Many older men have to face a loss of libido and general sexual functioning as a result of prostate cancer surgery and medication.[64] The affects of hormonal treatment may lead to very obvious changes in a man's body such as hot flushes and breast enlargement, and these changes may have a profound effect on how a man perceives himself. A man may have lost his 'role' as breadwinner as a consequence of a cancer diagnosis. All these factors may have led to a loss of the sense of masculinity that can have far reaching and negative consequences.[27] One important way of caring for someone who is experiencing these side-effects (or is likely to) is to carefully explain the possible outcomes and to acknowledge what he may be facing. Some men require a more in-depth counselling to deal with this important aspect of treatment, others seem to adjust to it without formal help. This may depend on the quality of the relationship a man is in and the ways that he has perceived himself as a man prior to his diagnosis, not to mention other life circumstances.

Gender and infertility

Infertility is a universal human concern, as is the anguish caused by infertility, whatever its cause.[10] When a woman fails to conceive, a wide variety of cultural explanations are given. This misfortune is often blamed on the individual's behaviour, on the 'natural' world, on the malevolence of other people or, on supernatural forces or Gods.[10] As Helman points out, lay explanations (of infertility) often draw on deep cultural images of what constitutes 'a woman' or 'a man'.[10] Infertility in women in the West, is thought to strike at the very essence of themselves. Indeed, it is sometimes thought that to be fertile is to be a woman.[75] One study showed that having a child post treatment for cancer denoted 'cure'.[76] In some communities, men are distraught when their wives fail to conceive and find it difficult to acknowledge their own sterility. Dignity and respect are enhanced by the number of children a man can father, and especially if they are sons.[77] Women are usually blamed for infertility in traditional societies and although the advances in assisted reproduction in the West have become more accepted and sophisticated, and male infertility has been addressed in recent decades, there remains a doubt that it could be 'a man's fault'.[78] It is against this background of insecurity that people have to come to terms with possible or real infertility as a result of having cancer.

Infertility caused by aggressive treatment regimens may be a source of distress in *both* men and women,[76] but healthcare providers are known to withhold information regarding this sensitive and difficult issue.[76] Of course the urgency to know details regarding infertility (including banking sperm) will depend on the age of the person and whether they have had children or as many as had originally been planned for. However, even older patients may be mourning the loss of the ability to have children, even when the family is complete. It is a mistake to assume that gay men and lesbian women are not concerned with having a family. Both may wish to have children and often want to keep their options open. Like everybody else, they too should have their needs assessed without making assumptions.

While young patients may think that starting a family is irrelevant when facing a life-threatening disease, there are indications that feeling healthy enough to be a 'good' parent after cancer was the strongest predictor of emotional well-being in the survivors of cancer.[76] The whole issue of fertility (or infertility) requires information 'counselling' with consent, and time to make decisions concerning sperm production and banking at the time of diagnosis when the latter is appropriate. Studies have shown that very few childless men bank sperm prior to treatment,[76] indicating that banking may be a particularly sensitive issue for *everyone*, including patients and health professionals. Sometimes the geography of hospital wards precludes privacy not only in obtaining informed consent but also in the production of sperm. The utmost care needs to be taken to make sure that men's needs are met. A quiet room, away from staff and patients may offer privacy if sperm cannot be produced in the seclusion of home. Often men are grateful for the offer of pornographic magazines to assist them in a situation that can cause embarrassment and long delays.

Straightforward talk that may help to normalize the act of sperm production is appreciated. A man who holds fast to stereotypical masculine ideals may feel particularly damaged by a negative reading of his sperm count. Indeed, particular attention to the words that are used to describe men's sperm may help those who can feel undermined by the whole process of sperm banking.

> I wish I had been directed to a clean toilet away from hospital staff. And I wish I had been allowed to leave my pot in an anonymous place so that I did not have to see the people who knew what I had been up to!

(24-year-old man)

The way that people spoke about my sperm was out of order. They said that it was 'poor quality', 'not good enough' and 'sub standard.' Why didn't they just say that it fell outside the given ranges?

(32-year-old man)

When men and women have their infertility verified, many ask for further counselling, sometimes months after the diagnosis. Counselling may involve working through the gendered aspects of infertility including the loss that is felt as a result and by both men and women. 'Masculinities' and 'femininities' are two important conceptual issues to bear in mind in this context. People's responses may not always be the expected ones. We think that people need time to come to terms with infertility before all the alternatives are put before them. These alternatives include adoption, *in vitro* fertilization, and surrogate motherhood. It is well to remember that certain cultures do not approve of such measures and this may be true of people in the West as well as in the East. For example, in Japan there has been both public and official opposition to the use of such procedures.[79] Many people in the West are likely to find this concept abhorrent but this may change as time goes on.[78]

This area of care has a great deal to say about the professional who is in a powerful position while looking after people who may feel undermined and vulnerable. We recognize how difficult it may be to provide a service that is fraught with difficult issues but both men and women must be treated with sensitive care bearing in mind that preconceived assumptions and the way that they are articulated, can so easily lead to distress.

Gender and body image, disability, impairment, and stigma

As Hellman[10] points out and as we have already indicated, in every society the human body has a *social* as well as a physical reality and this caveat might be borne in mind in the case of all the examples we have given above. The social body provides people with a framework for perceiving and interpreting physical and psychological experiences.[11] The ways that our bodies are shaped, how large or small we are, and the way we adorn them, are all ways of communicating information about our positions in society, that includes information about our age, gender, social status, occupation, and membership of certain groups, whether they are religious or secular.

The term 'body image' is used to describe all the ways that people conceptualize and experience their body consciously or not.[10] The culture that we live in teaches us to perceive and interpret the many changes that can occur over time in our own bodies and in the bodies of other people. We learn how to differentiate between old and young bodies, a sick body from a healthy one, a fit body from one that is disabled, how to perceive some parts of the body as public and others as private, and how to view some bodily functions as socially acceptable and others as 'unclean'.[10] Nowhere is this more true than in the context of cancer where 'healthy' bodies are often transformed into mutilated, 'disabled' and sick, ones that are likely to be stigmatized and held to be morally reprehensible.[8] However, the way that 'body image' is perceived is, we believe, contingent on the social or gendered relations we have with people. For example, the ways that we 'deal' with a disfigured face as a result of cancer may be influenced by our core beliefs. They in turn, may have been influenced by the ways in which we view bodily perfection and this in turn can be influenced by the socio-economic and political status of a society.[10] It may also rely on the power and gender relations between people. A man or woman who is entering into the employment market after disfiguring surgery may find it more difficult than a person who does not have this obstacle to get through. On the other hand, the quality of care people get from their doctors and other health personnel will have an impact on any kind of mutilation.

The concepts of 'disability' and 'impairments' are important here. Oliver (1990)[80] describes 'impairment' as a body lacking in a limb or limbs or some other bodily mechanism while 'disability' refers to the many social disadvantages imposed by society on people with physical impairments. 'Disability' is a social construction that helps to create a large number of people who are dependent, economically unproductive, marginalized, and ignored. Ramps for wheelchairs, for example may not be installed in hospitals; hospital toilet seats may be too low for comfort; patient 'call buzzers' may be out of reach or even absent. Thus, 'impaired' people may not be 'disabled'; disability may not be an *inherent* aspect of the individual, but determined by the meanings we ascribe to the person's bodily state and the state of dependency, our attributes engender. Although this may not be a gendered phenomenon *per se*, disability may very well be perceived in gendered terms as well as in terms of, for example age, social class, and ethnicity. People are known to be given different treatments according to their sex, sometimes leading to dangerous outcomes.[73, 74] Women may be encouraged to be carried to a part of the hospital where she requires treatment, simply because she is a 'cancer patient' and a female who requires help because of her sex. A man may be asked to walk because he is considered 'strong and stoical'. Both these examples may have both good *and* bad connotations and will depend on context. However, it is the *gendered* aspect of the latter that is important here.

Stigma too is a social phenomenon and an important concept in cancer care.[10] Stigma may be linked to gender. We have noticed the ways in which men and women are offered rehabilitation in differing ways. This is despite no obvious reason other than the fact that men are assumed to be able to take on more strenuous and perhaps more therapeutic interventions than women. The degree of stigma may also be dependent on the socio-economic position of the person and their family and just as importantly, stigma may depend on the types of rehabilitation and treatment that are available and provided within the hospital environment. All these factors may help to obliterate, cause, or perpetuate the ways in which men and women can blame themselves in terms of individual behaviour.[10] When people are faced with a lack of amenities that might help recovery, they can easily be led to believe that it is within their own remit to recover, to 'fight' to win the 'battle of cancer'.

Nowhere is the concept of 'body image' and stigma quite so researched and documented as in the area of reconstructive breast surgery. Their impact is usually assessed in terms of individual response. However this will depend on the person's social context; on the relationship she has with partners and friends and the quality of those relationships. In other words, it will depend on the *meaning* that the loss and reconstruction of her breasts will hold for her.[81] This requires the telling of a story, listening, and empathy. Meanings for women may depend on her age, her ethnicity, her social class, and/or marital status, or her 'gender'—that is, on the ways she 'lives out' her sexuality and how she perceives herself as a woman in those contexts that are most important to her.[1, 82]

> My lost breast left me bereft ... I was no longer a woman ... I know that I am old and I no longer have a sexual partner, but my body is important to me ... I still feel a sexual being.
>
> (70-year-old single woman)

While for many women, the loss of a breast is about her sexuality, it may equally be about *having cancer*, or both.

> The loss of my breast had a huge fall out ... I was concerned for my husband, my sex life and the ways that people would view my body and myself. Most of all it was about having a cancer that could kill me before my time ... that was the worst thing ... the possibility of not seeing my children grow.
>
> (35-year-old married woman)

When we speak about 'body image' we include 'body language'; bodily gestures and postures, 'symbolic boundaries'.[10] Clothing, for example is important in the signals it gives about rank and occupation. Consider the white coat of the doctor whether 'male' or 'female', and the bow tie of the surgeon professor. They do not just have practical connotations (such as cleanliness) or fashionable preferences, but they also serve a social function, indicating membership of their prestigious and powerful occupational groups. We know that when the white coat is removed, people with cancer may reveal themselves in more forthright ways.[38] This in itself does not necessarily have gender connotations. Both male and female doctors wear white coats and both men and women may feel more at ease in the presence of professionals who do not wear 'a uniform' or the opposite as the case may be. However, 'the white coat' syndrome lends itself to the 'masculine' ethos of hospital life; the ways in which there is a need to belong to a 'club'; to separate out from the 'other'[10] and to build a wall between doctor and patient that will possibly help to maintain medical autonomy and avoid emotional involvement. While we understand the need for professionals to maintain boundaries, we also know that when patients are made to feel 'the other', it can be undermining in the context of being ill and may help to establish certain (gendered) responses in people who are sick.

We, as health professionals, tend to be concerned for women with regard to side-effects of treatment such as hair loss. The distress caused by both may also apply to men.

We know that this will depend on many factors including the fashion of the day when it comes to losing hair, religion, and culture. Sikh men and women hold great store by their hair. However the meaning that hair holds for older sections of the Sikh community may not hold for younger members who have been born in the 'host' country (*see* under Ethnicity). A study carried out in the 1980s[38] revealed that white young British men who had received treatment for testicular cancer, felt that the 'skin head' look was 'normal' (*ibid*) but stressed that they could change their minds as the fashion changed or as they grew older. Indeed older men went to great lengths to cover up their baldness in the social context of work where there was a need for 'normality' and secrecy concerning their illness (*ibid*). We think that these contextual issues may apply to women too. The ways that people respond is never 'static'. 'Body image' will rely on emotional state, the kind of a disease the person has, surgery and medical treatments, and/or obesity or weight loss as a result of cancer treatment. It may also and importantly rely on other social factors such as the person's age (although not always in ways that we would expect).

Summary

- Be reflexive. The ways in which we, as health professionals, hold onto stereotypical assumptions may have an enormous impact on the ways in which 'men' and 'women', males and females respond and adjust. *Listen* to their needs.

- Take on the notion of difference *and similarity* both between and within the sexes. While each person is unique, they are living in a social context. Remember that age, social class, ethnicity to name but a few factors, may be interacting with 'gender.'

- Tailor your responses to men and women with cancer by allowing people to 'direct' their own care plans in relation to 'gender'.

Homeless people

Introduction

While homeless people and especially those who are sleeping rough may present themselves to cancer centres relatively infrequently, largely because they are likely to die of other disease-related problems such as alcohol abuse, we think this is an important group to focus on. This is because homelessness has its own unique problems. It is also an area where cancer researchers have seldom delved. For this reason we want to set the scene by briefly 'mapping' out the contexts from which they come. We will be turning to work that has been carried out in other areas of health and illness in relation to homelessness so that cancer carers and researchers have some guidance for the problems that are inherent in this group.

There will be many overlaps between the categories of 'homeless' people, 'asylum seekers and refugees'. Many of the issues raised here may, of course, apply to all people and their carers and friends who are going through a cancer experience and who are in subordinate positions in society, isolated, lonely, or unable to articulate their thoughts and needs. Likewise, the contents of the previous chapters and the underlying message that we are conveying (i.e. that 'adjustment' to cancer is a process and not a pathology and that our quest is to prevent serious distress in the context of cancer) will be of relevance to homeless people. A great deal of our background material is gathered from data that reflects the 'hard to reach' population in the United Kingdom and especially London for this is where the majority settle. We hope, nevertheless, that our observations will be relevant to other contexts in the UK and other countries, although there will be many differences too.*

Defining 'homelessness'

'Homelessness' is a broad term that relies on poor data for its definitions.[83] However in 2000 an estimated total of 172 760 households were recognized as homeless by local authorities in GB (shelter website:www.shelter.org.uk) representing roughly over 410 000 people. Of this number it is estimated that 49% of 'homeless' households were from ethnic minorities. Street homelessness, thought to be the most extreme and visible form of homelessness, is estimated at 10 000.[84]

Homelessness and health

There is a general consensus that the health of the homeless is poor in comparison with the general population[83] and people who sleep rough have worse health status than that of any other section of the population.[85] Whether homelessness provokes health problems or makes existing problems worse is not clear. It should not be forgotten, however, that the concept of homelessness varies in relation to health according to gender, ethnicity, relative and absolute poverty, personal behaviour such as smoking or not smoking, and other factors such as a person's living environment[83] and in many cases health problems may be wholly unrelated to 'homelessness'.

Pre-existing poor health status is important in the context of cancer care, since a cancer diagnosis may be but one more serious condition amongst many. Homeless people are likely to enter the hospital system with not only physical health problems but with mental health problems too.[86] 'Depression, anxiety, or nerves' have been shown to be eleven times higher than in the general population among people sleeping rough and eight times higher amongst single, homeless people in accommodation.[83, 85] Suicide rates have been found to be thirty four times more likely in people who sleep rough[83] than in the general population. Older women have higher levels of major mental health illness such as schizophrenia than men and younger women.[87] Diagnosis is difficult because behaviour that might be classified as dementia (not knowing the day or who the monarch is) may be due to homelessness itself where there may be no access to the media and there is a distinct absence of a regular routine that could underlie disorientation in anyone.

A bad diet, stress, cold, damp, inadequate or no sanitation; no place for storing food and few preparation facilities, all help to increase the risk of physical health problems.[83]

Infectious diseases such as tuberculosis, anaemia and arthritis, dermatological problems, and problems associated with alcoholism such as cirrhosis, damage to nerve muscles and brain are all more likely to be found among homeless people especially in those sleeping rough and who are single.[83] There are also concerns about HIV levels and hepatitis infection among young, single, homeless people who may use intravenous drugs or work in the sex industry.[83] It is important to remember however, that not everyone by any means falls into these categories. It would be a mistake for health professionals to assume this to be the case.

In general, men and women experience similar categories of physical illness. However, 75% of homeless American women reported gynaecological problems and 32% had arthritis compared with 26% of men. Anaemia was also more common in homeless women, occurring in 35% of the sample compared with 18% of homeless men.[88]

Homelessness and cancer

It is against this backdrop that those who have cancer and those who care for them have to grapple, with all the likely responses experienced by anyone with the disease, but with the added almost insurmountable burdens described above. Indeed it would be easy to make the assumption that those burdens might eclipse an interest in health behaviour such as screening for cancer despite the increased prevalence of most risk factors for cancer in the homeless population[89] that resemble risk figures of those in lower social class groups.[90] Contrary to expectations, however, studies have shown that homeless women are very positive about receiving cancer screening examinations and have been found to access screening at rates comparable to the general population in the USA.[91] Seventy-seven per cent homeless people within Los Angeles County have been shown to believe in the benefits of cancer screening. Seventy-nine per cent were not fatalistic about cancer, 63% believed that early detection was efficacious and 83% did not think it would be difficult to get screened.[89] However, cancer screening rates of those surveyed were lower than the rates in California for certain procedures including endoscopy, mammography, and cervical screening. This may have been a result of the unavailability of free services.[88]

Homeless people are known to present with disease that has become debilitating or painful.[83] This may be due as much to the inaccessibility of services, only exacerbated by the pressures of day to day living as to the possible health beliefs and behaviours of people in this group.[83] However it is known that head and neck cancer is prevalent in the homeless population but by no means confined to the latter. This may be a result of heavy drinking and smoking, poor oral hygiene, and other factors related to sleeping rough.[92]

General distress is reported amongst people with head and neck cancers.[92–94] Only socio-demographic variables (and not medical ones) predict quality of life after radiography in patients with the disease. This is not surprising since major surgery and/or radiation may cause grave disfigurement[92, 95] making people feel less sexual, less attractive, and may cause a general loss of identity[92, 95–98] that in itself can cause intense grief both in the private sphere of family life and in the public world of work.[92] Intensive monitoring in terms, for example, of adequate nutrition is crucial. Continual assessment is required as people learn to swallow, speak, and even kiss again.[95] Social support is of the utmost importance. This includes support from health professionals and family members whose involvement can be a determining factor in adjustment, morbidity, and even survival [92, 99].

Of course these pointers are particularly poignant in the context of the homeless for whom social support may be less accessible. 'Families' are not necessarily evident but this is not to say that this group does not access support from those who share similar circumstances. Homeless people are likely to gather a coterie of fellow homeless people around them for support *(Cook personal communication)*. It is important that people's personal strengths and social support networks are recognized in planning any services[88] and that health personnel are receptive to these networks. Like any other group, homeless people may wish to include another when seeing a doctor or when they are in hospital receiving treatment.

The possible 'gap' in access to formal support makes the task of rehabilitation and general follow-up all the more important, requiring outreach work that is not generally part of the structure of hospital life (personal communication). When people are trying to survive despite the lack of basic needs such as food, shelter, and money, they are unlikely to comply with the rigidity of hospital out-patient appointments[100] despite the fact that they may be no less interested in cancer services and cancer care than other people. This will mean that they go without 'in house' support from health professionals.

Homelessness: psychosocial factors

Health professionals may assume that the homeless are irresponsible or unconcerned regarding their health. As we have seen above however, services may either be unavailable or primary care may be a 'shifting' concept.[83] Often homeless people move from one place to another, negating any continuity of care. There are of course problems with regard to sufficient access to GP services, acute beds, mental health services, waiting times, and other services such as the ambulance service for the entire population of the UK.[83] Considering this, it is particularly important to think about the added problems experienced by homeless people in getting access to and using health services. Just as in the case of people in lower socio-economic groups, homeless people may be short of travel funds, sometimes have problems with reading and writing and often (like people in general) do not know what their rights are in terms of healthcare and other benefits.

Added to these 'obstacles', homelessness engenders feelings of repulsion and resentment in people, both lay and professional, who are known to perceive them as 'down and outs', 'bed blockers', and 'beggars' who undeservedly take services away from 'stalwart' members of our society[101] (personal communication with Jane Cook). Indeed homeless people are known to experience 'downright hostility' from GPs and their receptionists or even refusal to NHS services[83] sometimes because many are dependent on drugs or alcohol. Apart from the ways this must undermine already vulnerable people, the danger of stigmatizing homeless people for certain 'unhealthy' behaviours (such as smoking, drinking, and taking drugs) even implicitly, may only help to turn people away from medical advice, exacerbating a situation in which people are unlikely to feel engaged with and familiar in hospital systems.[83] It is worth remembering that homeless people may lack the so-called social skills, and find it difficult to cope with authority.[83] They may be unable to express themselves in the ways that are understood by health professionals. There is evidence that illiteracy makes it difficult for homeless people to deal with bureaucracy and this may preclude a chance to complain about the ways in which they are treated.[83]

Although progress has been made in identifying and addressing the needs of people with cancer who belong to ethnic minority groups (who are often classified as 'homeless'), progress has been slow in the homeless population. It is practically non-existent in relation to people who have attained or are seeking asylum. Homeless people with cancer form a relatively small population and this argument is made in defence of giving it top priority in terms of interest and investigation and the 'special' services that homeless people may need. There is a tendency to think that we not only may offend certain groups by highlighting their needs, but that we must respond to the 'whole population' and not to special plead on behalf of minority groups. (This and other 'barriers' are arguments that are also voiced in the context of ethnicity in relation to health).[31] We are not suggesting that resources are taken away from other populations; rather that this group is recognized in terms of cancer care and subsidized as necessary. As for offending people, offence might be taken in the ways that they and other groups such as asylum seekers, refugees, and ethnic groups are sidelined.

Homelessness and support

The caring of this particular group calls for innovative strategies and a multidisciplinary approach. We would suggest that an outreach team is established especially in those areas where this population is most likely to be found, for example inner city areas such as central London, UK. This of course, will require extra resources and will mean training health personnel to venture out to homeless cancer patients in an effort to support them.

It is important to remember that homeless persons may have their own 'key' worker; one that they will know. It is essential that key workers are kept involved from the start to the finish of treatment and during follow-up, both for the patient's sake and also for the backup it will provide for hospital personnel dealing with members of this group. The 'key worker' will act as advocate and help in areas such as when the person wishes to make a complaint. Key workers are in a position to help to clarify the existing local services for homeless people and their opening hours. There are various agencies that might enable joint assessments. For example, there may be mental health services in the vicinity of the patient's current residence. Clarification of who is ultimately responsible for final decisions is essential[100] and it helps to have a policy for adequate discharge planning from hospital (or prison). It is essential however, that one key person takes overall responsibility for the person with cancer and that this is established at the outset.

If the caveats described above are carefully taken into consideration and acted upon, we believe that a cancer experience will be eased. However, we also believe that homeless people (like many others) will not necessarily behave in a conventional way in relation to medicine. As with all people, it is important to approach a problem in a way that is led by the person in question. Offering routine types of counselling to this group may not be useful. However, this does not preclude an effort to 'contain' the person's dilemma.

We believe that the reticence shown on behalf of the 'hard to reach' may rest on 'ignorance' on the part of health professionals including funders of research monies as to where to start in the process of discovery. Unknown areas of experience are as frightening for us as health providers as they are for people who are entering the health system sometimes for the first time. All too often we concentrate on 'safe' populations in an effort to collect data that we can disseminate, not always in the name of patients, but for our own self-aggrandizement.

Summary

- Be aware of the assumptions you may be making regarding this population.
- Take into account that this population is likely to come to a cancer hospital with other physical and mental health problems.
- Be prepared for verbal abuse and an unorthodox approach towards institutions and bureaucracy in general. Try not to take responses personally but be aware of your boundaries and be aware that you as health professional are entitled to protection at all times.
- Do not expect this population to comply with conventional 'rules' in relation to their care.
- A lot of homeless people cannot read or write and may be inarticulate when it comes to talking about disease and illness in the context of cancer. Many will need help with complaints they may wish to make.

While people in prison are, for all intents and purposes, 'homeless' they will usually have their own medical structures although tertiary care is often sought. We want to bear in mind that prisoners are often sidelined in research and there is a paucity of material that would throw light on how they experience cancer. Our clinical work suggests that they feel isolated and stigmatized and their distress is as important as anyone else's in this particular context. We hope that the caveats that we present here may help health professionals to apply them to prisoners (and other 'invisible' groups).

- Many homeless people are not aware of their rights.
- A key worker is usually available and should be contacted and liased with throughout the person's cancer experience. They will know of the services at hand that cater specifically for this group of patient.
- Make sure that everyone knows who is ultimately responsible for a homeless cancer patient.
- Be innovative! Form an outreach team if necessary.

Ethnicity
Introduction

'Ethnicity' is a concept that is rarely given credence in cancer care and research,[102] although this is changing.[103] Few studies indicate the importance of addressing the difficulty of defining 'cultural differences' or 'ethnicity' nor the importance of variables such as gender, class, and health policies and how they may be impacting on responses. One of the reasons for this paucity may be that the incidence of cancers which predominate in the white ethnic majority is lower in minority ethnic groups.[104] However, this belief is based on the mortality data and not on the numbers of people living with the disease.[102] Furthermore the rate of cancer is expected to increase as a result of demographic changes such as ageing and increasing exposure to environmental risk factors in the West.[104] While the white, literate majority make up figures in this context, the beliefs and needs of minority groups are more often than not, negated. It is conceivable that 'ethnicity' has been sidelined because it has been difficult to make sense of given its complexities. 'Race', 'ethnicity', and 'culture' have often been used interchangeably and in ways that confuse meaning.

Defining 'race', 'culture', and 'ethnicity'
Race

The bioscientific concept of 'race' rests on an expectation of biological difference between human populations.[105] For example, skin colour is used in systems of classification based partially on phenotype assuming that people can be allocated to racial groups on the basis of a shared biology. This essentialism leads to 'medical racism'.[106] In the way that essentialism focuses on 'the person' and deflects us away from social structural issues such as the socio-economic climate of a society, so too does the assumption that a shared biology underpins existence while racial groups are categorized as 'superior' or 'inferior'.[106] This approach has been discredited by genetic research. All humans belong to the same species and genetic intra-racial variation is actually much greater than genetic inter-racial variation.[105] There remains a tendency, however, to believe that minority 'racial' groups are carriers of problematic cultures and 'exotic' illnesses, and dangerous to their own health.[107]

Culture

'Culture' refers to the ways of life of the members of a society or groups within a society.[108] 'Ethnicity' and 'culture' appear to be interchangeable and both are difficult concepts to define. However, while 'culture' is often spoken about in terms of 'higher things' such as art, literature, music, and painting,[106] the elements considered to be about 'ethnicity' are, for example language, religion, work, diet, or family patterns.[109] People who belong to an ethnic group can and do adopt aspects of other cultures, the latter being a constantly changing phenomenon.[105]

Ethnicity

The concept of 'ethnicity' holds within it the ways that people identify themselves as belonging to a social grouping because they differ culturally in fundamental ways.[105, 108] What holds people together or creates internal divisions within the concept of 'ethnicity' are real or probable or in some cases mythical, common origins, values, and conventions.[106] Moreover, 'ethnicity' when understood as a sense of belonging to a real or imagined community, applies as much to white as black or 'Asian' people. This is important as 'ethnic' is usually symbolic of minority groups from 'other' countries and almost never of the 'white' majority.[102]

Ethnic categories such as 'black' or 'white' can often be meaningless[102] and it would be a mistake to think that we can categorize people just because they have their origins in 'other' parts of the world. (For example, 'black' or 'Asian' people are thought to have a keen sense of family; the latter providing care when people are sick. 'White' people are depicted as living in nuclear families without a wider social network the assumption being that they are in need of support when they are ill. Inequalities of care will ensue if we do not attend to the words that we use and the assumptions that underlie them.) When we use the term 'Asian' we in Britain refer to people who have origins in Pakistan, Bangladesh, India, Sri Lanka, and East Africa. However, the US defines 'Asian' people as coming from China, Japan, and Korea.[110] In the UK, the term 'Asian' also assumes ethnic homogeneity to people who have little in common but that they are from the Indian sub-continent. Many northern Indians however, have different customs from their southern counterparts. Muslims and Hindus view the world through their religion in quite different ways while living together and 'white' people can include, Irish, Scottish, and Welsh people who live in different contexts, with differing customs, beliefs, and needs.

Ethnicity and essentialism

Essentialism is a way of conceptualizing 'ethnicity' as an innate and unchanging 'truth'. It is as if, for example, the Irish have an innate capacity to drink and talk. Ethnicity must however, acknowledge the fluid nature of contemporary ethnic identities. We may think of ourselves as belonging to an ethnic group yet our 'ethnicity' may be common to different groups and indeed we may perceive ourselves as having multiple ethnicities. Many Irish people, for example, do not drink and enjoy eating bagels that are the staple diet of the Jewish Community.[106] Categorizing people can therefore inadvertently lead to wrongful decisions regarding both treatment and discharge and may lead to all kinds of assumptions being made that prove to be without foundation. For all these reasons, danger lies in essentialism and stereotyping. This is especially the case when we consider how health workers who have been sensitized to the concepts of 'culture', may inadvertently be encouraging stereotyping with expectations to conform to certain ways of behaviour but without the patients' agreement.[111]

Ethnicity and social class

Essentialism does not take into account the importance of the dynamic and shifting nature of people's identities that may interact between class, ethnicity, gender, and religion. Even these interactions can be more complicated than they seem.[102] For example, a relationship between social class and health beliefs has been established in the white majority ethnic group (*see* under Social Class, pages 152-7). However social class classifications can be misleading with respect to ethnic minorities (as indeed they can in the 'white' majority) and are known to be insensitive to the social and material circumstances of people from minority ethnic groups.[106] People from 'Asian' communities who work in small businesses are automatically placed in social class two. However minority ethnic businesses are very often marginal and owned by people who are relatively poor. Migration can dramatically change a person's economic circumstances. A person who was once well off in his own country, may be poor as he struggles to establish himself in his host one. Unemployment is known to be higher amongst certain minority groups[112] and there is a difficulty in quantifying numbers of people who declare unemployment, but who may be working. The latter may be especially distressed at times of illness, especially if they are responsible for subsidizing family life but are unable to declare this.

Ethnicity: West versus East

Bearing these caveats in mind, work on ethnicity and culture[103] has revealed the many ways in which people's perceptions differ in terms of symptoms, including pain,[113] what constitutes 'normal' and 'healthy',[114] and the ways in which the symbolic meaning of cancer differs between oriental and Western cultures.[115]

'Oriental' perceptions regarding causation rests on weakness, genetic predisposition, and lifestyle choices of individuals.[115] 'Indians' consider cancer to be a result of past sins or 'karma'.[116] Differences lie in the ways that people of differing cultures, self-disclose and feel uncomfortable regarding answering questions about sex and 'subjective experiences' regarding cancer.[117] While these kinds of responses are attributed to people in minority ethnic groups they may also apply to the white majority. Coping mechanisms have been shown to differ between, for example 'African-American', 'Latinos', and 'Japanese Americans'. The former are shown to be fatalistic about cancer while the latter are likely to endure it stoically and avoid overt acceptance of the condition. 'Anglo-Americans' apparently use more active coping strategies such as being positive.[118] This may be due however, to the ways that people respond to certain well worn 'discourses'; what people say they do is not always borne out in reality.[119]

'Hope' is a concept that is held to have great significance in a Western cancer context, but is shown to have quite different meanings in some Asian groups. 'Punjabis in the UK' found questions in a well-known quality of life questionnaire regarding 'hope' as derisory. It was often met with 'defensive laughter about the stupidity of the concept because it was 'not for them to hope'.[120] It is not clear as to whether this is a result of their position in the West or whether it is part of their overall world view, nor is it clear that some Western people might also find the concept of 'hope' as useless in the context of a life-threatening disease. In India health professionals are regarded with trust, allowing people to relinquish personal control.[121] There, the family is shown to play a significant role in each stage of diagnosis and management while they support their sick relative.[116] This may be the case in some 'Indian' *and* 'white British' families in the Western countries, but may also be an example of how the ways in which the structure of healthcare lends itself to the ways in which people behave in the context of illness. In the USA, where healthcare is privatized and expensive, resident 'African-American', 'Asian', and 'Latino' groups, place a higher value on interdependence and strong family ties than middle class non-Hispanic whites.[118]

Awareness regarding diagnosis also varies cross culturally as do 'response styles'. In India, cancer patients are unaware of their diagnosis while doctors and family collude in secret keeping.[121] 'Indians' often respond with what they think they ought to be feeling rather than how they may actually be feeling[121] and 'Asians' may prefer an emphasis on sincerity or modesty.[113]

There are cultural differences in manifesting and expressing depression including somatization, guilt feelings, and suicidal ideation. For example, somatization or ways in which depression is expressed, differ between 'non-European' and 'European' cultures.[122] Muslims have difficulty with the concept of depression: feeling depressed shows a lack of respect to Allah.[123] Despite this some Muslims may feel in need of support when facing a life-threatening disease. Fatalism, a coping mechanism that is associated with dependency and hopelessness in the West, is a concept used by Muslims as part of the underpinning of their faith. Their 'fatalism' however, may lead health workers in the West to think that the patient is turning his head to the wall 'without the will to live'. However, it would be a mistake to equate 'fatalism' with despondence amongst 'Asian' groups. Atkin *et al.* (1998)[124] have shown that parents with children with an inherited disease couple notions of 'Allah's will' with a duty to struggle and the belief that Allah grants strength to cope at times of adversity.

Being a person with cancer is a complicated state of being. Our fragmented worlds cannot indicate certain truths anymore than we can begin to think that responses are 'fixed' or that they mean the same thing in every situation and amongst each ethnic group.

Ethnicity, religion, and death

Western systems have medicalized death; it has become an unnatural event[125]; quantity of life expectancy takes precedence over quality especially where resuscitation involves heroic, aggressive, uncomfortable, and painful forms of treatment. This factor affects everybody and in many cases there is no doubt that medicine has a great deal to answer for in terms of people's distress in the last days of life. This is notwithstanding the hospice movement that is underpinned by a seemingly egalitarian ethos where people make choices and die in peace and relative comfort. A 'haven' of peace and comfort does not always stand up however. Personal experience led some people across ethnic groups to say that they found the atmosphere of hospices 'depressing and grey due to the constant presence and reminder of death'. As far as hospice day centres were concerned, South Asians found that they had little to offer them especially those who did not speak English. Interestingly however, a few Asian women found that the social anonymity of the centres were preferable to an Asian support group where they had to think about their 'spoiled identity' as part of the community, reproduced within the group. Hospices did however, also stand out as examples of good practice due to their 'hospitality of care, one to one medical and nursing care, a homely and family friendly atmosphere where children were welcome and family had easy access to the patient on the telephone, a regard for individual religious preferences and a 'space' to pray regardless of religious denomination.[66] We wonder why these examples cannot be transported to mainstream care. If we know that they 'work' in one context, why are they held back in another? The cancer plan of 2000 recognized 'the willingness to listen and explain' as an important feature in 'allowing' patients to make decisions and participate in their own treatment plans. Plainly this is not always the case despite time passing and despite the good intentions of cancer plans made by policy makers.

Alarmingly, studies that have investigated ethnicity in the context of advanced cancer have found that very few ethnic minority groups know about the hospice movement as a place where people went to die[7, 126] compared to their 'white British' counterparts. Despite a general sense of foreboding regarding the Macmillan nurse who symbolized death to white study participants, South Asians in the study knew little about them either. Their lack of awareness was attributed to stereotypes such as 'fatalism' and 'closed awareness' as well as paternalistic attitudes and a lack of experience of these services.[7]

When asked, South Asians found the notion of going to the hospice for respite or terminal care as counter to their ideals of family obligations and caring across internal differences of religion, language, and culture. However, the distinction between hospice admission for symptoms and pain control as opposed to terminal care was seen to be acceptable and non-threatening in both minority ethnic and white families. Despite reservations, the study investigators found no instances of a South Asian patient refusing admission to a hospice for symptom control and/or pain relief and even used hospice care at the end of life when it was offered.[7]

Investigators have pointed out that 'the sparse literature on palliative care in relation to ethnic minority communities, constructs these communities in terms of a reductionist notion of "culture" as fixed and an innate attribute to the exclusion of agency and choice'.[7] In contrast they report that the white majority community is perceived in terms of individuality, autonomy, and choice; culture is not discussed. All these factors are important and we in the West may do well to take heed of the variations in people's beliefs and needs, including our own. These do not just apply to 'other people' but also to the ways that practices surrounding illness, death, and dying may differ between and within the social classes and of course, may be influenced by other variables such as gender and age.

To an extent all death and funerary practices are influenced by the cultural belief in an afterlife. Cultures that believe in reincarnation are likely to have very different attitudes to mourning to those without this belief, who see death as a final event rather than as part of a more cyclic process.[10] In any case there are many ways of caring for the dying and of grieving. People's beliefs will differ but it seems to be the case that dying is a 'social' act as well as a biological one.

We tend to carry out the work of death and dying in ways that relate to white British people in a context of 'a' Christian religion. It is important to remember, however that there is no such thing as a single 'Hindu', 'Muslim', 'African Caribbean', or 'Christian community' of people thinking similar thoughts and behaving in similar ways, all or even some of the time. There may be wide differences in traditions and ritual practices relating to illness, death, dying, and bereavement *within* a religious faith. To understand the nuances that abound in religious beliefs, requires sensitive questioning and an engagement with the concept of *diversity* within the groups as well as between them.[127]

For example, African Caribbeans are members of the Anglican, Methodist, or Pentecostal churches but in recent years a minority of the African Caribbean community have moved away from conventional religion and are now members of the distinct movement of Rastafarianism.[128] Within many African Caribbean communities, family members, friends, and community leaders are an important component of caring for the sick and dying.[129] In these cases, accommodation for large numbers of people is required. On the other hand, some families may prefer to restrict carers depending on their experience in the context of cancer. Prayer is important at this time, sacrament less so. Rastafarians may also wish to pray by the bedside, but last rites do not exist. Both African Caribbeans and Rastafarians offer last offices, and while there is no strong religious reason why others may not handle the deceased, respect and sensitivity by healthcare professionals are appreciated.[128] If death occurs at home, the laying out of the dead relative is performed by family and friends.[129] Many older African Caribbeans have strong beliefs that a body should remain intact after death and should not be disfigured in any way. Post-mortems are usually permitted by family members, but only at the request of a coroner.[129] Rastafarians view post-mortems and organ donation as distasteful.[128]

Among Orthodox Jews the '*chevra kadisha*' or Burial Society of each community made up of volunteers, carries out the ritual of caring for the dead person and preparing it for burial. When people have immigrated from societies where either the family or traditional death attendants usually take care of the dead are absent, people may find the impersonal approach of undertakers difficult to accept, especially when they do not understand the cultural background of the family who is grieving. Death rituals also differ in terms of the funeral and in the ways people mourn generally. The Irish 'wake' involves watching the corpse by relatives for several days and nights and sometimes involves a 'party' of feasting and drinking. Greek Cypriots weep and wail and mourn for a defined period while wearing black. Orthodox Jews in Britain and elsewhere hold a shib'ah that is a precise structure of mourning lasting seven days after the funeral which is held almost immediately following death. For the Jewish people as for others 'social death' takes place slowly, the whole process lasting for one year until finally the tombstone is laid. For Jewish people who have immigrated, and no longer have family around them, the impersonal undertaker might be difficult to understand and accept, especially when the latter are unfamiliar with the cultural background of the grieving family. Bereavement practices of Hindu immigrants to the UK have changed over the years compared to those practised in India. The open display of the dead, cremations, and the subsequent scattering of the ashes in a holy river are no longer possible.[10] However, compared to Christian burials in England, there is a communal approach and emotions are more volatile.

There are other requirements that apply to other religious groups and we suggest that these are taken seriously bearing in mind that it is a mistake to assume that beliefs hold steadfast. Even the strongest faith is contingent on many factors and often negotiated.[111] Pheffer[82] suggests that we refrain from using 'faith' or religion as an independent variable (as is often the case in research) but rather, a dependent one that is but one of the many factors when men or women negotiate an 'event' such as a medical examination. A strictly orthodox Jew for example, may refuse to shake hands with a male doctor because faith dictates that she should not but she will take her clothes off in order to undergo an intimate examination.[82]

Ethnicity and diet

Just as there are religious duties that apply themselves to illness, death, and dying, so too are there dietary requirements for people of certain religious affiliation.[130] Hospitals are likely to take into account that people of white ethnicity may be vegetarians and they are likely to accommodate their requirements regardless of religion. Dietary requirements of people of ethnic minority groups are not given as much attention in the context of hospital life. Of course, people who are ill do not necessarily want to eat.[7] However, some ethnic minority families may feel obliged to bring in cooked meals from home when food in hospital is inappropriate because certain needs have not been attended to. On the other hand, some people prefer to provide for their sick relative and bringing in cooked meals from home can, in itself, be a sign of fulfilling obligations of caring and affection.[7] This may be the case for people of all ethnicities but we think it is a good practice to take into consideration the many diverse ways in which people eat; food (as opposed to diet) having great symbolic value.[7]

Rastafarians, Muslims, and Orthodox Jews are forbidden to eat pork. In the Islam religion, the only meat permitted is from cloven-hoofed animals that chew the cud, and it must be *halal*—or ritually slaughtered. While we do not underestimate the ways in which hospital chefs rarely serve exotic dishes it is worth remembering that Muslims may eat only fish that have fins and scales; shellfish, shark, and eels are therefore forbidden. Orthodox Jews do not eat fish with fins and scales, birds of prey, and carrion. Only animals that chew the cud, have cloven hooves, are ritually slaughtered, and are *kosher*, may be eaten. Meat and milk dishes are never mixed within the same meal. Sikhs are not allowed to eat beef, but pork is allowed though rarely eaten. Meat must also be slaughtered in a special ritual way known as *jhatka*. Hindus are forbidden to eat beef. Milk and its products may be eaten, since they do not involve taking the animal's life. Fish and eggs are infrequently eaten. Many Rastafarians follow strict vegetarian diets[131] and their dietary restrictions are similar to Judaism.[130] As with many other religious groups, alcohol is strictly prohibited.

Racism and ethnicity

One of the most disturbing findings that has come out of empirical work regarding ethnicity and cancer is the concept of institutionalized *racism*[7, 126] that is often extremely subtle. It is important to remember that 'racism' is not just evident in situations involving black and ethnic minority groups with Asian origins. It may cut across to asylum seeking and refugee communities from countries such as Bosnia. Indeed a lack of awareness and understanding by health professionals about the cultural background of some refugee groups who have origins that are not black or Asian, has been found.[132]

When we stereotype people and assume that they behave in certain ways because of an association with their country of origin, we are guilty of 'racism'[111] and this inevitably will lead to inequality of care. There is a widespread assumption that cancer services are underutilized by ethnic minority patients because of 'cultural barriers',[133, 134] although there is little evidence to substantiate these claims. These barriers include a belief that women, for example are unable to understand an invitation to screening (written in English) (HEA 1994), a belief that they do not understand risk because incidence of and mortality from breast cancer is lower in their country of birth than in the UK (House of Commons Health Committee 1995:33) and a belief that ethnic minority groups practice 'closed awareness'—a means of turning away from difficult information. GPs and consultants are known to cite 'communication problems' as reasons for patient's seeming 'ignorance' concerning their disease and an unwillingness to discuss the illness and prognosis openly as one of the reasons for not referring South Asian patients to specialist palliative care services [7, 126, 133].

There is nothing to suggest however that South Asian patients might not report or postpone reporting symptoms due to cultural reasons or taboos related to the disease.[7] Delay is likely to be associated with discrepancies in the services provided. When a white population was compared with South Asians, it was found that the majority faced significant problems during the initial phases of diagnosis and treatment, compared to the 'terminal phase' although very few South Asians were aware of hospice services. This lack of awareness was related to the exclusion of South Asian communities on the basis of 'culturalist' assumptions and stereotypes about 'fatalism' and 'closed awareness' as well as paternalistic attitudes. Both groups identified problems that related to significant delays in diagnosis after reporting symptoms to a GP [7, 135] and people of all ethnic groups often faced anxious prolonged waiting times related to specialist appointments, various investigations, and crucial test results with little professional support. Often people of all ethnicities find it difficult to define whether they are simply not being 'cured', or well enough to work, and not yet defined as 'terminal'. Quick assessments of people's needs are often difficult to come by. This can lead to conflict between users and social services, often resulting in the use of precious savings in order to adapt homes and elicit home help.[7]

This way of delivering health services is exacerbated by the fragmented nature of all services and the variable quality of assessments. Chronic health problems may then be defined in ways that result in definitions that will curtail any extra benefits such as the Disability Living Allowance and the Attendance Allowance that a person may have had. These mishaps may be possible outcomes for *all* people with cancer and do not apply only to ethnic minority groups. Generally it has been found that people who are working class or lower middle class patients and carers feel less able to proactively engage with services. This is not to say that they are 'hopeless and helpless' however. While they may feel undermined, some people employ strategies to engage with their illness and treatment and ways that enable them to be taken seriously.[7] Other patients are known to give support, pass on 'tips' concerning treatment, and often they simply persevere through sheer 'bloody mindedness' in a struggle to survive [7, 25].

Structural factors can, then, cut across ethnicity and social class. Not withstanding this, the ways in which people are cared for by hospital staff has been shown to differ according to ethnic groups. This is disturbing and not only leads to inequality of care but a pervasive form of racism that may be invisible or unspoken. When white patients and their carers,[7] families, and friends, were compared to South Asians[7] or African Caribbeans[126] going through a terminal cancer experience, or who had died,[126] few differences were found in their responses and many reported examples of excellent care. However, the South Asians[7] and African Caribbeans were more critical of what they defined as discrimination against 'terminally ill' people by the NHS[7, 126]. While district nurses were found to care for white, African Caribbean, and South Asian patients in the final year of life, those with white ethnicity fared better, receiving more reassurance and support compared to the other ethnic groups.[126]

... another white nurse came to give me an injection. I said feebly, 'please give the commode, I can't control'. She paid no attention and moved on. Another one came and ... I said, 'please give me the commode'. She also paid no attention and moved on. Then the third one came, different one not the same and even she did not pay any attention. That night ... after all I am a human being and I felt that they were insulting me ...

(Elderly Indian woman[7])

I pleaded with our GP to come. He wouldn't come. He said my father was an old man so there was no point. I told him he was un-caring. He wouldn't speak to me or my stepmother. He sent the district nurse instead. I wrote a letter to the FHSA but I haven't heard yet.

(Carer of African Caribbean patient with cancer[126])

All people who are caring for cancer patients need to be mindful of the ways that 'racism' does not just depend on the quality of care given according to the origin of the patient but may also be present regardless of the origin of *the carer*.[7, 126] For example, carers of patients of the same ethnic background may not be anymore sympathetic or engaged with their patients.[7] Interestingly, nursing staff are known to experience a conflict in their professional roles and identities when patients with the same language make undue demands on their time and skills.[7] The usefulness of promoting staff awareness and support regularly to all who come into contact with patients and their families, may provide untold dividends. Not only is it likely to support hospital staff, but patients too will feel that their concerns are addressed.

Racist attitudes can extend themselves to the ways in which we sometimes assume that certain ethnicities are associated with particular diseases. This may lead to misreadings of symptoms. In a study of Asians and white people, four out of the thirty-seven South Asian cases and none of the white patients had symptoms that were perceived to indicate tuberculosis, causing distress and delay in cancer treatment.[7] Sometimes South Asians including those who are well educated, articulate, and speak good English, are told less about their medical condition and cancer treatment,[7] causing anxiety, confusion, and distress for patients and their families and carers. As mentioned above, explanations for this include professional stereotypes about 'Asian culture' and an assumption that 'Asian' patients are reluctant to know details about their illness and treatment when in reality their needs are likely to be the same as others[7]; a greater deference towards medical specialists and thus a reluctance to question them, and feelings of 'partial citizenship'.[7] Partial citizenship can have undermining consequences when people believe that they are asking and being given favours by people in their 'host' country rather than 'owning' rights.

They are doing their best (the palliative care team) ... we are very grateful to them. We must take from the system only what we need. After all, we are living in their country ...

(Asian daughter, carer to her 81-year-old mother[7])

These structural factors can be held responsible for the so-called 'delay' in many cases. However, 'delay' may result from people's biographical stories and have nothing to do with ethnicity or culture or the structure of healthcare. When a Muslim woman from Pakistan, who had recently arrived in the UK, failed to go to the doctor with symptoms, this had nothing to do with her 'ethnic' origins, but result from longstanding difficulties within the family and a reluctance to exacerbate problems.[7] When Peter, a 45-year-old self-employed white British builder confessed 'ignorance' concerning his family history of cancer and had delayed in presenting symptoms, it transpired that he had had a heart problem and the family had been at pains to protect him from what they thought was news that would affect him and cause further problems.[35] Delay may also rest on people's health beliefs and needs. These have seldom been given high priority in cancer research and care. It seems incomprehensible to us that this important area should have been sidelined, for without in-depth knowledge of how people perceive the disease, it is difficult to know how to service people's needs and to give information that is relevant. However, a few studies have looked at this important subject and especially in the context of ethnicity.

One study asked women from nine ethnic groups including white women how they experienced healthcare, what they thought about health promotion, what they knew about breast cancer, and various approaches to encouraging early presentation.[82] They were asked about the causes, signs and symptoms, diagnosis, and treatment of the disease.[82, 136] Many women found it difficult to accept that breast cancer can be painless,[136] and found it difficult to imagine that it was generally, a disease of older age groups. Some claimed that even young babies have 'lumps' and that it is 'God's will.' Causality was sometimes linked to marriages between close relatives.[82] Non-medical reasons are often given for compliance to screening regardless of ethnicity. A Sylheti speaking woman had been screened because her letter, emblazoned with official logos, represented a command and not an invitation. Others regarded the difficulties of transport and a fear of looking foolish in new and unfamiliar situations. Others had a preference for a female doctor and did not want to risk embarrassment.[82]

We tend to think that 'Asians' have wide networks of family and friends who 'take care of their own'.[7] This dangerous myth glosses over variations in family forms as well as the ways that social change has effected ethnic minority patients and their carers.[137] Old family care patterns had become established for reasons that include a required need to show solidarity and support, both emotional and financial, especially where there is no welfare state. These forms of support may become much weaker or disintegrate altogether in the British context.[138] Many Asians for example, live alone or in small family groups in their 'host' country, but like their white counterparts, may have many people paying hospital visits from the community. When large numbers of visitors appear to indicate strong support systems but in reality they do not, a patient's needs become invisible and this often negates the burden of care that may rest on one or two key individuals.[7] It may also lead to early and inappropriate discharge.[7]

While we are indicating a need that may be overlooked, namely a need for care that can easily go unheeded, it is worth remembering that often people in Asian communities perceive the notion of 'receiving help' as a charitable act putting them into a lower caste/class status within the community. This might be seen by both the patient and their family and the community at large as a moral failure, the latter perceiving it as a means of profiting through adversity.[139] This 'shame' may also be experienced by people in lower socio-economic groups and is an example not only of how sensitivity is called for at all times but of how all 'social' and personal factors including gender and age influence the needs for and access to services that may be more important than ethnicity *per se.*

While we have focused on racism in the context of ethnicity, people from lower social classes and who are 'white' may be receiving treatment that is below standard simply because of their socio-economic status. All these factors are reminders of how health personnel need to be mindful of the social aspects of a cancer experience and not least of the ways in which our own assumptions and behaviour can impinge on the ways someone might adjust.

Ethnicity and giving support: communication, advocacy, and interpreters

The impact of inadequate communication cannot be underestimated in all situations and for all categories of people, notwithstanding the inherent power structures that operate between doctors and their patients (see page 150). 'Effective' communication improves health outcomes[140] and it has been argued that doctors have responsibilities to their patients that can be fully met only by effective communication.[141] Needless to say, people from ethnic minority groups may speak English, but many do not, even when they have lived in the 'host' country for many years. This barrier is borne out in the ways that non-English speaking people, especially elderly patients are found to be particularly disadvantaged in access to services. We have already seen how information regarding hospice care and optimal primary care is withheld. This extends itself to information leaflets. Even when they are translated, they are not always in the language in which the patient is literate.[7] Many people with minority ethnic status have to rely on family members to translate information. Sometimes it is the patients themselves who have to pass on difficult information to their families, and this does not preclude very young people.[7] Not only is this unethical, but it may also be dangerous. Those close to the sick person may want to hide or to distort painful information, and they may not have a full understanding of what the doctor is telling them. When asked to do this, people take time off from jobs, from studies, or other commitments to do the job of translating.[7] This then results in inconvenience and even financial hardship. Sometimes it is the resident 'Indian' or 'Greek' nurse for example, or even those who are doing domestic jobs in hospitals, who are called to translate important information. This too is dangerous, since an 'Indian' nurse may not speak the required 'Indian' language and even when she does, the tricky nuances of medical advice may be missed, edited, or consciously obliterated.

Added to this, professionals and/or domestic staff who are called in to do this kind of 'extra' work are often resentful of the demands made on their time and skills.[7] This will transmit itself to the sick person and carers and cause further distress. Importantly, this kind of work or emotional labour may also be putting an enormous burden on people whose remit does not include this important aspect of care.

Appropriate and specialized *interpreters* (rather than generic training for interpreters in the field) and *advocates* are of paramount importance in this context, but it is important to distinguish between their roles. It is often assumed that language provision is all that is required to make services to non-English speaking people understandable. Likewise many interpreters have found that instead of merely addressing communication difficulties, they have had to extend their remit to include 'advocacy' roles of promoting better health and making healthcare systems more accessible.[31] Added to this is the notion that nurses themselves are advocates of the patient. Be that as it may, nurses are not always in a position to understand their needs and the needs of the family.

By 'interpreter' we are alluding to someone who finds out from the patient the answers to the staff's questions and relays to the patient the staff's wishes or directives.

An interpreter

- He/she is impartial in any communication or negotiation.
- He/she does not represent the interests of either party in the communication as his/her role is to 'encode' messages and information from the service provider (all health personnel including doctors and nurses) to the service user(patients, relatives, and friends) and vice versa.
- He/she often provides a specific service that is confined to communicating with a service provider and user at a specific point in time.

(taken from[105])

It may be useful to explore the possibility of collaboration between medical institutions and the relevant voluntary sector.[7] Interpreters ought to be involved from the early stages of diagnosis so that a sense of continuity and trust is established. We would advocate that as well as having specialized training, an interpreter has a continued rather than a piece meal relationship with the patient and one who appreciates the complexities of medical information. It is important that both interpreters and advocates have social skills and emotional awareness. They are every bit as important as technical linguistic skills. Empathy is always required and an ability to cope with emotional demands is essential.[7] This means setting boundaries early on in the encounter.

An advocate's role is the opposite from that of the interpreter's although many of the caveats given above are relevant. Advocates find out from the staff, answers to the patient's questions and communicate their wishes.[31] By advocacy we mean a way of 'helping people say what they want, obtain their rights, represent their interests, and gain the services they need'.[31] The fundamental emphasis of advocacy is that it sees things from the users perspective and recognizes the unequal power relationship between users of health services and service providers including doctors *(ibid)*. Advocates working for minority ethnic people relay cultural, religious, social, and linguistic messages about people to professionals and where necessary, may challenge discrimination and racism *(ibid)*. Both users and providers may find it difficult to express their views and be understood, not to mention the structural barriers that are placed in front of ethnic minority people in terms of healthcare. This is true of all people who are ill and come from differing social class backgrounds (see page 153), gender orientations (see page 158), and differing religious groups. The difference here is one of ethnicity and all its inherent 'problems'.

An advocate

- puts the needs and interests of the service user first;
- works to clearer and more defined outcomes, with the aim of helping the patient and/or carer to achieve their rights and obtain the very best from services;
- is proactive in meeting the needs of the patient and/or carer;
- often provides services across boundaries and may not be confined to one interaction with a specific service provider.

(taken from[105])

Often advocates run the risk of being used by both the patient, carers, *and* the medical profession. There may be a conflict of loyalties and demands. Well-defined roles within the context of cancer care, will help to solve this conflict.[7] If skilled interpreters and advocates are made available routinely, the cancer experience of the non-English speaking population will at least, in part, be eased. However there are other considerations to take into account.

While 'counselling' is a Western concept, and its usefulness depends on an individual's socio-economic background and cultural orientation,[142] gender, and age, non-English speaking patients and carers have very limited access to a counsellor or a clinical psychologist. Bilingual professionals within the field are rare.[7] One study found that both white and South Asians had found it useful when it was offered.[7] Interestingly, counselling has featured as one of the least favoured services by the white ethnic majority, especially when people were elderly.[7]

'We don't need counselling, we went through a World War. I think counselling is rubbish ... overrated industry to keep people employed ... counselling is a waste of time ...'

White carer of husband with cancer[7]

This quote might alert us to the ways that people's needs and our ways of offering help, do not necessarily 'follow' what we in cancer care may perceive as 'good' practice.

We agree with Jafar Kareem[143] when he suggests that the cause of an individual's distress is very difficult to define. It is not always the case that it is part of the patient's inner psychic reality or 'pathology'. In the same ways in which we have attempted to emphasize the social context of the person and not the 'pathology within', he suggests that socio-political and economic factors over which the individual may have little or no control, affect our inner worlds whatever our ethnicity.

It is also well to remember that certain cultural constraints may be at play when people are distressed. These constraints are *not innate* but part of the ways that we are expected to be and act. For example, the British appear to be guided by control, suggesting that crying in public is unacceptable, that stoicism and a brave face must be presented at all times.[144] We know that this is not true in all cases. We have already spoken of the ways in which women are *expected* to express emotion when they are ill and men are applauded for their stoicism in the face of disease. We also know that each does not necessarily live strictly to those ideals, especially when they are engaged in relations that allow or restrain certain responses.

For example, Hindu Indians come from a culture in which time is circular; expression is never frowned upon. Crying, dependence on others, excessive emotionality, volatility, and verbal hostility both in males and in females are not in any way considered as signs of weakness.[144] Since feelings and emotions are expressed readily and easily, there is little danger of hurting people's feelings or stepping on sensibilities and vulnerabilities.[144] We urge caution, however. These cultural mores may be palpable but this does not mean that some people may feel exactly the opposite when they are facing a life-threatening disease. They may be second generation immigrants who have grown up in Britain or in the USA and feel differently about the ways they wish to respond. Some may feel that the context of a medical institution restrains them or not as the case may be and according to the relations between themselves and hospital personnel.

In any case, when a person or their family are from an ethnic minority group and are showing signs of distress that requires extra support, we recommend that the reality of racism and discrimination are acknowledged. Remember that the power relationships between therapist/counsellor/doctor/nurse, patient, and carer may reflect the imbalance of power felt in the wider community or between different gender relations in the society in which they live. Be aware of the ways in which counsellors and therapists like others, are capable of projecting prejudice and discrimination in the reinforcement of stereotypes of inferiority, causing untold damage while espousing equality and freedom.[145] This is not necessarily overcome by culturally matching the therapist to the person in need of 'counselling.' A culturally sensitive counsellor is more effective than their cultural background.[146] However a person may prefer someone to help them who is of the same cultural and ethnic background. Although this kind of request may be difficult to fulfil, the fact that this question has been addressed will signify to the person that they have been taken seriously. Most people are more than willing to take on board the difficulties that are faced in recruiting personnel and the resources or the lack of them that will 'allow' or impede tailored care. This is especially the case when it has been discussed with the sick person and/or the family.

We think that it is important to take into account the structures within ethnic communities which serve to strengthen and support their members and draw upon these strengths when working with an individual. Adopt a flexible approach to their values, beliefs, and traditions that might be therapeutic such as the use of traditional healers and alternative medicines that might be used in conjunction with western treatments. Listen to and accept the person's own way of viewing their difficulties and problems and most importantly, the meanings they attach to them. Incorporate religious, ethical, and spiritual elements when appropriate and required. At times it is wise to re-evaluate the aims of the given therapeutic process in terms of personal and social interventions. Be aware that an individual may be greatly helped by their family members, if indeed they are present. Let the person who is ill, dictate the goals and course of therapy. Identify a 'problem' and the time keeping elements of the 'counselling' together. Strict 'contracts' may not always be adhered to.[147] As Webb Johnson and Nadirshaw[147] point out, these recommendations are not exclusive to any given ethnic group but can be applied to everybody. Indeed we would wholly endorse that sentiment. We would even go one step further and endorse these views in the light of *everyday practice* without 'reserving' them for a counselling intervention.

We think that multicultural therapeutic competencies are extremely difficult to acquire and people who need a more in-depth intervention than we have recommended above, will require specialist treatment by people who are well versed in counselling minority ethnic groups. It is essential that a 'bank' of competent and specialist therapists are documented and accessed when needs fall outside the routine clinical practice of health personnel, counsellors, and psychologists in hospital departments. This is especially pertinent in the case of inner cities and where it is known that ethnic minority communities are living. The ways in which we respond to the needs of under served people, will go some way towards providing equal services to all.

Summary

- Many of the summary points under 'Homelessness' and in 'Asylum Seekers and Refugees' will apply in this population.
- Be aware of the stereotypical assumptions we, as health professionals, make regarding ethnicity such as 'people from Asian countries look after their own' and practice 'closed awareness.' There are no 'fixed' ways of responding or behaving and this applies to people with cancer.
- Be aware that we are *all* ethnic. Sometimes the 'white majority' may be in the minority.
- Remember that there are differences and similarities between and within ethnic groups. Age, gender, and socio-economic factors may impinge on the

ways people are cared for as well as attending to the concepts of ethnicity, culture, or religion.

• Information must be accessible and relevant. Remember people from ethnic minority groups may have less personal contact with cancer information providers and cancer services in general.

• The importance of trained and specialized interpreters and advocates cannot be stressed too strongly.

Refugees and asylum seekers

Introduction

While many of the caveats that we have presented above will apply to asylum seekers and refugees, many will have had to face obstacles that are unique to their own experiences. We want to emphasize that policies pertaining to these groups are likely to change. We therefore want to set the scene as to what asylum seeking and being a refugee means in the UK and at this point in history. As with the indigenous homeless population there has been little research that illuminates the ways that an immigrant might be affected by a cancer diagnosis. We believe however, that if the context of the person is taken into account, health workers will be in a better position to research and start to make inroads into catering for their psychosocial needs.

Defining 'refugees' and 'asylum seekers'

'Refugees' are defined by the fact that people are applying for or are given refugee status; who gain the right to stay in this country indefinitely and who have had their application refused and are appealing.[148] There were 71 700 asylum applications in the UK in 2001.[149] In 1998 it was estimated that 230 000 refugees were living in the UK and numbers are likely to rise. In the whole world it is estimated that there are 12–15 million refugees.

As with indigenous homeless people, data on the number and characteristics of asylum seekers are poor and numbers who are experiencing homelessness is non-existent.[83] Many remain in induction centres until their application is supported when they will be moved to an Accommodation Centre.[150] It is likely however, that refugees and asylum seekers experience of homelessness will reflect that of other homeless people from ethnic minorities in that they may sleep in the houses of friends or bed and breakfast hotels rather than sleep rough or use provision such as night shelters or hostels.[150]

Asylum seekers, refugees, and health

On arriving at a port of entry in the UK an asylum seeker is referred to the port medical inspector if they 'look ill' or if they plan to stay more than six months.[150] They are given chest X-rays before admission, but in practice only a small proportion are screened, due to a lack of funding and insufficient staff. Only cursory examinations take place, putting individuals and public health at risk.[150] Recent research has shown that 17% of asylum seekers have a physical health problem severe enough to affect their life, and two thirds have experienced significant anxiety and depression.[151]

Because asylum seekers are not a homogenous group, many will come from countries where access to health is difficult due to conflict and lack of resources.[150] Many will have been deprived of medical attention because of imprisonment of professionals who have been involved in treating dissidents in the country of origin.[83] Often medical professionals in the host country are not trained in the many difficulties experienced by people who have had to go through the changes described above.[83]

Threats to health are diseases linked to poverty and overcrowding, whether communicable, degenerative, or psychological.[150] Health problems that are specific to asylum seekers originate from their experience in their own home lands such as torture or from the ways in which they have escaped. There is evidence, however, that the health status of new entrants may worsen in the two to three years after entry to the UK.[152]

Diseases experienced by asylum seekers and refugees are also experienced by other deprived or excluded groups and are linked to poverty and overcrowding, whether communicable, degenerative, or psychological (*ibid*). However, health problems that are specific to them include mental health problems,[83] tuberculosis, hepatitis, or parasitic and nutritional diseases and these will vary between refugee groups.[153] Often tests for tuberculosis have not taken place meaning that the condition goes undiagnosed. It is important to remember, however, that not all asylum seekers and refugees have these conditions. Often it is the relatively healthy members of a population who find their way out of their homelands. As with the white majority, men are more reluctant than women to access healthcare.[154] Although this appears to be a gendered response, it is worth remembering that the most important barriers to healthcare in this group include language, cultural differences, difficulty in finding information on health services, no continuity in hospital care, and a general lack of knowledge from the perspective of healthcare professionals.[150] These caveats apply to 'ethnicity' in general while gender, age, and class are also taken into consideration.

Asylum seekers, refugees, and mental health

Many asylum seekers have suffered the atrocities of torture without developing any serious psychological sequelae beyond a natural increase in anxiety and nightmares. Others show more severe levels of anxiety and depression, guilt and shame as a result of their previous experiences and current situation.[150] Long standing mental illness is sometimes evident or linked with their experiences.[154] Those suffering from psychological affects of torture are not always referred to specialist centres,[149] and it is important to remember that many have suffered abuse at the hands of people in authority and are fearful of them.[150]

'Cultural bereavement' and coping with 'deeply disruptive change'[155] are widely experienced by migrants in general. However refugees and asylum seekers do not have choice.[148] This makes their status all the more difficult. Refugees have had to leave their countries often travelling great distances, in hiding, sometimes in the back of lorries and without food, because of persecution and imprisonment. They may have endured torture and/or seen their families enduring torture, rape, sexual assault, landmine injuries, beatings, or malnutrition and even violent death. Many will be suffering from depression, stress, anxiety, or racial harassment.[156] Many asylum seekers entering this country will not have an established community of people from the same country to support them[83] and many including children have no other relatives in the UK.[148] Many are known to grieve and worry about relatives who have been left behind in their country of origin.[151] Some will have had to pay traffickers to enter the host country putting them in debt for indefinite periods. Many will contract diseases in the host country especially in relation to mental health, perhaps as a result of cultural change and a general sense of not belonging[83] or the uncertainty about their claim for asylum[150].

Asylum seekers and refugees: registration and information

All asylum seekers and refugees are entitled to the full range of NHS treatment free of charge, including the right to register with a general practitioner (GP). A number of initiatives have been instigated to promote access to mainstream GP services but there are deficiencies in the structure of healthcare for these populations, starting with primary care and through to secondary and/or acute services.[148] Indeed it is probable that all the caveats mentioned above in the sections titled homelessness and ethnicity, will apply to this group. It is known however, that 93% of survey respondents said they had been given no information on how to register with a GP and 97% said they had been given no information on how to use hospital services.[157] Female asylum seekers face particular unacknowledged difficulties.[158] Screening and health promotion programmes tend to have a low uptake, but while this may be due to cultural differences it is more likely that the structural elements of health provision preclude asylum seekers and those from ethnic minority groups in many ways.[159]

Like homeless indigenous people, refugees encounter problems registering with a GP and when they are registered with their GPs, it is often on a temporary basis, because of a sometimes erroneous belief that this population is highly mobile—up to 70% were found to remain in one area for a year.[105, 151] This prevents access to past records that in itself, takes away financial remuneration to undertake preventive interventions such as cervical smear tests.[148] Asylum seekers and refugees may be asked for passports when trying to register with GPs[160] and this is particularly worrying since some asylum seekers and refugees are unlikely to have one.[148]

Relatively little is known about this group in relation to GP's attitudes. One study[161] has reported that health professionals are anxious about treating patients with special needs who seemed to take up a disproportionate amount of time. Not surprisingly, language barriers are known to exist and health authorities have little knowledge about the languages spoken in their districts and the importance and extent of interpreter services.[148] Moreover, these are not likely to be available out of working hours and in acute consultations.[162]

Asylum seekers, refugees, and discrimination

Some boroughs in London have explicitly identified that African refugees suffer from discrimination, racial abuse, unemployment, and isolation due to a perceived high prevalence of HIV among their communities.[31] A drop in status is experienced by both men and women as a result of their experience, but men are known to be more acutely affected by this. Men granted refugee status are less likely to find work and this may lead to further changes in status, sometimes within the family, which can cause further distress.

Exemption of charges are the asylum seekers right. However, lengthy forms must be filled (usually in English and/or Welsh)[150]. People need to be given advice and assistance to complete the forms, making clear that the certificate is only valid for six months, when it can be renewed.[163] They need to be widely publicized so that they are aware of them at the time of application. As with all people who are illiterate, health advice cannot be read by many who are seeking asylum, especially women.[150]

This is an important factor. Innovative ways are required if we are to access people and give information to them after arriving in the host country where language will inevitably be a problem. For example, Somali culture focuses more on oral communication: story telling is an important way of disseminating information.[164] It is against this backdrop that refugees and asylum seekers have to face a cancer diagnosis. This makes it all the more important that healthcare professionals *listen* carefully to everybody in their care,[150] including indigenous people of all ethnicities who may rely on less conventional ways of assimilating information.

Asylum seekers and support

As in the case of ethnic minority groups, the roles of interpreter and advocate are of paramount importance. (*See* pages 190–1 under Ethnicity.) All the caveats that we have presented regarding this resource apply in this context. It is important that the use of family, friends, and other asylum seekers, as informal interpreters, should be discouraged. It denies patients confidentiality rights, especially as they relate to family or community. However there are not enough translation services in the UK and in particular in the area of mental health[150] that cater for people who are from other countries and who have empathy for the many horrendous problems they may have experienced. This requires thought and resources if an optimal service is to be provided.

Treatment for psychological problems

As in the case of some ethnic minority groups, one of the most important barriers to healthcare, is language. This especially applies to those people who are known to have psychological and emotional difficulties since their needs have to be explored verbally.[148] The added burden of having cancer makes communication in that context particularly important if serious distress is to be prevented, resulting possibly in long-term psychological and social problems. It is important to remember that every culture has its own framework for mental health and mechanisms for seeking help when there is a crisis.[165] This means that treatment requires specialist diagnostic and counselling skills.[151] Counselling may not be a resource nor conceptually evident in some cultures and many asylum seekers often have different ways of coping with psychological trauma.[150] For example, refugees from Mozambique[166] and Ethiopia[167] actively try to forget their experiences as their usual means of coping with difficulties. Many simply wish to tell their story which in itself can be therapeutic.[168] However, it should not be assumed that this is an umbrella solution since recounting trauma can be extremely distressing for many.[169] It is suggested that therapeutic skills that are used in day-to-day work are all useful in this context too.[170] However, the understanding and evaluation of appropriate therapy for this group in general is in its infancy (*ibid*). Special skills and appropriate training are needed and it is important that cancer health professionals recognize this and act accordingly. A 'do it yourself' approach may be dangerous for both the person with cancer and their families and for providing psychosocial care for this group.

As with indigenous homeless people, we suggest that close ties are kept with key workers. Although health workers are unlikely to encounter large numbers of asylum seekers and refugees with cancer because they are more likely to be young, numbers alone should not be the determining factor when assessing priorities. The health of all minority groups should be integrated as far as is possible into other aspects of learning, development, and priorities. Everyone is entitled to fair access to healthcare and the right to opportunities for better health—this is the underlying principle of the NHS and is re-emphasized in the current Government policy.

Summary

- All of the summary points mentioned under 'Homelessness' and 'Ethnicity' will apply here. (*See* pages 172–93.)
- Be aware of people's personal histories. Many will have gone through horrendous obstacles before arriving in the 'host' country, the effects of which may be long lasting.
- Be aware of the difficulties encountered in the context of medical care in the host country.
- Be aware that people have differing ways of communicating psychological (and physical) pain. Specialist diagnostic and counselling skills are called for.

Conclusion

We have not been able to touch on all domains in cancer care, nor on all conceptual issues surrounding the 'social'. For example, the field of genetics and cancer, or children and cancer are important areas of concern and there are many more. Likewise there are many conceptual issues that we have not been able to cover and when we have it has not always been in depth. Although we have touched on the conceptual issue of 'communication' for example, brevity of space has precluded a careful and critical look at this concept as it includes the doctor–patient relationship, ethical issues of consent, and informed decision making.

By looking at marginalized groups and their circumstances we have highlighted the danger of using messages of 'self-responsibility' and 'fighting' disease. We have attempted to show how these messages and the assumptions that we can so easily make about people do not sit easy alongside the reality of their lives. Sometimes it seems that we have posed more questions than given answers. Seldom do we espouse one way to go about 'good practice'. This we know is difficult, for we all want quick and easy answers. But ambiguities reflect the fragmented reality of our lives. We live in worlds that are forever changing. Gobalization is a growing phenomenon. Nothing is fixed or 'static' but fluid and always in flux. In many ways a social class divide is hidden and may not exist in relation to many aspects of people's lives; in others it is starkly obvious and especially in ways that health services have been delivered to differing sections of society. Young people may have different needs from older ones regardless of their ethnicity. Men and women may be more similar than we assume. Differences in response may be as much to do with the ways in which we, health professionals impute our stereotypical ideals on to the care we give than to biological difference. More and more ethnic groups are living amongst us and will have differing *and* similar needs to the indigenous population who have their own ethnicity. Homeless people, asylum seekers, and refugees face many similar difficulties as lower social class groups with white ethnicity. They also have their own unique sets of problems. We hope that readers will find it possible to use the tools of a sociological approach to enhance ways of caring, and to apply them to everyday practice. The more we are able to look at the wider picture of our lives and the ways in which we, as health practitioners, go about our tasks, holding in view the structural aspects of medicine and how they may impede (or enhance) patient care, the more it will be possible to offer an optimal service.

References

1. Moynihan C. (2002). Men, women, gender and cancer. *European Journal of Cancer Care* 11:166–72.
2. Blair A. (1993). Social class and the contextualization of illness experience. In: A Radley (ed.), *Worlds of illness. Biographical and cultural perspectives on health and disease*, London: Routledge, pp. 27–48.
3. Comoroff J. (1982). *Medicine: symbol and ideology*. Edinburgh: Edinburgh University Press.
4. Greer S, Moorey S, Baruch J, Watson M, Robertson BM, Mason A, *et al.* (1992). Adjurant psychological therapy for patients with cancer: a prospective randomised trial. *British Medical Journal* 304:675–80.
5. Watson M, Haviland JS, Greer S, Davidson J, and Bliss JM. (1999). Influence of psychological response on survival in breast cancer: a population-based cohort study. *Lancet* 354(9187):1331–6.

6. Petticrew M and Bell RH, D. (2002). Influence of psychological coping on survival and recurrence in people with cancer: systematic review. *British Medical Journal* **325**:1066–9.

7. Chattoo SA, W Haworth M, and Lennard R. (2002). *South Asian and white patients with advanced cancer: patients' and families' experiences of the illness and perceived needs for care.* Cancer Research UK and Department of Health.

8. Sontag S. (1991). *Illness as metaphor.* London: Allen Lane.

9. (2003) Cancer patients forced to wait months for scans or radiotherapy treatment. *The Guardian.*

10. Helman C. (2000). Cultural definitions of anatomy and physiology. In: *Culture health and illness,* Oxford, Boston: Butterworth Heinemann, p. 12–31.

11. Douglas M. (1973). *Natural symbols.* London: Penguin.

12. Stacey M. (1991). *The sociology of health and healing.* London, New York: Routledge.

13. Annandale E. (1998). *The sociology of health and medicine: a critical introduction.* Cambridge, Oxford. USA: Polity press.

14. Knowles JH. (1977). The responsibility of the individual. In: JH Knowles (ed.), *Doing better and feeling worse: health in the United States,* New York: Norton.

15. Crawford R. (1977). You are dangerous to your health: the ideology and politics of victim blaming. *International Journal of Health Services* **7**(4):663–80.

16. Marsland D (1981). Education: vast horizons, meagre visions. In DC Anderson (ed.), *Breaking the spell of the welfare state,* London: Social Affairs Unit.

17. Johnson T. (1972). *Professions and power.* Oxford: Macmillan.

18. Lash S, and Urry J. (1994). *Economies of signs and space.* London: Sage.

19. Annandale E. (1998). The theoretical origins and development of sociology of health and illness. In: E Annandale (ed.), *The sociology of health and medicine: a critical introduction,* Cambridge, Oxford, USA: Polity Press in association with Blackwell Publishers pp. 3–32.

20. Annandale E. (1998). Professional powers: the formal health-care division of labour in transition. In: E Annandale (ed.), *The sociology of health and medicine: a critical introduction,* Cambridge, Oxford, USA: Polity Press in association with Blackwell Publishers, pp. 223–50.

21. Elston M. (1991). The politics of professional power: medicine in a changing health service. In: JCM Gabe, M Bury (ed.), *The sociology of the health service,* pp. 58–88. London: Routeledge.

22. Silverman D. (1987). Communication and medical practice: social relations in the clinic. London: Sage.

23. Annandale E. (1998). Accomplishing health and healthcare. In: *The sociology of health and medicine: a critical introduction,* pp. 193–222. Cambridge, Oxford, USA: Polity Press in association with Blackwell Publishers.

24. Loyd-Bostock S. (1992). Attributes and apologies in lettters of complaint to hospitals and letters of response. In: J Harvey, T Orbuch, and A Weber (ed.), *Attributions, accounts and close relationships,* New York: Springer-Verlag.

25. Costain Schou KC and Hewrison, J. (1999). *Experiencing cancer: quality of life in treatment.* Buckingham, UK: Open University Press.

26. Annnadale E. (1998). 'Race', ethnicity and health status. In: E Annandale (ed.), *The sociology of health and medicine: a critical introduction,* pp. 160–92. Cambridge, Oxford and USA: Polity Press in association with Blackwell Publishers.

27. Moynihan C. (1998). Theories of masculinity. *British Medical Journal* **317**:1072–5.

28. Holton R and Turner B. (1990). *Max Weber on economy and society.* London: Routledge.

29. OPCS. (1995). *Occupational mortality.* London: Department of Health.

30. Cartwright A and O'Brien M. (1976). Social class variations in health care. In: M Stacey (ed.), *The sociology of health and healing*, London: Unwin Hyman.

31. Silvera M, Kapasi R. (2000). *Health advocacy for minority ethnic Londoners.* London, UK: King's Fund.

32. Annandale E. (1998). The experience of illness in healthcare in contemporary society. In: E Annandale (ed.), *The Sociology of health and medicine: a critical introduction*, p. 263. Cambridge, Oxford, USA: Polity press in association with Blackwell publishers.

33. Radley A. (1999). Ideas about health and staying healthy. In: A Radley (ed.), *Making sense of illness: the social psychology of health and disease.* pp. 36–60. London, Thousand Oaks, New Delhi: Sage Publications.

34. Bernstein B. (1974). Social class, speech systems and psychotherapy. *British Journal of Sociology* **15**:54–64.

35. Moynihan C, Burton S, Huddart R, *et al.* (2002). *Men's understanding of genetic disease.* London: Cancer Research UK.

36. Cornwell J. (1984). *Hard earned lives.* London: Tavistock.

37. Martin J and White A. (1988). The financial circumstances of disabled adults. *OPCS surveys of disability in Great Britain Report 2*, London: HMSO.

38. Moynihan C. (1987). The psychosocial problems of testicular cancer patients and their relatives. *Cancer Surveys* **6**(3):477–510.

39. Viney LL and Westbrook MT. (1982). Coping with chronic illness: the mediating role of biographic and illness-related factors. *Journal of Psychosomatic Research* **26**(6):595–605.

40. Hines S. (2001). Coping with uncertainties in advanced care planning. *Journal of Communication* **51**(3):498–513.

41. Acheson ED. (1990). Edwin Chadwick and the world we live in. *Lancet* **336**(8729):1482–5.

42. Nazroo J. (1997). *The health of Britain's ethnic minorities: findings from a national survey.* London: Policy Studies Institute.

43. Gallagher BJ. (1980). *The sociology of mental illness.* Engelwood Cliff, NJ: Prentice-Hall.

44. Davis H and Fallowfield L. (1991). Counselling theory. In: Fallowfield H and Davis H (ed.), *Counselling and communication in health care*, pp. 23–57. Chichester, New York, Brisbane, Toronto and Singapore: John Wiley and Sons.

45. Moorey S and Green S (2002). *Cognitive behaviour therapy for cancer patients.* Oxford: Oxford University Press.

46. Rough sleeping: Report by the Social Exclusion Unit. (1998). London: HMSO.

47. Thomas C, Morris S, McIllmurray MB, Soothill K, Francis B, and Harman JC. (2001). *What are the psychosocial needs of cancer patients and their main carers?* Lancaster: The Institute for Health Research, Lancaster University.

48. Kandrack M, Grant K, and Segall A. (1991). Gender differences in health related behaviour – some unanswered questions. *Social Science and Medicine* **32**(5):579–90.

49. Verbrugge L. (1985). Gender and health: an update on hypotheses and evidence. *Journal of Health and Social Behaviour* **26**:156–82.

50. Doyal L. (2001). Sex, gender and health: the need for a new approach. *British Journal of Sociology* **323**:1061–3.

51. Harrison J, Chin J, and Ficarrotto T. (1992). Warning: masculinity may damage your health. In: *Men's lives.* New York: Macmillan.

52. Lloyd T. (1996). Men's health review. *Men's health forum.* London: Royal College of Nursing.

53. Martin E. (1987). *The woman in the body.* Milton Keynes: Open University Press.

54. Moynihan C, Bliss J, Davidson J, Burchell L, and Horwich A. (1998). Evaluation of adjuvant psychological therapy in patients with testicular cancer. *The British Medical Journal* **316**:429–35.

55. Connell R. (1995). *Masculinities*. Berkeley: University of California Press.

56. Schofield CA, Connell R, Walker L, Wood JF, and Butland JL. (2000). Understanding men's health and illness: a gender relations approach to policy, research and practice. *Journal of the American College Health* **48**:247–58.

57. Bendelow G. (1993). Pain perceptions, emotions and gender. *Sociology of Health and Illness* **15**(3):272–94.

58. Bendelow G and Whitehead M. (1987). *The health divide: inequalities in health in the 1980s*. London: Health Education Commission.

59. Bendelow G. (1992). *Social contexts of pain perceptions*. Plymouth: ESRC.

60. Miller J and Bell C. (1996). Mapping men's mental health. *Journal of Community and Applied Social Psychology* **6**:317–27.

61. Meyer TJ and Mark MM. (1995). Effects of psychosocial interventions with adult cancer patients: a meta-analysis of randomized experiments. *Health Psychology* **14**(2):101–8.

62. Charmaz K. (1994). Identity dilemmas of chronically ill men. *Sociological Quarterly* **35**(2):269–88.

63. Eakin EG and Strycker LA. (2001). Awareness and barriers to use of cancer support and information resources by HMO patients with breast, prostate, or colon cancer: patient and provider perspectives. *Psycho-oncology* **10**(2):103–13.

64. Lintz K, Moynihan C, Steginga S, Norman A, Eeles R, Muddart R, *et al.* (2003). Prostate cancer patients, support and psychosocial care needs: survey from a non-surgical oncology clinic. *Psyco-onchology* **12**:769–83.

65. Gray RE, Fitch M, Davis C, and Phillips C. (1997). Interviews with men with prostate cancer about their self-help group experience. *Journal of Palliative Care* **13**(1):15–21.

66. Chattoo S, Small N, and Rhodes P. (2001). Too ill to talk? *User involvement and palliative care*. London, New York: Routledge.

67. Dunphy K. (2000). Dying in West Herts – Does gender make a difference? In: *Conference – 'men and cancer'*. Berkhamstead, Herts. The Hospice of St. Francis.

68. Jenhins V, Fallowfield L, and Saul J. (2001). Information needs of patients with cancer: results from a large study in all cancer centres. *British Journal of Cancer* **84**(1): 48–51.

69. Leydon G, Boulton M, Moynihan C, Jones A, Mossman J, Boudioni M, *et al.* (2000). Cancer patients' information needs and information seeking behaviour`: in depth interview study. *British Medical Journal* **320**:909–13.

70. Yates P and Stetz K. (1999). Families' awareness of and response to dying. *Oncology Nursing Forum* **26**(1):113–20.

71. Ember C and Ember M. (1985). *Cultural anthropology*. Englewood Cliffs. NJ: Prentice Hall.

72. Shepherd G. (1982). Gender and homosexuality. In: Capland P. (ed.), *Mombassa as a key to understanding sexual options*, The Cultural Construction of Sexuality.: Tavistock.

73. Lock M. (1982). Models and practice in medicine: menopause as syndrome or life transition? *Culture, Medicine and Psychiatry* **6**(3):261–80.

74. Marshall J and Funch D. (1986). Gender and illness behaviour among colorectal cancer patients. *Women and Health* **11**(3-4):67–82.

75 Becker G. (1997). *Disrupted lives*. University of California Press.

76 Schover L, Rybicki L, Martin B, and Bringlesen K. (1999). Having children after cancer. A pilot survey of survivors' attitudes and experiences. *Cancer* **86**(4):697–709.

77. Palgi P. (1966). Cultural components of immigrants' adjustment. In: David HP. (ed.), *Migration, mental health and community services*, pp. 71–82. International Research Institute.

78. Pheffer N. (1985). The hidden pathology of the male reproductive system. In: Homans H. (ed.), *The sexual politics of reproduction*. pp. 30–44. Aldershot: Gower.

79. Macer D. (1994). Perceptions of risk and benefits of in vitro fertilization, genetic engineering and biotechnology. *Social Science and Medicine* **38**:22–3.

80. Oliver M. (1990). *The politics of disablement*. London: Macmillan.

81. Potts L. (2000). *Ideologies of breast cancer: feminist perspectives*. London: Macmillan.

82. Pheffer N. (2004). Screening for breast cancer: candidacy and compliance. *Social Science and Medicine* **58**:151–60.

83. Pleace N and Quilgars D. (1996). *Health and homelessness in London: a review*. London: King's Fund.

84. Siddal R. (1994). Homelssness – in another world. *Community Care Supplement* (**April**):15–16.

85. Bines. (1994). *The health of single homeless people*. New York: The Centre for Housing Policy, University of York.

86. Susser E, Lin S, and Conover S. (1991). Risk factors for homelessness among patients admitted to a state mental hospital. *American Journal of Psychiatry* **148**(2):1659–64.

87. Marshall E and Reed J. (1992). Psychiatric morbidity in homeless women. *British Journal of Psychiatry* **160**:761–8.

88. Breakey W, Fischer P, Kramer M, Nestadt G, Romanoshi AJ, Ross A, *et al.* (1989). Health and mental health problems of homeless men and women in Baltimore. *Journal of the American Medical Association* **262**:1352–7.

89. Chau S, Chin M, Chang J, Luecha A, Cheng E, Schlesinger J. *et al.* (2002). Cancer risk behaviours and screening rates among homeless adults in Los Angeles county. Cancer epidemiology. *Biomarkers and Prevention* **11**(5):431–8.

90. Weinreb L, Goldberg R, and Perloff J. (1998). Health characteristics and medical service use patterns of sheltered homeless and low-income housed mothers. *Journal of Gerneral Internal Medicine* **13**(6):389–97.

91. Long H, Tulsky J, Chambers D, Alpers LS, Robertson MJ, Moss AR, *et al.* (1998). Cancer screening in homeless women: attitudes and behaviours. *Journal of Health Care for the Poor and Underserved* **9**(3):276–92.

92. Whale Z. (1998). Head and neck cancer: an overview of literature. *European Journal of Oncology Nursing* **2**(2):99–105.

93. Williams M. (2001). An investigation of psychological distress in patients who have been treated for head and neck cancer. *British Journal of Oral and Maxillofacial Surgery* **39**(5):333–9.

94. Sehlen S, Hollenhorst H, Lenk M, Schymura B, Herschbach P, Aydemir U, *et al.* (2002). Only sociodemographic variables (and not medical ones) predict quality of life after radiography in patients with head and neck cancer. *International Journal of Radiation Oncology* **52**(3):779–83.

95. Davis R and Roberts D. (1999). Nursing care of the patient with head and neck cancer: review article. *Oncology Nurses* **4**(1):9–15.

96. Piff C. (1986). *Let's face it*. London: Sphere.

97. Specht L. (2002). Oral complications in the head and neck radiation patient. Introduction and scope of the problem. *Supportive Care in Cancer* **10**(1):36–9.

98. Espie S, Freedlander E, Campsie L, Soutar DS, and Robertson AG. (1989). Psychological distress at follow up after major surgery for intra oral cancer. *Journal of Psychosomatic Research* **33**(4):441–8.

99. Krishnasamy M. (1996). Social support and the patient with cancer: a consideration of the literature. *Journal of Advanced Nursing* **23**:757–62.

100. Cook J and Marshall J. (1996). Homeless Women. In: K Abel, M Buszewicz, S Davison, S Johnson, E Staples (ed.), *Planning community mental health services for women*. London and New York: Routledge.

101. Martin P, Wiles R, Pratten B, Gorton S, and Green J. (1992). *A user perspective: views on London's acute health services*. London: King's Fund and Greater London Associations of Community Health Councils.

102. Pheffer N and Moynihan C. (1996). Ethnicity and health beliefs with respect to cancer: a critical review of methodology. *British Journal of Cancer* **74**(Suppl XXIX):66–72.

103. Parker R and Hopwood P. (2000). *Literature review: quality of life of black and ethnic minority groups with cancer.* London: Cancer Research UK.

104. Ethnicity and health: *A guide for the NHS.* (1993). London: Department of Health.

105. Arorea S, Coker N, Gillam S, and Ismail H. (1991). *Improving the health of black and minority ethnic groups.* London: King's Fund.

106. Pheffer N. (1998). Theories of race, ethnicity and culture. *The British Medical Journal* **317**:1381–4.

107. Annandale E and Ahmad W. (1996). The trouble with culture. In: D Kellehor and S Hillier (ed.), *Researching cultural differences in health* pp. 190–219. London: Routledge.

108. Giddens A. (1993). *Sociology.* Cambridge: Polity Press.

109. Bradby H. (1995). Ethnicity: not a black or white issue. A research note. *Sociology of Health and Illness* **17**:405–17.

110. Bhopal RS, Phillimore P, and Kohli H. (1991). Inappropriate use of the term 'Asian': an obstacle to ethnicity and health research. *Journal of Public Health Medicine.* **13**:244–6.

111. Gunaratnam Y. (1997). Culture is not enough. D Field, J Hockey, and N Small (ed.), *Death gender and ethnicity* pp. 166–86. London: Routledge.

112. Jones T. (1993). *Britain's ethnic minorities: an analysis of the labour force survey.* London: Policy Studies Institute.

113. Warnecke R, Ferrans C, Johnson T, Chapa-Resendez G, O'Roushe DP, Chavez N, *et al.* (1996). Measuring quality of life in culturally diverse populations. *Journal of Community and Applied Social Psychology* **20**:29–38.

114. Marshall P. (1990). Cultural influences on perceived quality of life. *Seminal Oncology Nursing* **6**:278–84.

115. Wellisch D, Kagawa-Singer M, Reid S, Lin Y, Nishikawa L, Wellisch M, *et al.* (1999). An exploratory study of social support: a cross cultural comparison of Chinese, Japanese, and Anglo American breast cancer patients. *Psycho-oncology* **8**:207–19.

116. Chaturvedi S. (1994). Exploration of concerns and role of psychosocial intervention in palliative care – a study from India. *Annals of Academic Medicine. Singapore* **23**:256–60.

117. Bullinger M, Anderson R, Cella D, and Aaronson N. (1993). Developing and evaluating cross cultural instruments from minimum requirements to optimal models. *Quality of Life Research* **2**(6):451–9.

118. Meyerowitz B, Richardson J, Hudson S, and Leedham B. (1998). Ethnicity and cancer outcomes: behavioural and psychosocial considerations. *Psychological Bulletin* **123**:47–70.

119. Wilkinson S and Kitzinger, C. (2000). Thinking differently about thinking positive: a discursive approach to cancer patients' talk. *Social Science and Medicine* **50**:797–811.

120. Farooq S and Gahir M. (1995). Soomatization: a transcultural study. *Journal of Psychosomatic Research* **39**:883–8.

121. Saxena S, Chandiramani R, and Bhargava R. (1998). WHOQoL Hindi: a questionnaire for assessing quality of life in health care settings in India. *National Medical Journal India* **11**:160–5.

122. Ramirez A, Bogdanovic M, and Jasovicgasic M. (1991). Psychosocial adjustment to cancer-cultural considerations. *European Journal of Psychiatry* **5**:9–18.

123. Goh CR, Lee KS, Tan TC, Wang TL, Tan CN, Wong J, *et al.* (1996). Measuring quality of life in different cultures: translation of the functional living index for cancer (FLIC) into Chinese and Malay in Singapore. *Annals of Academic Medicine Singapore* **25**:323–34.

124. Atkin K, Ahmad W, and Aknionwu E. (1998). Screening and counselling for sickle cell disorders and thalassaemia: the experience of parents and health professionals. *Social Science and Medicine* **47**(11):1639–51.

125. Konner M. (1993). *The trouble with medicine*. London: British Broadcasting Corporation Books.

126. Koffman J and Higginson I. (2001). Accounts of carers' satisfaction with health care at the end of life: a comparison of first generation black Caribbeans and white patients with advanced disease. *Palliative Medicine* **15**:337–45.

127. Eisenbruch M. (1984). Cross-cultural aspects of bereavement II: Ethnic and cultural variations in the development of bereavement practices. *Culture Medicine and Psychiatry* **8**:3125–3.

128. Green J and Green M. (1992). *Dealing with death: practices and procedures*. London: Chapman and Hall.

129. Koffman J. (2001). Rituals surrounding death in the black African Caribbean community. *Palliative Care Today* **10**:7.

130. Helman C. (2000). Diet and nutrition. In: C Helman (ed.), *Culture, health and illness,*. pp. 32–49. New York: Oxford University Press.

131. Karmi G. (1996). *The ethnic health handbook: a fact-file for health care professionals*. Oxford: Blackwell Science.

132. Coker N. (2001). *Racism in medicine: agenda for change*. London: King's Fund.

133. Karim K, Bailey MJ, and Tunna K. (2000). Non white ethnicity and the provision of specialist palliative care services. Factors affecting doctors' referral patterns. *Palliative Medicine* **14**:471–8.

134. Boomla L. (1994). *What local factors best explain low mammography uptake in East London and the City Health Authority*. London: London School of Hygiene and Tropical Medicine.

135. Spellman P and Smith I. (1999). *The cancer journey to secondary care of patients with suspected cancer of the colon or lung: a perspective from general practice*. Leeds: Nuffield Institute for Health, University of Leeds.

136. Pheffer N. (2004). "If you think you've got a lump, they'll screen you." Informed consent, health promotion and breast cancer. *Journal of Medical Ethics* **30**: 327–30.

137. Smaje C, and Field D. (1997). Absent minorities? Ethnicity and the use of palliative care services. In: D. Field, J Hockey, and N. Small, (ed.), *Death, gender and ethnicity*. London: Routledge.

138. Ahmad W. (1996). Family obligations and social change among communities. In: W Ahmad (ed.), *Race and community care*. Buckingham: Open University Press.

139. Katbamna S, Bhakta P, *et al.* (1998). *Experiences and needs of carers from the South Asian communities*. Leicester: Nuffield Community Care Studies Unit, University of Leicester.

140. Stewart M. (1995). Effective physician-patient communication and health outcomes: a review of the literature. *Canadian Medical Association Journal* **152**:1423–33.

141. Meryn S. (1998). Improving doctor patient communication. Not an option but a necessity. *The British Medical Journal* **316**:1992.

142. Asylum seekers: (2002). *Meeting their healthcare needs*. London: British Medical Association.

143. Kareem J. (2000). The Nafsiyat intercultural therapy centre. In: H Jarl (ed.), *Intercultural therapy*. London, USA, Australia: Blackwell Science.

144. Laungani P. (2002). Understanding mental illness across cultures. In: S Palmer (ed.), *Multicultural counselling*. pp. 129–56. London, Thousand Oaks, New Delhi: Sage Publications.

145. Lago C and Moodley R. (2002). Multicultural issues in electic and integrative connselling and psychotherapy. In; Thousand Oalls, New Delhi: Sage Publicaations.

146. Wade P and Bernstein B. (1991). Culture sensitivity, training and counselor race: effects on black female clients' perceptions and attrition. *Journal of Counselling Psychology* **38**(1):9–15.

147. Webb Johnson A and Nadirshaw Z. (2002). Good practice in transcultural counselling: an Asian perspective. In: S Palmer (ed.), *Multicultural counselling*. London, Thousand Oaks, New Delhi: Sage.

148. Jones D and Gill P. (1998). Refugees and primary care: tackling the inequalities. *The British Medical Journal* **317**:1444–6.

149. Heath T, Jeffries R, and Lioyd A. (2002). *Asylum Statistics, United Kingdom*. London: HMSO.

150. Asylum seekers: meeting their healthcare needs. (2002). British Medical Association Board of Science and Education, London.

151. Carey Wood J, Duke K, Karn V, and Marshall T. (1995). *The settlement of refugees in Britain*. London: HMSO.

152. Health of Refugees and Asylum Seekers. Report by London Health Observatory, London. (2002).

153. Dick B. (1984). Diseases of refugees – causes, effects and control. *Trans R. Soc. Tropical Medicine and Hygiene* **78**:734–41.

154. Burnett A. (2002). Meeting the health needs of refugees and asylum seekers in the UK: an information resource pack for health workers.: NHS Department of Health.

155. Loizos P. (1981). *The heart grows bitter: a chronicle of Cyprus war refugees*. Cambridge: Cambridge University Press.

156. Unsworth C and Goldenburg E. (1998). Psychological sequalae of torture and organised violence suffered by refugees from Iraq: trauma related factors compared with social factors in exile. *British Journal of Psychiatry* **172**:90–4.

157. Gammell H, Nahiro A, Nicholas N, and Windsor J. (1993). *Refugees (political asylum seekers): service provision and access to the NHS*. London: College of Health.

158. Burnett A and Peel M. (2001). Health needs of asylum seekers and refugees. *British Journal of Cancer* **322**:544–7.

159. Islington Refugee Working Party. (1992). *Report on questionnaire survey*. London: Islington Voluntary Action Council.

160. Grant C and Deane J. (1995). *Stating the obvious: factors which influence the uptake and provision of primary care services to refugees*. London: Lambeth, Southwark and Lewisham Health Authority.

161. Ramsey R and Turner S. (1993). Refugees' health needs. *British Journal of General Practice* **43**:480–1.

162. Hicks C and Hayes L. (1991). Linkworkers in antenatal care: facilitators of equal opportunity in health provision or salves for the management conscience. *Health Service Management Research* **4**:89–93.

163. (2000). Refugee council briefing. *Access to health services for asylum seekers and refugees*. Refugee Council.

164. (1998). Promoting the health of refugees. In: *Health education authority expert working group on refugee health*, London: Immigration Law Practioners Association.

165. Bracken P, Giller J, and Summerfield D. (1995). Psychosocial responses to war and atrocity: the limitations of current concepts. *Social Science and Medicine* **40**:1073–82.

166. (1997). Guidelines for providers of counselling training to refugees and guidelines for refugee community organisations providing counselling. In: London, Evelyn Olfield Unit. Refugee Mental Health Forum.

167. Summerfield D. (1996). *The impact of war and atrocity on civilian populations: basic principles for NGO interventions and a critique of psyochosexual trauma projects*. London: Relief and Rehabilitation Network Overseas Development Institute.

168. Cienfuegos A and Monelli C. (1983). The testimony of political repression as a therapeutic instrument. *American Journal of Orthopsychiatry* **53**:43–51.

169. Summerfield D. (1995). Assisting survivors of war and atrocity: notes on 'psycho-social' issues for NGO workers. *Development in Practice* **5**:352–6.

170. Turner S. (2000). Therapeutic approaches with survivors of torture. In: Littlewood J (ed.), *Intercultural therapy*. Oxford, USA, Canada, Australia: Blackwell Science, pp. 180–192.

Chapter 5

Clinical context

General practice. 208
Diagnosis. 211
   Speed of diagnosis. 211
   Eliciting key concerns 212
   Concerns associated with early phases of treatment. 213
Surgery. 214
   Hospital admission. 215
   Preparation for surgery 216
   Continuity of care. 217
   Psychiatric drugs 217
Radiotherapy 226
   Preparation for radiotherapy 227
   Main areas of radiotherapy information 228
   Side-effects of radiotherapy. 229
   The role of radiographers. 229
Chemotherapy and hormone therapy. 231
   Preparation for chemotherapy. 232
   Side-effects of chemotherapy and hormone therapy. 234
Common treatment difficulties 242
   Fatigue. 242
   Nausea and vomiting. 245
   Pain 247
   Depression. 253
   Intense fear 255
   Worry. 258
   Insomnia 260
Rehabilitation 262
   Mobility 263
   Activities of daily living 264
   Psychosocial rehabilitation. 264
   Rehabilitation teams 265
Recurrence. 266
Palliative care. 267
   Psychosocial issues for people who are dying 268
Bereavement care 277
References 282

Many cancer treatments are notoriously challenging, though fortunately there is a lot 'that healthcare staff can do to minimize their patients' distress. This chapter looks at some of the main clinical areas of oncology and considers how these services can deliver optimal supportive care.

Supportive care is ultimately tied to the clinical situations that patients and professionals find themselves in. For healthcare professionals this 'clinical context' involves the challenge of providing different cancer treatments at different stages of the patient's illness. The more professionals are aware of the psychosocial effects of surgery, radiotherapy, and chemotherapy, the better equipped they are to minimize their damage to the individual patient's quality of life. However, residual problems often only become apparent after active treatment has ended, so as cancer increasingly becomes a chronic illness for many, there must be a corresponding emphasis on cancer rehabilitation. Finally, this chapter takes a brief look at the supportive care of people who are dying, and the mourning of those that they leave behind.

Healthcare staff who show sensitivity to these concerns can have an enormous impact on how safe and supported people with cancer feel as they endure the uncertain and exhausting demands of treatment. Ultimately, the way cancer treatment is delivered either helps or hinders people's adjustment to their illness the rest of their lives.

In several places we illustrate the psychosocial impact of cancer treatments by describing some of the main issues facing people with particular types of cancer or particular types of treatment (i.e. *Focus on* breast cancer, head and neck cancers, CNS tumours, pelvic radiation, bone marrow transplants, lung cancer, and prostate cancer). These discussions are far from an exhaustive list but serve to reveal the varied psychosocial concerns associated with different disease sites and treatments. Few cancers are exclusively treated in one way so our focus on different cancer sites merely exemplifies different facets of particular cancer treatments.

General practice

Although individual family doctors rarely have more than a handful of patients being actively treated for cancer at any one time, their role in supportive care and accessing other services cannot be overstated. They are the first port of call for most patients with suspicious symptoms and, even when the diagnosis may have been made elsewhere (e.g. through national screening programmes), it often falls to the GP to tell their patients they have cancer. Indeed, it will be the family doctor who will continue to care for the patient in the months or years after active cancer treatment has finished, and frequently it is the primary care team who will support the dying patient at home, and their family, through to bereavement.

Family doctors are usually the only healthcare professional the patient has known for any significant length of time, and in many communities the family doctor continues to assume symbolic and social importance. They have a significant role in health promotion, encouraging people to desist from lifestyle behaviours that raise the risk of cancer, especially smoking, poor diet, and excessive sun exposure. They also have a responsibility to ensure that their patients are aware of the early signs and symptoms of cancer so that they report them at the earliest opportunity. Family doctors are the gateways to specialist cancer services although they are sometimes criticized by patients for assuming too strict a gate-keeping role. Their difficulty is that amidst the many benign lumps and vague symptoms a GP sees there will be the odd one that is malignant and requires specialist attention. This may present particular difficulties among patients who are generally anxious about becoming ill and who repeatedly consult their doctors for reassurance.

When a patient is referred to a hospital specialist for suspected cancer, the family doctor must sensitively assess how much the patient wants to know about their suspicions. Not all patients want to know that they are being investigated for cancer although increasing numbers of people do (*see* Chapter 6—Disclosure of Diagnostic Information). However, it is important that all patients are prepared for the possibility of more sinister news, even if tests are ostensibly being conducted 'to be on the safe side'. If the possibility of cancer is discussed, time should be taken to explore the patient's understanding of the disease and its treatment so that any frightening misconceptions can be corrected. Likewise, in preparing patients for hospital attendance, whether for tests or an admission, discussing what it may involve can help to allay natural anxiety about the unknown.

General practitioners require good communication with the hospital healthcare team. They need timely up-to-date information from cancer care teams regarding diagnosis, prognosis, treatment, follow-up plans, and what further care is expected of the primary care team. Terse descriptions of cancer treatment protocols are rarely adequate without further information. Similarly, the family healthcare team needs systems in place to ensure that such information is relayed to the right person in the practice with the appropriate level of urgency. When a patient is diagnosed with cancer at a hospital, the GP should be informed as soon as possible so that a member of the primary healthcare team can contact the patient to discuss the diagnosis and offer their support. This simple caring act is deeply appreciated by most patients, and is an important opportunity for the family practice to respond to the immediate concerns and questions of the patient and family. The communication skills required to elicit patients' concerns are described in Chapter 6.

Primary healthcare teams often have a good working knowledge of the patient's family and are therefore in the best position to monitor the emotional well-being of family members, especially the main carer, while offering them information and support. However, the patients' and their family's previous contact with their GP is likely to shape their expectations of their doctor's role. Unless the primary care team make it clear what they can offer, their patients may be uncertain about what to expect of them. Similarly, family doctors sometimes misinterpret why a patient is consulting them; therefore disentangling whether the patient is seeking information, support, or medical intervention is a key skill.[1]

Discharge from hospital care is often a difficult time for people with cancer, especially as many patients will not have a follow-up appointment with their hospital doctor for some weeks. There is often an alarming sense of being cast adrift from their reassuring contact with medical personnel (*see* Chapter 2—Ending Treatment). However, this feeling of separation can be softened if patients and their families are offered a follow-up appointment with their family doctor in which they can review what they have been through and be reassured that they will continue to have the support of the primary healthcare team. In this regard, patients often hugely value follow-up support from district nurses.

Patients and their families should be given the name of the person within the practice whom they can contact at short notice over the ensuing months, whether to discuss treatment options, support needs, or symptom advice. Ideally, cancer patients should have preferential access to this doctor or nurse within the practice, and as in any other area of cancer care, patients should be encouraged to report their physical (e.g. pain) and psychosocial symptoms and concerns so that they can be promptly addressed. This 'key worker' within the primary care team should keep a record and clarify to other members of the primary care team what the patient has been told and what they understand about their condition and treatment plan. Clearly, explicit communication pathways must be established to ensure that vulnerable patients can obtain information and medical support when someone else is deputizing for their nurse or doctor (i.e. during 'out-of-hours', holidays, etc.).

Members of the primary care team not only co-ordinate the patients' overall care, but are also the patient's advocates ensuring that the best possible care is obtained from hospital and other services.[2] They have a key role in helping patients and their families interpret information that has been gleaned from hospital doctors, as well as supporting them as they adjust to the many implications of their disease (*see* Chapter 2). Indeed, GPs sometimes find themselves having to break bad news that has not been effectively delivered in the hospital setting (*see* Chapter 6—Bad News). The practice, especially the district nurse, should have sound knowledge of other agencies (social care, emotional support, specialist palliative care, information resources, support groups, etc.) so that patients and their carers have easy access to supportive care services, although a comprehensive up-to-date directory of these services can be maintained on a more regional basis.

District (community) nurses and palliative care nurses, often known as Macmillan nurses in the UK, provide expert community care for the dying and are supported by highly specialized palliative care services based in hospitals or hospices. However, although community (district) nurses typically spend more time than doctors with the patient and their family, their expertise and knowledge are not always sought, and communication between nurses and doctors, at least in the past, has sometimes been characterized as deficient.[3] Similarly, some GPs tend to retain control over all aspects of their patients' care and, despite not achieving good symptom control, are reluctant to let palliative care specialists 'interfere'.[2] This again points to the need to ensure there is excellent communication and liaison between primary care and hospital services so that optimal care can be delivered to the patient and their family. More promisingly, however, GPs in the UK are continuing to diversify their skills, with many acquiring training in oncology or palliative care before becoming GPs. Finally, primary care continues to play a crucial role in the support of families whose loved one has died of cancer (*see* Bereavement Care, page 277).

Diagnosis

It takes little imagination to see that the diagnosis of cancer can be a catastrophic moment in someone's life and that the period surrounding the diagnosis of cancer is one of the most stressful times for cancer patients and their families (*see* Chapter 2—Shock of Diagnosis). In one study, over 80 per cent of women with breast cancer retrospectively rated the diagnostic period as more stressful than both the treatment phase in hospital and the period at home following it.[4] Although we discuss how best to communicate 'bad news' in Chapter 6, this section addresses other clinical issues pertaining to diagnosis.

Speed of diagnosis

There can be little doubt that waiting for test results, when one fears that the result may be cancer, is a tortuous experience. It is certainly associated with very high levels of anxiety.[5] Intuitively, one might assume that this wait should be minimized, and in the case of follow-up test results it almost certainly should. But with a first diagnosis of cancer, this 'waiting game' has been rarely studied, and the picture may not be as simple as it seems.[6]

Breast cancer offers an interesting opportunity to study how the speed of giving women their diagnosis affects them emotionally. Since the introduction of fine-needle aspiration biopsies there has been an accelerating shift in the UK towards offering same-day ('one-stop') diagnostic clinics for breast cancer. This trend has been driven more by intuitive reasoning than research evidence.[7] More traditional clinics for breast cancer continue to operate by offering a diagnosis within a recommended maximum of five days from the day on which diagnostic 'triple assessments' (physical examination, imaging, and cytology/histology) are administered. It would be important to know which type of service is psychologically preferable.

Preliminary evidence suggests that if a cancer diagnosis is made too quickly, patients may not have had sufficient time to prepare themselves for this possibility. A randomized controlled trial of 791 breast patients compared those who received the one-stop service with those having to wait an average of six days for their results.[5] In every other respect the clinics were identical. Eight weeks after their diagnosis was given, the 78 women who were diagnosed with cancer were compared. The 44 women who had had the same-day service reported significantly higher levels of depression than the 34 who were diagnosed in the delayed two-stop system.

Another study measured the levels of distress in women with breast cancer while waiting three days for their biopsy results.[7] This investigation found that the levels of anxiety when biopsies were taken were maintained over the next three days, with highly anxious women remaining anxious, and more composed women remaining calm. However, many patients who had surmised from their doctors that they had 'suspicious symptoms' appeared to use the delay as a 'preparatory period' which 'allowed them time to reflect, adapt to the prospect of having cancer, and think of questions they wished to address upon return to clinic.'[7] Qualitative studies support the value of psychological preparation time.[8]

As discussed in Chapter 1, when people are prepared for an event it is less likely to be experienced as shocking and traumatic. Yet the period of waiting for a test result is often described as tortuous. The clear benefits of a rapid diagnosis to those given an all-clear must be therefore weighed up against the need for people to prepare themselves adequately for the possibility of a cancer diagnosis. Further research is needed to ascertain the optimal balance though it is likely that it will depend on the individual.

Whatever the speed of diagnosis, there may be advantages in the patient having met a member of staff (e.g. a clinical nurse specialist) prior to the diagnosis so that, whatever the result, they have had at least some time to consider a few of the implications of the diagnosis, as well as having the chance to prepare their psychological resources, per-haps even formulate some appropriate questions and, most importantly, to have already established a supportive relationship with someone.[9] Such an approach is similar to 'pre-test counselling' which has long been used in the UK in the context of testing for HIV infection.

However, in practice there is often an understandable but unhelpful tendency for healthcare staff, from family doctors to diagnosticians, to minimize the likelihood of cancer until the diagnosis is finally given. This does little to prepare the patient who ideally needs some indication that cancer may be on the agenda. Telling the patient that the tests one is putting them through are 'very unlikely' to reveal cancer may even amplify the shock of diagnosis if cancer is subsequently found.

Eliciting key concerns

Following their diagnosis, all patients will naturally have profound concerns about their illness and treatment, their prognosis and future life, and their loved ones. These con-cerns are the subject of Chapters 2 and 3. Above all, patients and families require a clear road map of what the next few days, weeks, and months have in store for them. It should be clear from the outset whose job and responsibility it is within the healthcare team to keep patients and relatives up-to-date with the treatment plan and its implications for the patient's day-to-day life. Information allows people to prepare themselves to adjust their expectations for what is to follow. Ambiguity and lack of information leads to fear and uncertainty in a situation where there is already more than enough stress.

Research has shown that the number and severity of patients' concerns in the first few weeks after diagnosis can predict the later development of serious emotional distress like clinical anxiety and depression.[10] However, patients rarely volunteer their concerns unless prompted, and relatively few concerns are identified by healthcare staff.[11] In an Austrian study, only a third of severely distressed patients were recognized as such, while over 40% of those with major social needs were not referred to a social worker.[12] An American study found that oncologists underestimated the severity of depression in over a quarter of 'moderately' to 'severely' depressed cancer patients, but also overestimated its severity in almost 15% of cases.[13] British studies were some of the first to document the fact that healthcare staff are generally poor at identifying emotional distress in their patients.[14]

It is therefore a key psychosocial role of healthcare staff to elicit these concerns and, where possible, resolve them.[11] In the context of busy clinics, large case-loads, and other demands on doctors and nurses, this vital role is sometimes perceived as an 'extra' task which is unrealistically time-consuming. However, assessing people's principal concerns does not require the clinician to resolve them all in the clinic, even though some concerns may be dealt with quickly (for example, by providing further information). The very act of identifying key concerns has value in itself because it frequently suggests a pathway to their resolution (e.g. referral to another member of the healthcare team), and helps to shape the areas of concern into more manageable chunks. Several studies have shown that oncologists and nurses can be taught to communicate in ways that efficiently elicit their patients' concerns rather than block them.[15, 16] Communication is the subject of Chapter 6, so here we consider particular concerns associated with the early phases of treatment.

Concerns associated with early phases of treatment

Excessive fear

Many people do not like hospitals and, for some, hospitalization can represent an intolerable level of danger or uncertainty. For these patients, the normal elements of preparation for surgery, radiotherapy, or chemotherapy, described below, are insufficient to relieve their anxiety. People with a history of anxiety problems, for example, sometimes experience paralysing fear and panic in the face of surgery.[17] The fears are commonly to do with being alone in an unfamiliar place, the possibility of dying during the operation or losing control during anaesthesia. Such situations can sometimes be resolved easily if the healthcare staff are flexible; for example, if they allow a trusted relative to stay with the patient as much as possible throughout the particular treatment, or take the time to provide more information before and during clinical interventions. But excessive anxiety sometimes requires a more specific intervention before treatment can begin, such as graded exposure techniques (i.e. desensitization to needles), relaxation training, cognitive-behaviour therapy, or the use of a low-dose benzodiazepine, and these sometimes require the involvement of a psychosocial specialist. (*see* Intense Fear, page 255)

Suicide risk

The results of cancer treatment are not always predictable. Sometimes a tumour cannot be removed safely, or is found to be more widely dispersed than first thought.

Where surgery has revealed a worse clinical picture than anticipated, the surgeon will need to communicate this devastating news to patients and their families, irrevocably changing the landscape of their lives. Even after careful preoperative preparation, the patient may find themselves overwhelmed by the losses that surgery may have left them with—of a part of the body, for example, a bodily function, their appearance, their fertility, or sexual response, etc. Similarly, radiotherapy and chemotherapy may not achieve the response that oncologists and their patients had expected and this reappraisal can be hugely demoralizing and disappointing for all. Moreover, the accumulated changes in lifestyle, role, and status over the course of the illness may all contribute to a damaging sense of hopelessness and despair.

While most people eventually find a way to adjust to the very different future that lies ahead for them (*see* Chapters 1 and 2), some patients consider suicide to be a more appealing option. In our clinical experience, most people with cancer entertain the possibility of suicide at some stage but usually fleetingly. However, these thoughts merit particular concern when they are combined with feelings of hopelessness about the future and other symptoms of clinical depression and demoralization. Therefore, if a member of the healthcare staff elicits these feelings, they should enable the patient to explore them further without being afraid that the patient will act on them. On the contrary, people usually find it a relief to talk through these frightening thoughts. Where there appears to be serious suicide risk the patient should be referred to a mental health specialist (*see* Chapter 6—Working with Someone Clinically Depressed or Suicidal).

Surgery

Surgeons are invariably involved in the early stages of cancer treatment. They are very much in the 'front line', both medically and psychologically. It is often surgeons who are required to deliver the cancer diagnosis, outline the treatment plan, and care for patients at this acutely distressing phase of the illness. It is to a surgical ward that most patients are first admitted, so first we consider the emotional impact of hospital admission. Having the power to save lives, surgeons are symbolically powerful figures for patients; amidst the fear and emotional chaos caused by the diagnosis they are rightly seen as key to the patient's safety and survival.

Most people understand what cancer surgery is for and what, in principle, it involves but it is essential that patients are given as much detailed information about the operation (and type of anaesthesia) as they wish and sufficient time in which to digest it. This is especially true where there is the likelihood, or even risk, of permanent functional disability (e.g. sterility, impotence, etc.) or disfigurement. Although patients may have signed their consent to treatment, surgeons and anaesthetists who show they are receptive to questions and happy to answer them are more likely to have patients who feel safe and cared for. It is often difficult to absorb and comprehend information on hearing it for the first time, so at least two preoperative interviews are essential to enable patients and their loved ones to ask further questions and clarify their understanding.

Hospital admission

> During my stay I seemed to see so many examples of love in action, of extra care taken by the nurses. S. [a member of the catering staff], racing round making extra cups of tea for everyone, and the nurses who took the old lady opposite to the phone and set up the foot spa for her. There was also a lot to make me think – the man who was in an unconscious state at the other end of the ward when I arrived, who was gone the next day. I heard the charge nurse say he had died. D. the lady initially in the next bed who had advanced ovarian cancer and was going to St G.'s [hospice] for respite care. C., the young man with only one leg and obviously advanced cancer, but so cheerful even though he was in hospital a lot. The lovely old lady, R. who took his bed, and had a nose tube and a constant drip feeding her as her cancer was obviously very advanced.

Hospitalization can be daunting for many people, especially those who have never been in hospital before or who are unused to sleeping away from home. The stress of hospitalization involves many challenges for people with cancer (*see* Table 5.1).

A number of studies of hospital inpatients have indicated that patients are concerned about fitting in with what they think is expected of them. They also worry about whether the medical and nursing staff like them.[19] Indeed, 'difficult' or 'bad' patients are seen by nursing staff to be those who complain, are emotionally dependent on the staff, or seek to be informed and involved, while 'good' patients are seen as those who are passive and accepting.[1] In one recent survey, nurses rated patients as 'popular' if they neither complained about pain nor were anxious, while those who were in most pain or coping poorly with their pain were described as 'demanding' or 'dependent'.[20]

TABLE 5.1 Concerns regarding hospitalization

Challenge	Example
Worries about the seriousness of one's illness. Uncertainty	Will I leave here alive? Will they discover the cancer is worse than they thought?
Unfamiliarity of the hospital environment	Sleeping in the same room as strangers, unfamiliar food, ward routines
Concerns about one's home life	Loss of income, concerns about loved ones
Indignity of condition	Having to have help with bedpans, the smell of fungating tumours
Loss of control	Entrusting one's life to strangers, having to conform to ward rules and conditions
Lack of support	Lack of people to talk with, missing one's loved ones

Adapted from Volicer BJ, Isenberg MA, Burns MW. (1977).[18]

The disturbing implication from these research findings is that hospital wards may be subtly encouraging their already vulnerable patients to be passive recipients of care, rather than active collaborators in their treatment. This, in turn, may lead patients to feel increasingly helpless and dependent, and may be one of the reasons why they appear to be loathe to trouble doctors and nurses either about their levels of pain,[21] or the psychological concerns they may have.[22]

Preparation for surgery

People are understandably anxious before surgery. It is not natural to have one's body cut open by other people, so there is valid apprehension about one's safety. By contrast, the clinicians who do the cutting may regard their procedures as routine and safe, especially the more experienced surgeons.

It may seem obvious therefore that clinicians should reassure patients as to the safety of the surgery, calm them down (e.g. with relaxation training), and provide sufficient information to prevent them worrying. Yet the evidence suggests that although simple reassurance and relaxation help to reduce preoperative anxiety, making patients easier to anaesthetize, it may paradoxically also lead to an increased hormonal stress response to surgery and a greater need for analgesia after surgery.[1] The implication is that reassuring patients may enable clinicians to keep patients' distress at a distance, but may not be particularly effective at reducing their distress. Rather, it seems that people are better able to prepare themselves if they can 'work through' their fears and concerns (i.e. by putting them into words), and obtain information that is relevant to these concerns.

Information reduces distress by enabling the patient to feel a sense of control over what is about to happen to them while in hospital. Being able to anticipate what is likely to occur helps to reduce anxiety. A meta-analysis of interventions designed to prepare people for surgery found that procedural information (what is likely to happen before, during, and after the operation) and behavioural coping instructions (how the patient can best respond) were consistently and strongly associated with positive post-operative recovery.[23] Another meta-analysis found that the use of preoperative psycho-educational interventions not only reduces post-operative pain and psychological distress but also has the cost-saving advantage of patients being discharged earlier than those receiving standard care.[24]

In addition to teaching people how to manage the physiological symptoms of anxiety (e.g. relaxation training), information and explanation should be provided in response to patients' individual concerns. It must *fit* with the patient's assumptions about what is about to happen. This allows 'reassuring information' to be relevant to the actual concerns of the patient, rather than what the clinician presumes to be their concerns. Indeed, unless it is responsive to the patient's concerns, crass attempts to reassure patients can be interpreted as an insensitive *lack* of understanding.[22]

Continuity of care

The other main factor in reducing the stress of surgery is continuity of emotional support from the medical and nursing team.[25] One study found that doctors on a cancer unit were less supportive and less likely to address patients' needs than doctors treating general medical patients.[26] However, support from a specialist nurse, who meets patients before and after surgery, can reduce their emotional distress and provide continuity of care.[27] It is much easier for people to ask questions to someone they have already met than someone new, so it is helpful if the patient can communicate with the same nurse over the course of the illness.[28] Specialist nurses can provide information about what is likely to happen, what the surgery will involve, what the wound will probably look like, what the post-surgical symptoms are likely to be, what the patient can do to maximize their recovery (e.g. exercises), and the nature of any adjuvant treatment that is likely to follow. In addition to providing information, they can also respond to the concerns of the patient, correct misconceptions, and help the patient to 'work through' their worries by putting them into words and formulating a plan. By listening to and acknowledging the patient's feelings of fear, loss, and anger, doctors and nurses can reassure them that their reactions are understandable and natural, given the circumstance. The patient (and other people designated as carers by the patient) will also be reassured to know that they can continue to have contact with a particular nurse or doctor in the ensuing months, should they have further concerns.

Psychiatric drugs[17]

Where patients are taking psychotropic medication to sustain their mental health (i.e. for conditions such as schizophrenia, bi-polar affective disorder, etc.), psychiatrists may be reluctant to allow them to stop their medication for protracted periods before surgery. It is recommended therefore that psychiatrists and anaesthetists co-ordinate their care, especially when the patient has acute psychiatric symptoms, before the operation. Much of their discussion will need to weigh up the costs and benefits of maintaining or discontinuing a particular drug. For example, stopping minor tranquillizers, such as benzodiazepines, needs careful consideration to avoid provoking a severe withdrawal reaction. Some serotonin specific reuptake inhibitors (SSRIs) can continue to be taken until the day before surgery provided the anaesthetist is aware of it and can plan accordingly, but SSRI anti-depressants vary and where there is doubt a discussion between the anaesthetist and the patient's psychiatrist is advisable. Major tranquillizers carry the risk of post-operative delirium when other drugs (such as scopolamine) are used. Lithium carbonate (often used in the treatment of manic-depression) can exaggerate the effects of certain muscle relaxants but is otherwise largely safe to continue until the operation.

Focus on breast cancer

Breast cancer is the most common cancer among women. In the UK currently one in nine women will develop the disease; in 2001, 13 000 women died from breast cancer.[29] In 2003 it is estimated that 211 300 American women were diagnosed with invasive breast cancer, along with 55 700 new cases of noninvasive breast cancer.[30]

Numerous studies have demonstrated the devastating effects of breast surgery on the quality of life of women[31–33] and the relatively few men who develop it.[34] In addition to the concerns described in Chapters 2 and 3, women with breast cancer carry additional burdens. The impact of damage to the breast to a woman's sense of her femininity and identity can affect all women, but it may be most acutely threatening to younger women who have yet to establish a long-term relationship or who may wish to have children one day. For older women the presence of any cancer compounds other losses they may already be adjusting to. Most breast cancer surgery also involves the removal of the axillary lymph nodes, resulting in lymphoedema in about a quarter of all cases,[35] much of which can have a colossal and permanent impact on women's quality of life. In addition, women often care for other people and, consequently, the anguish of diagnosis may be as much to do with concern for their dependents as it is with their own personal survival. However, their nurturing position within the family can lead to ambivalence about obtaining support from others (see Chapter 3).

Sexual and relationship difficulties can also affect women of any age (see Chapter 3—Sexual Problems), though in younger women these may be the result of an early menopause. Destruction of the ovaries (female castration) can have a positive impact on survival in those with hormone dependent cancers. However, an early menopause can also be the result of systemic chemotherapy given to patients whose cancers are not hormone dependent (though the cessation of periods may produce no benefit unless the cancer is hormone sensitive). The physical and psychological side-effects of an early menopause can be devastating, particularly for those women who want to have further children, or even just one child. Hot flushes can result in broken nights and poor sleep for patients and sometimes their partners, and potentially cause more distress than the loss of a breast[36] (see Chapter 3—The Menopause). Unfortunately, young people who have developed breast cancer and whose treatment has involved an early menopause sometimes see taking hormone replacement therapy as too dangerous, regardless of the real risks involved.[37]

Research supports the value of trained breast care specialist nurses in preventing the development of psychosocial problems,[27] though concern has been expressed that relatively few nurses in the UK who offer counselling to their oncology patients have acquired appropriate counselling qualifications and less than half receive formal supervision.[38] The use of an 'advocacy' style of nurse counsellor intervention, in which the nurse prepares the patient for the consultation with the surgeon by developing a list of questions she would like to ask, also offers promise as a model of nursing support.[39]

Mastectomy versus breast conservation

> Today, I decided to wash my bra. Before putting it to soak, I had to take the prosthesis I am now wearing out of the little extra pocket in the left cup. As I fingered this warm false gelatinous tit with its fake nipple, I took a sudden violent dislike to it. I can't imagine ever getting used to the sight of my missing breast.

Breast cancer treatment has changed rapidly over the past two decades. Surgical techniques that conserve as much of the breast as possible (wide local excision or 'lumpectomies') have been shown to be as safe as mastectomy for the majority of women. Lumpectomies were also expected to reduce the psychological impact of losing an entire breast. However, the many studies that have compared the psychosocial outcome of women treated by mastectomy or lumpectomy have fairly consistently found little difference between the two techniques in terms of either psychological well-being or sexual functioning.[40] The one consistent difference that these studies did identify was that women receiving lumpectomies reported fewer body image problems than those receiving a mastectomy,[41] though it has been speculated that this advantage may be offset by these women being more concerned about the cancer recurring in the preserved part of their breast.[42]

A more recent meta-analysis of 40 studies[43] has suggested that, due to methodological problems (especially the methods of assignment to one treatment or the other), many of these studies may have masked the positive effects of breast-conserving surgery. These advantages, albeit modest, include psychological and social adjustment to cancer, and marital and sexual functioning. The meta-analysis confirmed the strong advantage of lumpectomies where body image is concerned but also, contradicting earlier speculation, that breast conservation gave a small but significant advantage as regards cancer-related fears. Thus, it may be that patients' and professionals' early doubts about the safety of lumpectomies are beginning to be put to rest. (*see* Chapter 6—Consent, Collaboration, and Choice)

Breast reconstruction

Reconstructive surgery, which involves a range of surgical procedures designed to recreate a breast shape, is adopted by roughly 30% of American, but as yet only between 5% and 10% of UK women who have had a mastectomy.[44] Techniques vary between inserting artificial implants (e.g. silicone) or tissue from other parts of the body, including the lat-dorsi procedure, and the transverse rectus abdominis myocutaneous (TRAM) flap procedure.

Whatever the procedure, the surgery is usually long and often involves several operations to achieve a satisfactory outcome. The result may visually approximate a normal breast but it has neither the sensation nor function of a normal breast. However, for those who have had a reconstruction, more than 80% in one study reported they were pleased with it. It was those who had had especially high expectations of the reconstruction, or who were having it to please others, who were most at risk of disappointment.[45] Reconstruction does not result in such high patient satisfaction or cosmetic outcome as breast conserving surgery, but it has been found to be preferable to mastectomy alone in one recent retrospective study.[46] For those women requiring a mastectomy, or for those who opt for one rather than a lumpectomy, the offer of breast reconstruction should always be made if at all possible.

What is less clear is whether the breast reconstruction should be immediate or delayed.[44] Should reconstruction optimally occur during the operation to remove the cancer, or are there advantages in delaying reconstruction until after the woman has completed any adjuvant treatment she is required to have? The stressful preoperative period is hardly the best time for anyone to be making such important decisions, dominated as it is by the overarching wish to survive; indeed, with quicker diagnoses for breast cancer there is a danger that women have insufficient time in which to make an informed decision. For many years it was felt that if a woman was given sufficient time to grieve for her lost breast, she would be able to incorporate more readily the reconstructed breast into her body image. However, the advantages of immediate reconstruction include improved cost-effectiveness, speedier recovery and reduced inconvenience for the patient, and a request for immediate reconstruction is now thought to indicate positive adjustment to the diagnosis, at least in the immediate post-operative period.[32] Further research on this topic, however, is needed.

Focus on head and neck cancers

Head and neck cancers represent some of the most psychologically devastating forms of the disease. In addition to all the psychological and social concerns described in Chapter 2, people with head and neck cancers often face severe impairments affecting some of the most deep-seated assumptions of normal life: the ability to speak, see, smell, taste, and hear clearly. The quality of a person's life is profoundly undermined when their ability to communicate with other people, or to enjoy a meal, is impaired or destroyed. Even where the ability to speak is intact, emotional expression can be limited as a result of surgery to the facial muscles, while changes to the voice can limit the individual's capacity to signal emotion.

Advances in non-surgical forms of treatment, reconstructive surgery, and improved prostheses have greatly reduced the extent of disfigurements and loss of function, but head and neck cancers continue to present many people with huge challenges in terms of psychosocial adjustment. The treatment itself is commonly long and unpleasant, frequently involving several operations and many adjuvant treatments. The impact of surgery is a function of how much disfigurement and motor and sensory damage the patient is left with,[17] as well as other long-term physical symptoms such as bleeding, dry mouth, coughing, hoarseness, nasal discharge, pain, and fatigue.[47]

Unlike other cancers, the disease and its treatment can leave patients with facial disfigurements that are all too clearly visible. The patient must adjust not only their own image of themselves, they must also adjust to other people's reactions to them. Facial disfigurements leave people feeling like social outcasts. Their deformity causes other people to be shocked by their difference, and socially awkward as to how to behave in their presence. Should the deformity be acknowledged? When should it be spoken about? Inevitably, social awkwardness leads to avoidance. Head and neck cancer patients are at a higher risk of suicide than other cancer patients;[48] and social withdrawal is common with some patients becoming highly reclusive.[47] Even medically cured head and neck patients have been shown to have significant psychological distress seven to eleven years after treatment.[49]

However, the severity of disfigurements does not always equate to the level of distress experienced by the patient, so healthcare staff must be wary lest they appear to trivialize the impact of a 'minor' disfigurement.[50] Interventions focus on helping people with facial disfigurements understand and handle the reaction of other people through social interaction skills training. In doing so they develop a repertoire of positive social skills (e.g. quickly putting other people at their ease, learning to present themselves, communicating with confidence, etc.).[51] By monitoring and adjusting their own reactions, and learning to value themselves once more, patients' self-esteem can improve. Specialist groups, workshops, leaflets, books, and videos can also help to normalize people's reactions to their disfigurement and to obtain emotional support during their social and personal adjustment.

Eating and drinking are social activities as much as biological ones. Having a meal with others is a form of social cement that is shared by people from every culture in the world. When people lose their ability to swallow and eat using their mouths they also potentially lose access to this important form of social contact. People may choose to eat on their own rather than 'inflict' themselves on their loved ones, or because they wish to preserve their dignity. Similarly, carers may feel it cruel and insensitive to eat in front of patients with eating and swallowing difficulties and, as a result, may ignore their own needs for adequate nutrition. Open discussions with the patient and family members may help to clarify and resolve these concerns.

Although many people with head and neck cancers have a history of heavy tobacco and alcohol use, this is not true of all patients. An assessment of these premorbid factors may be important for rehabilitation, reducing further health risks, and in order to prevent severe nicotine- and alcohol withdrawal symptoms. However, it is essential that, in addition to the enormous physical and psychosocial challenges facing them, people with head and neck cancers do not face discrimination or prejudice from healthcare staff who may regard them as having brought the cancer upon themselves. Some of these patients may already be suffering intense self-blame and guilt. In this regard, signs of self-neglect, non-compliance with medical care, and loss of motivation may indicate depression and should therefore always be investigated further.

What can healthcare staff do beyond providing medical care and expertise?

- Acknowledge the often massive psychosocial challenges facing the patient;
- guide patients regarding appropriate rehabilitation strategies (e.g. encouraging patients to look at and care for their surgical wounds);
- provide a 'secure base', a person with whom patients can express their distress, and explore and practise ways of reintegrating into the social world. The backup of speech and language therapists, audiologists, specialist head and neck nurses and dieticians, as well as psychosocial specialists is essential;
- consider specialist interventions such as social interaction skills training;
- in view of the distressing nature of supportive care for people with head and neck cancers, it has been recommended that healthcare staff working in this area particularly require support for themselves[47] (*see* Chapter 7).

Communication in the context of speech difficulties

- Do not be embarrassed to ask the individual to repeat what they have said. They would probably prefer to say it again and be understood, rather than for others to pretend to understand.
- After a couple of attempts at understanding, suggest to the person with a speech difficulty that they say it another way, using different words which may be easier to articulate, or write it down, spell it out, or use pictures and gestures.
- Give people time to speak and do not finish sentences for them.
- People with speech problems are not deaf so do not raise your voice.
- If an individual is using an artificial larynx or 'voice-box' on the telephone they may wish to alert the listener to this fact to avoid them assuming it is a hoax call. They could say: 'My voice may sound like a robot because I have to use a machine to talk to you'.
- By openly acknowledging their problems, people with head and neck cancers can often pre-empt the social awkwardness of others. 'You may have noticed that my voice sounds a bit strange (that I dribble when I speak ...). This is because ... ' It is of course up to the individual how much detail they wish to convey about their problems.
- Other people, including family members, may worry that it is painful or tiring for the person with a speech problem to speak, so they therefore avoid making unnecessary conversation or asking questions. This can result in the individual feeling increasingly isolated and frustrated. It is always preferable to ask the person concerned whether speaking is tiring or uncomfortable.

Focus on ostomies

The impact of colostomies and urostomies on body image and normal daily living has attracted relatively little research yet can sometimes cause overwhelming distress. Any important change to the body usually leads to an emotionally painful adjustment but this is even more pronounced where there is also a change in how the body functions (*see* Chapter 2—The Body). The diversion of faecal and urinary waste into a visible bag contravenes most people's assumptions of cleanliness and dignity. Even when they are able to be reversed, urostomies and colostomies require patients to learn a number of practical skills connected with cleanliness, how to cope with accidents and what clothes to wear, as well as having to endure occasional pain or discomfort. Moreover patients must learn to manage their ostomies in the context of their partners and families, at best a socially difficult process. For some it can remain a continuing source of loss.

> Grief amounting to bereavement still surrounds my attitude to my colostomy. I have found it hard to come to terms with my altered body image and the outward scarring.

The limited research on the psychological impact of stomas indicates that surgery results in significant distress in just under a quarter of patients.[52] People who believe that they are no longer complete people, that the stoma rules their lives, and that they are no longer in control over their body, are particularly at risk for post-operative distress.[53] Preoperative information and discussion, using simple diagrams, is critically important in preparing patients for what will be involved in living with an ostomy. Discussing possible sexual difficulties and concerns is especially helpful and where there is a partner, they should ideally be involved too. A visit by a trained ex-patient who has learned to manage their ostomy can also be helpful and informative to patients before surgery.[54]

> The nursing staff were wonderful: the Stoma Care Nurses gave me all the advice, support and encouragement I needed to learn to deal with my sudden colostomy. The doctors were also very supportive, especially the Senior Registrar, a lady who visited me almost every day and whose sympathy and empathy helped me through some of my low moments.

Focus on CNS tumours

Compared with other disease sites, cancers of the central nervous system (CNS) are rare, though most show a steep decline from diagnosis to palliative care. While primary brain tumours rarely metastasize to other parts of the body, between 25 and 45 per cent of brain tumours are secondary cancers, with lung cancer being a common primary.[55] The majority of adult primary brain tumours occur in the glial cells and are known as gliomas, while the majority of these gliomas arise from astrocytes, the cells supporting neurones. These astrocytomas vary in their malignancy (classified as 'high grade' or 'low grade') with the most aggressive type being referred to as a glioblastoma multiforme (GBM). The outlook for most people with CNS tumours is poor and among those people with a glioblastoma the two-year survival rate is only around 5 to 10 per cent,[56] though younger patients generally survive longer than older ones.

Central nervous system disease can result from …

1. primary brain tumours (astrocytomas, meningiomas),
2. damage of the spinal cord by impingement from adjacent secondary cancers in the spine (primaries in this area are rare, but secondaries are common);
3. brain metastases (e.g. from primaries in the lung, melanoma, breast, etc.) or
4. treatment complications (e.g. corticosteroids, brain radiation, etc.).

Treatment for CNS tumours commonly involves a combination of surgery (where possible), radiotherapy and chemotherapy (in the case of brain metastases whole brain radiation is common). Steroids (glucocorticoids) are often used in the treatment of CNS tumours, whether primary or metastatic, and may be administered in very high doses.[55]

CNS tumours can cause progressive damage to a person's personality, motor functions (loss of mobility can lead to other medical complications), and cognitive abilities (including language), as well as other unpleasant and potentially dangerous symptoms such as fits (seizures). The measures taken to treat these symptoms can also have harmful effects on the individual. Whole brain radiation may lead to organic mental syndromes involving tiredness, somnolence, headaches, nausea, and vomiting; while taking steroids can result in substantial weight gain, especially causing a round face, or Cushingoid faces, which can alter the appearance dramatically. Fluid retention and weak muscles (proximal myopathy, causing difficulty particularly in climbing stairs) often result, as well as hypomania, more commonly depression and sometimes psychotic symptoms such as delusions and hallucinations.[55] In the context of such wholesale personal disintegration, it is little wonder that many people who experience these adverse effects become anxious, hopeless, and depressed.

Cognitive assessment

Careful specialist assessment is necessary to disentangle the symptoms and causes of delirium, dementia, and depression (see Table 5.2), all of which are common among people with CNS tumours. Withdrawal, for example, may be a symptom of depression or delirium but other features can help distinguish these conditions. Assessment can be further complicated as delirium can occur in the context of dementia and/or depression. (*see* Chapter 6—Working with Someone Acutely Confused or Cognitively Impaired).

Table 5.2 Differentiating delirium, dementia, and depression

Delirium	Dementia	Depression
Often rapid onset	Gradual onset	Variable onset
Decreased awareness, disorientation for time and place	Little clouding of consciousness	Normal awareness
Sleepiness	Usually alert	Sleep disturbance
Withdrawal	Possible withdrawal	Withdrawal common
Poor concentration and memory	Impairment of intellect, memory, or language Concentration can be impaired	No frank cognitive deficits though concentration is often impaired
Tearfulness, agitation, restlessness, emotional lability	Little general mood disturbance	Hopelessness, despair, self-blame and self-criticism, or helplessness

The effect of CNS cancers on patients and their families is profound. For those who have been successfully coping with a primary cancer in some other part of the body, the emergence of brain secondaries is shattering and frightening. Both they and those suffering with a primary CNS tumour face the combination of a poor prognosis with the uncertainty of not knowing how the tumour will affect them. Fears of loss of control, dignity, and the ability to communicate are common and understandable. The burden patients anticipate placing on family members can feel intolerable, leading to thoughts of suicide. Although the family may be willing to assume it, this encumbrance is very real and the family is rarely prepared for the months ahead. Levels of distress, exhaustion, and frustration among family members are thus high. This is especially true where there are communication difficulties which can result in isolation for both the patient and the family.

Rehabilitation

As many brain cancers are associated with progressive functional decline in any area, the focus of rehabilitation efforts must be flexible and respond to frequent reassessments of the patient's changing disability and prognosis. In response to rehabilitation programs, patients with brain tumours have been shown to make gains that are comparable to those made by people with traumatic brain injury or stroke.[57] Rehabilitation efforts focus on mobility, activities of daily living (hygiene, dressing, and self-care), neuropathic bowel and bladder management, skin care, and pain management (*see* Rehabilitation).

Although the use of psychotropic medication, especially neuroleptics, for neuro-oncology patients may be helpful, their use can be complicated by existing damage to the brain caused by both the tumour and its treatment.[55] Psychosocial and rehabilitation care should also be considered. Apart from providing helpful emotional support, an effective therapist can …

- help patients learn problem-solving techniques;
- normalize the patient's reactions to their illness;
- prepare the patient for the likely course of the disease;
- teach psychological techniques of symptom relief (e.g. relaxation in pain relief);
- teach patients to use memory aids such as lists and calendars, as well as visual and auditory prompts to enhance their ability to attend to details; (cognitive retraining);
- encourage the use of memory prostheses (e.g. carrying a notebook around, visual reminders around the home, etc.);
- find alternative methods of communication (e.g. some patients unable to speak may still be able to sing or whisper);
- support patients preparing for their death (e.g. eliciting their wishes regarding resuscitation, the funeral, writing their will, etc.).[55]

Radiotherapy

Radiotherapy is given to about 40% of people with cancer yet despite it being a common treatment, the public continue to regard it with fear and suspicion.[58] Radiotherapy is commonly used as an adjunct to surgery (adjuvant radiotherapy) or as a palliative measure, but it can also be deployed as the primary treatment for some cancers, including Hodgkin's disease, throat cancer, and prostate cancer. It is used in emergencies (e.g. for the treatment of spinal cord compression) or, more rarely, prophylactically (e.g. for the prevention of brain metastases in the context of small cell lung cancer).

There are two main modes of radiotherapy delivery: external beam radiotherapy (teletherapy) and brachytherapy where the radiation source (a radioactive isotope) is implanted within the body (e.g. vagina) as close to the tumour as possible. The latter usually involves hospital isolation and can last for several hours or days, while the former generally lasts a few seconds but may range between a single treatment to treatments which are delivered daily over two or three weeks, but sometimes up to six or even seven weeks.

Radiotherapy departments are often under pressure to treat as many patients in as short a time as possible. Efficiency, however, can compromise the quality of patient care when it is taken too far. Radiotherapy, especially when given over several weeks, can have far-reaching consequences for a patient's personal and social life (e.g. home-management responsibilities).[59] Radiographers (radiation therapists) have daily contact with their patients and are therefore ideally placed to develop a caring and supportive relationship that can have a major impact on the patient's overall adjustment. Preparation for radiotherapy is as important as regular monitoring of the patient's current physical, psychological, and social concerns. Likewise, the end of radiotherapy often rekindles feelings of uncertainty about the future; it is therefore helpful to prepare patients for the end of treatment and to use this opportunity to reassess their psychosocial needs.

Preparation for radiotherapy

The importance of clear information about radiotherapy and chemotherapy cannot be overstated. The public generally harbour intense dread towards these treatments. The word 'radiation' is associated with atomic warfare, radioactive fall-out, and accidents at nuclear power stations. Some of the public's fears about radiotherapy may simply be very out-dated (e.g. that radiotherapy is only used for the palliation of symptoms,[60] or is a desperate measure used in hopeless cases). Other fears may have substance but are overstated (e.g. that radiotherapy causes cancer as well as cures it; that radiotherapy inevitably causes skin burning). Indeed, the use of plastic moulds to immobilize the patient's head during radiotherapy (especially in head and neck cancers) can cause anxiety in many and severe claustrophobia in a few (see Intense Fear), so special care must be taken to prepare patients for what is to come. But the most common source of anxiety is likely to be fear of the unknown.

As with surgery, information about radiotherapy should always start with the patient's pre-existing assumptions and fears, rather than what the clinician presumes these concerns to be. Only after the clinician has elicited the patient's understanding and initial concerns about radiotherapy should further information be offered. Radiotherapy patients primarily need information about how the treatment works and what side-effects they may expect, given their particular treatment. It is essential that the possible long-term consequences (e.g. oedema, skin changes, etc.) are clearly explained before radiotherapy begins, and other related treatments (e.g. restorative dentistry for people with head and neck cancers) are planned and discussed from the outset.

Preparing patients for radiotherapy enables them to feel more in control and involved, and less apprehensive about the unknown.[61] Although levels of anxiety usually decrease rapidly once the treatment has begun, the first appointment is one of high anxiety for most patients.[62] Patients will be left alone, under a huge intimidating treatment machine, in a room that frequently contains nothing that is reassuringly familiar. Simple steps to make the room more 'friendly' can include the use of curtains, pictures, and music, while a short tour of the room prior to treatment can help orientate people and enable staff to respond to their concerns and questions. A sound system that enables patients to continue to communicate with radiographers outside the treatment room might also benefit particularly anxious patients.

Although in the UK, for example, there appears to be sufficient written information about radiotherapy available within treatment settings, not enough of it is available in languages appropriate to local communities.[63] Preparatory booklets have been shown to reduce anxiety in radiotherapy patients,[64] though written information is usually very general and offers a poor substitute for face-to-face explanations given by doctors and radiographers.[65] Unlike surgery, most people have little understanding of radiotherapy or what it will be like to experience treatment. Not everyone find reading easy and, for some, it may seem too technical and daunting to have to read about how radiotherapy works.

People appreciate having a simple, reassuring model explained to them, backed up with written information. Simply stating that radiotherapy kills cancer cells is less helpful than explaining that:

- the body is made up of cells;
- cancer cells are more sensitive than normal cells to (ionizing) radiation;
- radiotherapy destroys the ability (i.e. damage to the DNA) of cancer cells to reproduce (i.e. mitosis);
- whereas normal cells can repair this damage, cancer cells cannot, so that giving daily radiotherapy over a number of weeks results in the cancer cells accumulating damage until they are completely destroyed, whereas most normal cells will recover.

This simple model can be rephrased in many ways, using a vocabulary that is appropriate to the patient. The essential point is that having a model allows people to imagine how their treatment is working and thus feel more in control over what they are going through. The use of information videos, which the patient and family can review at home, can be helpful in this respect.[66]

Information recall is generally poor when information is given to people under stress, so explanations and information should be ideally offered on more than one occasion; for example, by the oncologist and also by the radiographer (radiation therapist). A recent study found that, of 100 patients undergoing radiotherapy who had given their written consent to receive the treatment, a quarter could not remember being told of the side-effects and of those who did remember, half were unable to remember the most frequent side effect (fatigue).[67] Thus brief pretreatment, mid-treatment, and end-of-treatment interviews conducted by radiographers ensure that patients acquire as much information about their treatment and its side-effects as they wish (backed up with written information), and that emerging physical and psychosocial concerns are addressed as soon as possible.

Main areas of radiotherapy information

- orientation to the radiotherapy department
- information provided by oncologists or radiographers on how the treatment works and how it is administered, the aims of the treatment, short- and long-term side-effects, etc.;
- written information, video information, and audiotape information reproduced in languages appropriate to the community served by the hospital;

- pre-, mid- and end-of-treatment assessments conducted by radiographers to assess physical and psychosocial concerns;
- continuity of contact with the treatment team as required after the treatment has ended (e.g. thereby giving patients the opportunity to ask questions about management of side-effects etc.).

Side-effects of radiotherapy

Clinicians may be familiar with the common side-effects of radiotherapy, but few patients will know what to expect unless they are told. People with cancer are continually trying to make sense of their bodily experiences and may therefore believe that some symptoms are caused by their radiotherapy when, in fact, they are not, or that other symptoms are attributable to extraneous factors, such as disease progression, when they are more likely to be caused by radiotherapy.[68] Thus, providing detailed information about side-effects is essential if misattributions are to be avoided.

In the past, information about possible side-effects has been withheld, based on the rationale that it may provoke impressionable patients to perceive symptoms where none exists, or cause patients to fear the treatment is not working if they do not experience a particular side effect. Such a position is not tenable if adequate support and information are made available.

The side-effects of radiotherapy will depend on the site, dose, and volume of treated area. Tissues that involve rapidly dividing cells (e.g. skin, hair follicles, lining of the intestine) are more vulnerable to immediate damage.[69] Fatigue, nausea, and weight loss are common though early attention to these side-effects by both staff and patient can minimize the likelihood that longer-term problems will develop.

Nausea is likely in patients receiving total-body radiation or radiotherapy to the abdomen. The cause is thought to be the release of serotonin in the gut when intestinal mucosal cells are damaged.[69] Conditioned nausea (i.e. learned through association) can also occur. While anti-emetic medication is often helpful in treating nausea, conditioned nausea can be overcome by the short-term use of a minor tranquillizer or relaxation training (*see* Common Treatment Difficulties—Nausea).

Certainly, the after-effects of radiotherapy can be long-lasting. Fibrosis of the treated area is a typical long-term side effect of radiotherapy. In one study, over half the breast cancer patients who had completed radiotherapy an average of eight years earlier reported that their irradiated breast felt firmer and harder than their other breast, thicker-skinned or especially sensitive.[33] Sexual difficulties are common following a number of cancer treatments (*see* Chapter 3—Sexual Problems), and permanent sterility can result from radiotherapy to the genital area.

The role of radiographers

Radiographers (radiation therapists) are highly trained in the physics of radiotherapy, radiation safety, and therapeutic applications of radiation. They have traditionally played an important, if undervalued, role in supporting patients through their treatment. Radiographers frequently have daily contact with their patients over many weeks and thereby have the potential to develop strong therapeutic relationships with them. This unique perspective enables radiographers to assess changes in their patients' mood over time, as well as the cumulative effect of radiation fatigue and other side-effects of radiotherapy.

Despite its potential, the radiographer's role as a source of emotional support goes largely unrecognized and undocumented, and consequently there seems to be considerable variation in practice. Pretreatment preparation interviews should be used not only to convey information about radiotherapy (including a simple explanation of how it works) and as an opportunity for patients to ask questions, but also to assess the patient's current psychosocial concerns. This assessment does not require an excessive amount of time and should be repeated mid-way through treatment as well as towards the end of radiotherapy when, additionally, patients may need preparation for the conclusion of their cancer treatment (*see* Chapter 6—Conducting a Patient-Centred Clinical Interview). Unfortunately, as a result of pressures on greater throughput radiographers too often lack the time to have meaningful conversations with their patients, let alone assess their personal and social needs.

Focus on pelvic radiation

> Radiotherapy caused fragility of my perineal skin, and vaginal stenosis made intercourse at first impossible, and later painful. I used a vaginal dilator for 2 years; now I occasionally experience discomfort, and sensations which I thought had gone forever are returning.

Intracavitary radiotherapy, or brachytherapy, for gynaecological cancers (e.g. of the cervix) involves women spending up to three days in an isolated hospital room, after an applicator has been inserted into their vagina and loaded with radioactive pellets. This is a difficult and challenging treatment for anyone because the patient is required to remain in one position for an extended period of time, causing intense discomfort and pain. It is not surprising that most patients find this form of treatment highly unpleasant and anxiety-provoking.

Brachytherapy can lead to radiation damage to the rectal wall and bladder. It is often given with external pelvic radiation which can lead to nausea, vomiting, and diarrhoea, while vaginal dryness is currently considered an inevitable consequence of treatment.[56] Changes to bladder function can include higher levels of pain, greater 'frequency' of urination and leakage,[70] as well as sexual difficulties, often only becoming apparent many months after treatment has been completed. Once again, careful preparation of the patient for the treatment and likely side-effects is essential. Although realistic information about the impending treatment may initially raise anxiety levels, the patient's fear can be abated if healthcare staff explain clearly what can be done to palliate any discomfort and difficulties, and how the patient can continue to exercise some measure of control over their needs (e.g. by using a call button beside the bed).

- Staff caring for women undergoing intracavitary radiotherapy should ensure that the patient has adequate pain control.

- Patients should be actively encouraged to report any pain and reassured that they will be regularly monitored.

- Sufficient distracting entertainment should be available to help patients pass the time.

- Preparatory relaxation training can help people cope with feelings of claustrophobia, and a regular schedule of visits by staff can reassure patients that they have not been abandoned.

- Every patient who has received pelvic radiation should be provided with a vaginal dilator (regardless of whether or not she has a sexual partner) and taught how to use it to maintain a healthy vagina.[70] Follow-up care should include an assessment of the effects of treatment on the individual's sexuality (see Chapter 3—Sexual Problems) and detailed information about self care.

Chemotherapy and hormone therapy

Of all the cancer treatments, drug therapy is the most notoriously challenging for patients. Chemotherapy treatments are frequently long and associated with noxious side-effects, a combination which can indeed have a destructive impact on people's mood, quality of life, and even family income. Not surprizingly, most patients approach chemotherapy with considerable anxiety and this can have the effect of exacerbating some of its side-effects; moreover, as we will see, some symptoms may even be sustained by psychological processes.

But if chemotherapy and hormone therapies are handled well by those providing them, and patients undergoing these treatments are adequately prepared and supported, most of what were sometimes intolerable side-effects are no longer excessively noxious to most people. And the performance of many of these treatments is better than ever.

During the past fifty years the advent of new chemotherapies, with or without other forms of anti-cancer treatment, has led to dramatic improvements in the treatment of a number of cancers, including acute childhood leukaemia, Hodgkin's lymphoma, and testicular cancers. Although cytotoxic drugs can be given on their own (e.g. for Hodgkin's disease), more often they are used as an adjunct to surgery and radiotherapy, either given before ('neoadjuvantly') or after ('adjuvantly') these other treatments.

They are also used to prolong survival (e.g. for small-cell lung cancer, stage IV breast cancer), and as palliative treatments (e.g. for large-cell lung cancer).[71]

Chemotherapy is beneficial only if it is more toxic to malignant cells than to normal cells, so treatments are given in cycles that are carefully timed to enable normal cells to recover before the next treatment. Cytotoxic drugs are often given in combination, the main rationale being to reduce innate or acquired drug resistance. By combining different drugs, each of which has its own toxicity profile, and using them at slightly lower doses than if they were given singly, the clinician can reduce the probability that any particular toxicity will become intolerable and prohibitive.[56]

Hormone drugs are given to patients whose tumours are sensitive to endocrine changes, and may be taken for five years or even longer. They are generally less toxic and better tolerated although this should not be overstated. Hormone therapies often have more subtle side-effects than cytotoxic treatments but they can still have a major impact on an individual's quality of life.

Cytotoxic and hormone drugs are systemic treatments that can cause widespread side-effects. Despite the advent of more effective treatments for some of these side-effects (e.g. the use of $5HT_3$ anti-emetics), the costs to the individual in terms of suffering may sometimes outweigh the benefits (e.g. prolonged survival) in cases where the cancer is incurable. This conflict may result in significant ethical and communication challenges for clinicians as they negotiate with patients to achieve the optimal balance between the quantity and quality of life.

Preparation for chemotherapy

> At the moment am progressing well and to date no news of when my chemo may start, the first treatment of which I am looking to with some apprehension. Once I know just how I'll react, then I'll be able to know how to deal with it, but it really is fear of the unknown.

In general, people with cancer are more likely than people without cancer to choose aggressive chemotherapy treatments with little chance of benefit.[72] However, unless they are provided with more authoritative information, patients will make treatment decisions based on public expectations and fears about chemotherapy, rather than on up-to-date facts.[73] For example, the public continues to associate chemotherapy with intolerable and unremitting nausea and vomiting yet modern anti-emetics are considerably more effective than they were even a decade ago. Drug treatments are often seen as experimental rather than standard treatment and consequently patients and families may have concerns about being used as 'guinea pigs'.[71] Sadly, some patients refuse even to begin chemotherapy, or, if they do, subsequently fail to continue with it.[74]

Since the prospect of chemotherapy is likely to elicit any number of common fears, clinicians should start by exploring the patient's understanding of the treatment in question and the nature of chemotherapy generally. In offering information, health-care staff should:

- provide a simple model of how chemotherapy works and explain that it is a systemic treatment designed to detect and destroy cancer cells;

- explain that there are many different types of chemotherapy but the one being offered is chosen because of the individual's particular disease, while the dose will be calculated according to the patient's weight, body mass, etc.; point out the advantages of the particular drug you have chosen, and the extent and cause of its side-effects;

- inform the patient that there are different methods of administration, given by highly trained nurses or doctors, and how and where the patient's own treatment will be administered;

- explain how long and how often the patient will have to have the treatment (i.e. a clear treatment calendar);

- explain why the patient must attend pre-assessment clinics (i.e. to check blood for an adequate number of *red cells* which protect against anaemia, *white cells* which deal with infection, and *platelets* which deal with clotting); explain why the patient should avoid infection and what to do if the patient develops an infection between appointments;

- describe probable side-effects and offer an explanation of interventions (e.g. anti-emetics) that can be used to remedy them;

- provide a description of nausea-prevention measures: e.g. drinking lots of fluid before treatment; drinking soda water or weak tea, eating ginger, or sucking on ice cubes or water-based ice-creams during and after treatment, and avoiding rich or fatty foods;

- stress the fact that patients on toxic chemotherapy pose no risk to other people;

- emphasize the importance of recruiting the help and support of other people over the course of the treatment, while attempting to maintain a normal lifestyle whenever possible;

- provide rehabilitation strategies, such as graded exercise to overcome fatigue, although written rehabilitation information also needs to be delivered towards the end of treatment;

- offer patients psychological techniques for managing the side-effects of chemotherapy. For example, some people find it helpful to visualize the chemotherapy working its way round the body destroying cancer cells (e.g. flushing out cells like a cleaning fluid, coating them with poison or other more violent imagery). In this way, people are often able to reappraise their side-effects in a more positive light, making them easier to endure.

There is good evidence that people with cancer rarely initiate a discussion about their worries with healthcare staff so during the preparation interview the patient should be invited (though in no way pressured), to share any fears and concerns they may have about chemotherapy (*see* Chapter 6—Eliciting Concerns). It is essential that all concerns are acknowledged and responded to with care. The prospect of a long, toxic, and debilitating treatment not only interferes with many aspects of the individual's life, but also impacts on family members and the financial security of the family (*see* Chapters 2 and 3).

Occasionally, people will admit to a phobia about needles and, where this fear is pronounced, the patient should be referred to a clinical psychologist or specially trained counsellor for a course of systematic desensitization (*see* Intense Fears). In view of widespread fears about chemotherapy, most patients will benefit from some form of relaxation training prior to the start of their treatment and, ideally, this should be offered as a routine part of the chemotherapy service. A recent meta-analysis[75] of 15 studies, examining the effectiveness of relaxation training among cancer patients undergoing non-surgical treatments, found a small but significant effect size indicating that relaxation prior to treatment can reduce side-effects such as nausea and pain. It also had positive effects on levels of depression and anxiety.

One randomized controlled study[76] has shown that a more extensive programme to prepare people for chemotherapy can reduce patients' distress and nausea before their chemotherapy treatment, and diminish the frequency of post-treatment vomiting, both immediately and later at home. The programme involved (a) a tour of the oncology clinic, (b) a videotape presentation of a patient coping with chemotherapy, (c) a question-and-answer session, and (d) a booklet summarizing what had been presented during the tour.

Side-effects of chemotherapy and hormone therapy

Cytotoxic drugs work throughout the entire body system. Like radiotherapy, they interfere with various stages of cell division and thus preferentially affect rapidly dividing cells, such as those found in a malignant tumour. But they also damage rapidly dividing normal cells such as bone marrow, hair follicles, and cells lining the stomach and mouth, giving rise to some of the most common side-effects of chemotherapy: reduced immune function, fatigue, hair loss, nausea, vomiting, diarrhoea and constipation, sore mouth, and the development of learned food aversions. In addition, chemotherapy is associated with premature menopause, weight loss and weight gain, anxiety, depression, irritability, sleeping difficulties, infertility, peripheral neuropathy, and sexual problems.

Many of these problems are underreported in both clinical literature and practice and only become evident when formal evaluations of quality of life are made.[74] Nausea and fatigue are considered to be the most oppressive side-effects of chemotherapy and are discussed separately below (See Common Treatment Difficulties) though they are not unrelated to one another and it has been argued that the treatment of nausea may help reduce fatigue.[77] The cognitive side-effects of chemotherapy appear to be rarely discussed with patients, yet many people given chemotherapy complain of concentration difficulties, often well after active treatment has finished. Cognitive symptoms should be monitored for possible neurotoxicity, especially when drugs such as interferon are used. Vincristine, cisplatin, paclitaxel, docetaxel, and many other agents can cause sensory, motor, and/or autonomic neuropathies.

The effect of hair loss can be an abhorrent and demoralizing prospect for a number of people. While baldness in men is socially acceptable, it is considerably less so in women. Some women choose to refuse chemotherapy rather than lose their hair. It is important to enable such women to articulate and explore the basis of their fears, and acquire a sense of control over their loss (i.e. encouraging women to have their hair cut short before treatment begins). Voluntary organizations, especially those run by ex-patients such as *HeadStart* in the UK which provides advice on headwear, may be especially valuable in normalizing and supporting women facing hair loss. The now international *Look Good... Feel Better* programme provides cosmetic advice that often helps restore women's confidence in their appearance.

Weight gain, especially during the treatment of breast cancer, is another common side effect of chemotherapy and hormone therapies that can have significant negative effects on people's self-esteem and body image (*see* Chapter 2). Even among women with early-stage breast cancer who are not receiving adjuvant therapy weight gain is common, though it is accentuated in those receiving chemotherapy or hormone therapy.[78]

The side-effects of hormone treatments have had less attention than those of chemotherapy. While generally considered safe compared with cytotoxic drugs, hormone interventions can still have significant effects on people's lives. Tamoxifen, for example, is associated with an increased incidence of uterine cancer though it is usually detected early by irregular vaginal bleeding, and thus cured. It is also associated with thromboembolic disease and, more rarely, disorders of the eye (cataracts and retinopathy),[79] though it is also thought to reduce the incidence of osteoporosis.[80] Tamoxifen not only induces menopausal symptoms in premenopausal women, but leads to a dramatic increase in hot flushes (or flashes as they are called in America.) In clinical practice, a number of women have attributed unexpected mood swings and increased irritability to their tamoxifen although these problems have not been formally reported elsewhere.

Premenopausal women having hormone therapy are more at risk of weight gain than postmenopausal women, as are those undergoing a longer course of adjuvant chemotherapy. Aromatase inhibitors (which prevent androgen from being converted to oestrogen) can also cause severe hot flushes, and megestrol acetate, now more rarely used in the treatment of metastatic breast cancer since the arrival of aromatase inhibitors, causes significant weight gain, noticeably increasing the appetite, as well as causing fluid retention and a number of deaths from thromboembolic disease.[81] Tamoxifen, by contrast, results in somewhat less weight gain. A combination of nutritional advice and a graded exercise programme can sometimes be helpful for those who can tolerate it (*see* Rehabilitation). Many women will have already gained weight during their adjuvant chemotherapy: temporary alopecia for five to seven months and no clothes that will fit can result in major problems with body image.

Hormonal therapy in the treatment of prostate cancer can lead to reduced, if not total loss of libido as well as other sexual problems such as impotence. Men also suffer with hot flushes that are similar to those experienced by women undergoing menopause. A reduction in foods that can stimulate hot flushes (caffeine, alcohol, and hot fluids) has been recommended.[82]

Focus on bone marrow transplants

Over the past three decades bone marrow transplantation (BMT) has emerged as an increasingly successful treatment for a progressively wider range of cancers and other diseases. While its use was once confined to haematological cancers where the bone marrow had failed, such as leukaemias and lymphomas, it is now occasionally being used to treat solid tumours such as ovarian cancer (though no longer breast cancer), and germ cell tumours. BMT involves three steps: the patient's bone marrow is removed or 'harvested' and subsequently treated; the patient is given intensive doses of chemotherapy with or without radiotherapy; and the harvested bone marrow is then infused back into the patient. Marrow may be harvested from the patient themselves (autologous BMT), a genetically similar donor (allogeneic BMT), or a twin (syngeneic BMT). Allogeneic and syngeneic BMT are mainly used when the bone marrow itself is diseased, as in leukaemias, while autologous BMT is used when the marrow is free of disease.[83]

The treatment is highly demanding of both patients and their families, involving long periods of hospitalization (often more than six weeks), much of it requiring the patient to be isolated from possible infection. Although it offers the promise of a cure for an increasing proportion of patients, BMT is also a potentially fatal treatment (e.g. due to infection, toxicity, or GVHD) with frequent long-term side-effects from treatment. These include fatigue, weakness, neurocognitive impairments (e.g. memory), sleep disorders, sterility, cataracts, pulmonary problems, and prolonged, if not chronic, graft-versus-host disease (GVHD) of the skin, gut, or liver.[83] Sexual problems, such as ejaculatory dysfunction, occur in about half of all patients undergoing BMT.[84]

In view of the risks involved, the decision to undergo BMT is no small matter and often occurs at a time of high stress for both the patient and their family.[83] Not surprisingly, some patients therefore may seem to be avoiding the seriousness of the decision, or testing out the resolve and competence of the medical team in various ways. On the other hand, because it often represents the only possibility of cure, patients can quickly become over-committed to having BMT without completely understanding its risks. Consequently, it is essential that BMT staff prepare patients and families carefully for what is to follow and regard the consent procedure as a gradual process involving a number of discussions, rather than a single event. It therefore may be helpful to reintroduce information about longer-term complications on more than one occasion.[83] When the donor is related to the patient, it is important to prepare the donor adequately since they are likely to identify strongly with the patient and feel a sense of guilt if the treatment is unsuccessful. Being a haematological match, they may also feel vulnerable about their own health.[85]

Unless there is a medical emergency, patients and families should be carefully prepared prior to the start of treatment. A clear 'road map' or treatment calendar which is explained in person and backed up in writing is essential, especially when long, demanding treatments are involved (e.g. for leukaemia). Families and patients should be allowed to visit the BMT unit, meet some of the staff, see an isolation room and preferably meet another patient who has undergone or is undergoing the procedure.[85] They should be encouraged to plan their hospital stay and consider what they wish to bring with them in order to make the environment more familiar (e.g. photographs, music, games, and other personal items). Wherever possible, a clinical nurse specialist, or other psychosocial specialist, should start to develop a relationship with the patient and family and begin to gather a picture of any concerns and vulnerabilities they may have which can then be addressed by the entire medical team as well as the psychosocial specialist.

The period of hospitalization, much of which is spent in germ-free isolation, can be especially stressful for both patient and family. The BMT unit may be a long distance from the patient's home, thus causing considerable domestic upheaval; and intensive contact with the medical team usually needs to be maintained for 100 days or more following the transplant. The intensive chemotherapy can result in both high levels of nausea and pain (due to mouth and gastrointestinal mucositis) as well as hair loss and other challenges. The complete dependency on hospital staff often leads patients to feel helpless and lacking control so, as far as possible, patients should be encouraged and given opportunities to make choices (Hospital Admission; Chapter 2—Relationship with the Healthcare Team; Chapter 6—Consent, Collaboration, and Choice).

Patients frequently complain of having too much time with their own thoughts, ruminating anxiously about whether they will survive and how their families would cope if they do not. Enabling patients to develop a daily routine which involves doing something meaningful for themselves not only fills up time but restores some sense of control (e.g. allowing patients to medicate themselves, providing them where possible with exercise facilities such as weights, arts and crafts, 'digital' contact with friends, and family, etc.).

Although they should have as much access to patients as possible, families often feel helpless while their loved one is in hospital. Without an active role, families are also hungry for information. Emotional support and information from staff is therefore essential if patients and family are to endure prolonged hospitalization. By the end of treatment, especially where there has been prolonged GVHD, families are frequently emotionally exhausted. Their relationship with the healthcare team is therefore extraordinarily important in order to sustain their resilience in support of the patient. Families should be centrally involved in preparations for discharge so as to ensure that they reinforce the patient's compliance with medical aftercare and are aware of the patient's anxieties about re-entering the world of the well. In addition, patients sometimes have difficulty integrating the experience of BMT with their life narratives (see Chapter 1) and communicating with other people what they have been through.

BMT units are frequently small, close-knit settings where staff, patients, and families experience an intensity of emotion. When the treatment fails, its impact extends beyond the patient and family to other patients, their families, and the BMT unit staff. All the aggressive treatments that the patient has endured have come to nought, and BMT quickly becomes a 'miracle that has failed.'[85] In view of the intensity of the relationship between patients and their healthcare team, and the fact that deaths do occur as a result of this treatment, BMT staff are at particular risk of 'burn-out' and may benefit from access to additional support (*see* Chapter 7).

Focus on lung cancer

Over 150 000 people in Europe are diagnosed with lung cancer each year,[86] and in 2003 almost 172 000 Americans were estimated to be diagnosed with the disease.[87] Lung cancer is the leading cause of cancer death worldwide, and in 1987 it surpassed breast cancer as the leading cause of cancer death among American women.[87] Tobacco use is the primary risk factor in 80% of cases[88] yet, despite this widely known link, it is estimated that 27% of the British adult population were still smoking cigarettes in 2001.[89] In spite of its high prevalence, the prognosis for lung cancer has not improved significantly over the past 20 years.[86] The five-year survival of all lung cancers is a grim 15% in the USA[87] and generally lower elsewhere. Eighty per cent of patients die within a year of the diagnosis.[90] Nowhere is the clinician's understanding of quality of life more important than in the treatment of lung cancer.

Small-cell lung cancer, comprising a quarter of all lung cancers, is generally responsive to chemotherapy and radiotherapy, but usually requires intensive treatment lasting from three to six months. The more common non-small-cell lung cancer is usually diagnosed at a late stage and, with the exception of surgery and radiotherapy for early stage disease, is almost exclusively treated with palliative intent since only a minority (20–30%) of patients respond to chemotherapy.[88] Nonetheless, despite its side-effects and the fact that it currently provides only a six-week survival advantage, chemotherapy does appear to improve quality of life compared with best supportive care alone.[91] Furthermore, newer chemotherapies (gemcitabine, doce-taxel, paclitaxel, vinorelbine) promise fewer side-effects and better quality of life.

Twice as many men develop lung cancer as women, though the number of women across the world developing the disease is growing. Whether it is the preponderance of men, the fact that they are mainly elderly, or the backdrop of a generally bleak prognosis, the fact is the concerns of people with lung cancer are rarely voiced and healthcare staff are slow to elicit them. A survey of 80 newly-diagnosed lung cancer patients, for example, found that their psychosocial concerns were more worrying to them than their physical symptoms yet were much less likely to have been dealt with effectively by the healthcare team.[90] The future trajectory of the illness and the impact of the illness on the family were rated as major concerns but fewer than 30% of patients who were worried about these issues felt they had been given an opportunity to discuss them with a professional.

Psychosocial distress among people with lung cancer is often related to physical symptoms associated with the disease, including pain, fatigue, and dyspnoea,[88] although the side-effects of treatment can also be severe and distressing (e.g. neu- tropaenia, fatigue and nausea). For example, dyspnoea (laboured, uncomfortable breathing) can result in significant levels of anxiety. Between 15% and 40% of people with lung cancer report dyspnoea at the time of their diagnosis,[92] and about 90% of patients with non-small-cell lung cancer experience at least moderate levels of dysp- noea through their illness.[93] Because breathing is a basic life function, difficulty in breathing can induce feelings of intense panic that can exacerbate the breathlessness. This sometimes results in people feeling anxious to be on their own and a general tendency to remain in the safety of the home. Behavioural techniques of teaching patients diaphragmatic breathing have been shown to be an effective adjunct to the medical management of dyspnoea by encouraging the use of abdominal muscles while inducing a state of relaxation.[93] It also provides family members with a useful role. Family members can encourage the patient to learn these techniques while set- ting goals which gradually develop their loved one's confidence to explore the world beyond the home. Having access to oxygen at home when dyspnoea is severe can help to relieve the feelings of panic.

Physical symptoms associated with disease progression cause significant distress. Cognitive impairment (memory loss, motor co-ordination, verbal memory, etc.) may be the first sign of disease or the effect of systemic chemotherapy, but is fre- quently a distressing omen of advanced disease (e.g. brain metastases). Weight loss and subsequent fatigue can lead to such functional decline that patients are no longer able to participate fully in their normal social roles. Not surprisingly, when such symptoms are poorly managed there is a higher likelihood of depression and a decline in the quality of the patient's life. However, depression may also be associat- ed with guilt and regret due to prolonged tobacco use. Family members sometimes also find it difficult to manage their ambivalent feelings towards someone who has smoked heavily and developed lung cancer. Therefore, although smoking cessation may be helpful in decreasing symptom distress (and promoting weight gain),[88] healthcare staff must be sensitive to the danger of increasing the individual's sense of guilt at such a vulnerable time. Finally, lung cancer frequently has damaging financial consequences for families, many of whom are poor, so the early offer of social work support is essential.

Focus on prostate cancer

Prostate cancer is the second most common cancer among American males, 80% of whom are over 65 years old,[82] and the fourth leading cause of death in men worldwide. It accounts for 33% of new cancer cases in American men,[87] though black Americans have a 32% higher incidence rate of prostate cancer than white Americans, and they have twice their mortality rates. Nine per cent of all prostate cancers are thought to be hereditary.

Improved detection rates, due to the prostate specific antigen (PSA) test, have led to a better prognosis in recent years. According to the American Cancer Society, over 90% of men with prostate cancer will survive five years and over 70% will survive ten years.[94] Nonetheless, it remains difficult to distinguish the indolent form of prostate cancer from the more lethal form. This is important because it is unclear whether active treatment of slowly progressing prostate cancer is justified in view of the poor quality of life that treatment sometimes inflicts.[82] In the past many men would eventually die of other causes and their prostate cancer had little effect on either the quality or quantity of their lives.

Indolent forms of prostate cancer are often not treated but instead a long period of surveillance ('watchful waiting') is begun. This is especially the case where the man is suffering with another illness and his life expectancy is less than ten years. But even the PSA test has shortcomings. Cancer may exist despite a normal PSA level (4 or less), and higher levels can be caused by other conditions (prostatitis, benign prostatic hypertrophy) and even needle biopsies. PSA readings can also vary according to the age of the patient.[82] PSA levels can become the source of obsessive worry and concern as men wait for their latest test result, sometimes plotting their fluctuating levels on a graph. For others, this sense of 'doing nothing' can be intolerable.[82]

Surgery in the form of radical prostatectomy is gradually being replaced with 'nerve sparing' surgery which results in less impotence and urinary incontinence. Radiotherapy (both external beam teletherapy and sometimes transperineal radioactive seed implants—brachytherapy) can also result in less urinary and sexual dysfunctions but increases the risk of bowel problems. Whole pelvis radiotherapy can also lead to increased levels of fatigue. Surgery and brachytherapy can cause urinary incontinence, leading men to feel anxious about social activity and humiliated at having to wear incontinence pads. Pain can also be a significant feature of prostate cancer, especially in advanced disease, and can contribute to other problems such as weakness, fatigue, and depression.

Hormonal treatments, which are sometimes given before surgery (neoadjuvant therapy), are used to decrease the production or effect of testosterone on prostate cancer growth. Such androgen deprivation therapy is the mainstay of metastatic prostate cancer treatment.[95] Hormonal treatments (including orchidectomy), however, frequently cause impotence and loss of libido, fatigue, anaemia, and osteo-porosis, as well as hot flushes that are similar to those experienced by menopausal women. The effect of androgen deprivation therapy on mood is as yet poorly understood, although depression appears to be high among men receiving this form of treatment.[95]

The psychosocial impact of prostate cancer is not hard to predict. Men with prostate cancer experience the fear and uncertainty associated with any other form of cancer, but additionally worry about the loss of their masculinity and potency. The later stages of the disease can lead to fatigue, weakness, and a general loss of vitality; the resulting dependence on family and friends and loss of autonomy can represent an intolerable shift in the self-image of some men. Similarly, loss of sexual desire and the ability to obtain an erection (affecting more than 40% of men treated with radical prostatectomy and hormone therapy) both impact on patients' sense of 'manhood', especially among men who were sexually active before their cancer. As Anderson has suggested, a person's sexual self-concept is likely to be an important predictor of how people adjust to the impact of cancer on their sexuality,[96] once again highlighting the importance of people's assumptions and expectations on how they experience such changes in their lives.

Growing evidence suggests that the needs of men with prostate cancer are poorly addressed. A survey of 206 Australian men attending prostate cancer support groups found that a third of them had moderate to high unmet needs in three areas: psychological concerns (e.g. fears of cancer recurrence and spread), sexual difficul-ties (e.g. changes in sexual relationships, loss of manhood, etc.), and medical infor-mation (e.g. benefits and side-effects of treatment).[97] A UK national survey of nearly 11 000 men with prostate cancer reported that 15% would like to have been more involved in decisions about their care, an alarming 17% of those with pain were not given any medication to alleviate this, and over half (56%) had not been told of any support or self-help group.[98]

The fact that their needs are often neither voiced nor identified by professionals is likely to be related to the fact that prostate cancer patients are all men. Older men are often less inclined to share their emotions and needs openly, seeing it as a matter of dignity and pride to maintain a stoic strength. If self-reliance and self-control broadly characterize many older men, it requires tact and diplomacy to ensure that such men are not needlessly suffering. However, it also suggests that healthcare pro-fessional should take the initiative in offering medical information and eliciting psychosocial and physical concerns. With such potentially disturbing consequences for the man's quality of life, it is imperative to make sure that men with prostate cancer are fully informed about different treatment options. Presenting supportive care in the form of a routine educational programme, for example, can ensure that the man's dignity is not undermined. Psycho-educational courses and structured prostate cancer support groups, both of which can help to normalize concerns, hold promise in this regard.

Finally, the families of men with prostate cancer also require adequate levels of support and information, particularly since some men prefer to maintain a stoic silence rather than worry their loved ones, while many elderly men have few other sources of support. A Swedish study of 342 men with prostate cancer found that nearly a quarter (24%) had no one to confide in.[99] Those with a spouse depended almost exclusively on her for their emotional needs, while among those living without a partner, eight out of ten men had no one to confide in. However, men who did confide their emotional concerns reported better general well-being.

Common treatment difficulties

A large number of unpleasant symptoms are associated with either cancer itself or cancer treatments. All physical symptoms have psychological consequences that, in many cases, can exacerbate the problem. Here we consider a few of the more common treatment difficulties associated with cancer so that healthcare professionals can assess and alleviate these problems before they become entrenched. (*see also* Chapter 3—Sexual Problems).

Fatigue

Fatigue is the most common and distressing side effect of surgery, chemotherapy, and radiotherapy, affecting more than 70% of patients,[100] yet it is a symptom that is often overlooked in discussions between doctors and patients.[101] As cancer treatments have become more intense and demanding, so has fatigue become more overwhelming and distressing,[100] to the extent that it is cited as one of the main reasons patients discontinue with treatment.[102] Several studies have found that radiotherapy-induced fatigue, for example, can continue for months or even years following the end of treatment.[103–105] One implication of this is that healthcare staff will increasingly need to ensure that disability assessment boards are educated about this frequently chronic disability.[101]

Whatever its cause, fatigue can have a debilitating effect on almost every aspect of a person's quality of life.[106, 107] High levels of physical and emotional exhaustion, and the resulting inability to live life normally, can contribute to hopelessness and despair,[100] and when this leads to clinical depression, the depression itself may cause further fatigue. One survey[107] of people with chemotherapy-associated fatigue found that more than 20% had stopped working completely as a result of fatigue, while 12%

reported that their primary carer had been forced to take unpaid leave or quit work altogether. Forty per cent of patients with fatigue had been offered no help by health-care staff, and the most common recommendation that professionals did make was for bed rest or relaxation, even though current evidence suggests that exercise may be more beneficial.

Despite a current surge of scientific interest in fatigue, relatively little is known about the relationship between its many possible causes.[108] Fatigue can be a symptom of the cancer itself or a result of other physical problems, most notably anaemia[109] and pain. On the other hand, fatigue is also associated with clinical depression, anxiety, sleep disorders, and simply the cumulative emotional distress of having cancer. In the case of radiation fatigue, it remains unclear whether the degree of malaise is related to the length of treatment, the cumulative dose, or the volume of tissue irradiated. Total body irradiation, however, is known to cause profound fatigue.[110]

Although fatigue is generally thought to increase in a linear fashion soon after starting radiotherapy, careful daily monitoring of (non-depressed) women receiving radiotherapy for breast cancer has found that fatigue levels reach a peak during the fourth week of treatment and then plateau.[111] The authors of this study speculated that physiological homeostatic mechanisms (i.e. the body adapting) may have been responsible for this levelling out of fatigue. There was no support for earlier evidence[112] that patients receiving daily treatments are able to recover some of their energy by the second day of the weekend.

Since a large number of factors may be involved, the cause of fatigue in an individual patient can be difficult to determine. Clinicians must rely on the patient's own report of their level of fatigue although, as with pain and psychological distress, patients are often reluctant to mention their fatigue to their busy clinicians, fearing their cancer treatment may be delayed,[100] or that nothing can be done about it.[107] In assessing someone's fatigue, it may be helpful to draw a distinction between *physical fatigue* (e.g. muscle weakness and lack of stamina) and *mental fatigue* (reduced alertness, feeling easily overwhelmed, vulnerable to distraction, etc.),[108] so that one may begin by ruling out more obvious physical (e.g. chemotherapy-induced anaemia) and psychological factors (e.g. depression).

There is, as yet, no optimal strategy for managing fatigue, although the U.S. National Comprehensive Cancer Network (NCCN) Fatigue Guidelines Panel has offered some recommendations for assessment and care.[100] These indicate the following:

Assessment of fatigue

1. All cancer patients should be regularly screened for fatigue.

2. Patients should be warned that they may experience fatigue as a result of cancer treatments. If they are not prepared, patients can worry that an increase in fatigue means the treatment is not working and the disease is progressing.

3. If a patient reports fatigue it should be quantified. Using 0–10 rating (endpoints: 'no fatigue' and 'severe fatigue') enables the clinician to monitor change and evaluate the effectiveness of any treatment.

4. Where screening reveals moderate or severe fatigue, a more focused history and a physical examination are indicated. This assessment should evaluate the five common clinical conditions known to lead to fatigue: pain, emotional distress, sleep disturbance, anaemia, and hypothyroidism.

5. If this initial evaluation of fatigue fails to reveal a primary cause, a more comprehensive assessment is indicated:

   (a) A review of medications and interactions should be undertaken. Medications with interactions that are associated with fatigue include: narcotics, hypnotics, sedatives, antihistamines, anti-emetics, antihypertensives, and anxiolytics.

   (b) A search for comorbidities (e.g. cardiac, pulmonary, renal, neurological, or endocrine disorders).

   (c) Evaluation of nutritional status including fluid and electrolyte balance.

   (d) Levels of daily activity (inactivity as a result of prolonged cancer treatment can lead to poor physical condition, muscle wasting, and loss of cardiorespiratory fitness).[113]

Treatment of Fatigue

1. If patients are educated about the fatigue that they are likely to encounter in their cancer treatments, they will be less distressed and better prepared to cope with it.

2. Non-pharmacological strategies and interventions can be particularly helpful in overcoming fatigue:

   • *energy conservation* (e.g. postponing non-essential tasks, delegating high-energy tasks, scheduling important activities for times of high energy, etc.);

   • *distraction* (e.g. reading, socializing, relatively passive recreation such as listening to music, etc.);

   • *stress management techniques* such as relaxation training. Participation in a support group has also been found to decrease feelings of fatigue;

   • *nutrition.* Patients who have difficulty taking in food as a result of nausea and vomiting may simply lack energy resources; in such cases referral to a dietician/nutritionist may be indicated;

   • *sleep* disorders can obviously be a cause of fatigue and should be assessed and treated appropriately;

   • *exercise* has been shown to be helpful in reducing fatigue. Physical inactivity among cancer patients may be a significant cause of fatigue.[113] A number of studies have consistently found that patients who exercise during cancer treatment report less fatigue and fewer mood and sleep problems compared with controls. Rehabilitative exercise programs should be individualized, begin with modest expectations and build up very slowly. Walking appears to be particularly safe and effective for many people.

3. Anaemia is a common cause of fatigue in cancer patients and has been shown to respond to erythropoietin alfa. Where depression is evident this should be treated (see Depression, page 253).

4. Corticosteroids have been used to increase energy levels in advanced cancer while the use of a psychostimulant (such as methylphenidate—Ritalin) has been found to be helpful in some patients with persistent fatigue,[106] as well as with patients with psychomotor slowing as a result of a primary brain tumour.[108] However, the NCCN Fatigue Guidelines Panel was unable to recommend specific pharmacological treatments until more research has been reported.

Fatigue management courses

Multidisciplinary fatigue management programmes hold promise because they aim to reduce the symptoms of fatigue while simultaneously supporting people to manage their symptoms. Such psycho-educational group programmes can reassure patients that fatigue is a common side effect of cancer treatments and is unlikely to be a sign of disease progression. A typical eight-week course ($2^{1}/_{2}$ hours per week, of which half an hour is exercise) might include the following topics:[114]

Activity diaries and setting baselines	Stress management
Belief systems about fatigue	Problem-solving
Pacing and goal setting	Communicating assertively
Sleep management	Overcoming depression
Graded exercise training	Dealing with setbacks
Nutritional advice	Strategies for the future
Positive and negative thinking	Small group work

Nausea and vomiting

Until recently, roughly 60% of patients developed nausea and 50% developed vomiting following cytotoxic chemotherapy[115]. These reactions are particularly common following infusions which contain cisplatin. Patients regard the control of nausea as more important than the control of vomiting (emesis) but doctors and nurses tend to regard emesis control as more important.[116] The 5-HT$_3$ anti-emetic drugs used these days are more effective than previously used drugs in controlling vomiting, especially when caused by chemotherapy that includes cisplatin, although nausea control is generally less successful. Furthermore, they may become less effective over repeated courses of chemotherapy, especially when nausea and vomiting have become a learned (conditioned) response. The addition of steroids (e.g. dexamethasone) increases the efficacy of 5-HT$_3$ and other anti-emetic drugs.[115] Non-pharmacological control of nausea therefore remains important.

Those more likely to experience severe nausea and vomiting include:[74, 117]

- people who have already experienced nausea or vomiting as a result of chemotherapy;
- people with a history of motion sickness;
- people who have experienced nausea and vomiting in response to foods or situations such as pregnancy;
- people who are particularly anxious;
- people who strongly expect to be sick.

A number of studies have indicated that providing patients with relaxation training enables them to cope more easily with the side-effects of chemotherapy; it can reduce physiological arousal, nausea and distress.[75, 118, 119] However, recent work has tended to focus more on the development of treatments for anticipatory nausea and vomiting. A number of patients feel nauseous or actually vomit while waiting for their treatment to begin or shortly after the infusion has begun, while others have been reported to vomit in response to cues such as seeing a clinic nurse while out shopping[119] or even simply imagining the chemotherapy clinic.[120] Similarly, the development of food aversions can affect as many as 50% of patients undergoing chemotherapy.[121] Anticipatory nausea occurs when people and objects in the vicinity of the chemotherapy clinic become associated with feelings of nausea. Subsequently, these people and objects alone can evoke the nausea, without the presence of an active drug. It is a clear example of classical (Pavlovian) conditioning.

Recent studies have shown that a patient's expectations that they will feel nauseous after an infusion of chemotherapy only become predictive after the individual has actually experienced nausea (i.e. after the first course), suggesting that expectations make a contribution to subsequent nausea but cannot on their own account for it.[122] The role of the patient's expectations in anticipatory nausea was explored in a prospective study of 100 breast cancer patients undergoing chemotherapy, 47% of whom subsequently reported anticipatory nausea.[123] Patients who expected to be nauseated by treatment, and who were by nature anxious people, were more likely to have developed anticipatory nausea and vomiting by the middle of their treatment. Once anticipatory nausea had begun, the effects of conditioning ensured that it usually continued.

The treatment of conditioned nausea and vomiting usually involves what psychologists call counter-conditioning or systematic desensitization (though other techniques such as distraction and biofeedback have been used).[117] This usually involves training the patient to achieve a state of deep physiological relaxation (sometimes the patient is also encouraged to visualize pleasant relaxing scenes). Once the patient has learned how to become sufficiently relaxed, they are exposed to cues associated with the chemotherapy clinic (e.g. smells, photos, a needle, their own memories, etc.). The patient continues to expose themselves to this conditioned cue, while keeping themselves as physically calm as possible, until they no longer feel nauseous or anxious in response to it. With practice, the patient becomes habituated to the stimulus (e.g. imagining themselves receiving an infusion) which now no longer evokes nausea. Often such treatments begin in another setting and only later are deployed in the chemotherapy clinic, though some success has been reported by clinicians modifying these techniques to include an element of hypnosis without the therapist having to be present during chemotherapy.[124, 125]

Apart from reducing nausea and vomiting (which enables some patients to complete their treatment), such techniques often have the added benefit of allowing patients to exercise some control over the experience rather than feeling passive and helpless. This may be one of the reasons why anxiety-reduction techniques often result in an improvement in mood, not just a lessening of anxiety.

Pain

Pain is a common and much dreaded symptom of cancer. While clinicians and researchers estimate that 90–95% of cancer pain can be effectively treated, half of all patients do not receive adequate pain relief.[126] Nearly a third of cancer patients are in pain when they are diagnosed and this proportion increases to between 65% and 85% as the disease becomes more advanced.[127] The prevalence of pain varies with the site of the disease; it is common in cancers of the lung, bone, and genito-urinary system, while comparatively infrequent (5%) among those with leukaemia.[128] Most pain is the result of the disease process, although up to a quarter of pain may be related to cancer treatment or other factors (e.g. secondary muscle pain). In one study of people with advanced disease, cancer itself was found to be responsible for only half of the pains reported by patients.[129]

There is little doubt that pain has profound and widespread effects on patients' quality of life.[130] Unrelieved pain can engender a sense of helplessness, hopelessness, and irritability,[126] and is a major risk factor for depression. Unalleviated pain has also been reported as one of the most likely causes of cancer-related suicide.[131] Sleep, mobility, anxiety levels, loss of appetite, impaired concentration, and many other problems can all be affected by pain. Effective management of acute post-operative pain, for example, not only speeds recovery by allowing patients to accomplish prescribed tasks such as coughing and walking, but may even prevent chronic pain.[132] In addition to the avoidable suffering caused by untreated pain, there are also significant financial costs to health services due to unscheduled admissions of cancer patients whose pain is poorly controlled.[133]

A lingering and common misconception about pain is that it is directly related to the extent of tissue damage. This outdated and mistaken view has been replaced, albeit slowly, by a multidimensional model in which pain is seen as an integration of physical, psychological, and cultural factors.[134] The pharmacological treatment of pain is well beyond the scope of this book, but we wish to highlight some psychosocial aspects of pain management that have received less attention. We start by examining why, despite significant advances in the management of cancer pain, large numbers of patients still fail to receive adequate pain control.

Pain is under-reported and under-treated

Cancer pain is often not reported by patients and not assessed by healthcare staff. An American study of 533 radiotherapy outpatients found that, of the 37% reporting pain, over a quarter had not received any analgesia for it[135] Almost identical figures were reported in a UK replication study that assessed all oncology patients attending a cancer hospital during a single week.[136] In a recent study of cancer patients attending general hospitals in Australia, nearly half the patients reported having experienced pain over the preceding 24 hour period and of these, over 50% described this pain to be 'distressing, horrible, or excruciating'. However, half of those in pain had spoken to no one about it.[127] Finally, in general practice, many cancer patients report being generally satisfied with overall pain management despite being in moderate to severe pain.[137]

If over 95% of cancer patients could be free of significant pain, as has been estimated,[138] why are so many cancer patients continuing to receive inadequate analgesia, are reluctant to report their pain, or fail to adhere to the treatment they have been given? The reasons are complex and still poorly understood but they appear to be due to a combination of (a) patient/public and professional beliefs, (b) a reluctance of patients to take opioids due to their side-effects (such as constipation and sedation),[139] and (c) the fact that doctors simply do not prescribe adequate levels of analgesia or fail to follow recommended guidelines.[140] Table 5.3 lists a number of patient concerns about taking strong analgesia. Many of these misconceptions are shared by families and the public,[141] as well as by healthcare staff.[142]

Ironically, patients may be most reluctant to 'complain' about pain when there is a good doctor–patient relationship and their doctor is perceived as 'doing their best'.[137] Perhaps not surprisingly, if patients do not ask for information about how to manage their pain or even tell staff they are experiencing pain, staff are inclined to believe that patients are satisfied with the information and treatment they have been given. This may be especially the case with older patients who are often less willing to report their pain or take action to relieve it, while healthcare staff are less likely to provide information about

Table 5.3 Common beliefs about strong analgesia[21]

Fear of addiction
Fear of developing tolerance (i.e. risk of uncontrolled pain later in the illness)
Fear of side-effects
'Good' patients do not complain about pain
Pain is inevitable in cancer
Talking about pain may distract the doctor from curing the cancer
Admitting to pain is equated with admitting that the disease has progressed
Fear of injections

pain to older people, or ask them about it, compared with younger patients.[127] Nurses often fail to give as much analgesia as has been prescribed due to concerns about addiction and respiratory depression, and an erroneous belief that the effectiveness of analgesics lasts longer in older people than younger people.[143]

Patient education

The answer probably lies in patient and staff education. In a UK survey of over 65000 NHS patients in the year 2000, 13% reported that they were not given enough medication to help with their pain, including 8% who were not given any medication at all. An astonishing 21% of the 5652 men with pain from prostate cancer reported inadequate pain relief; 17% had been given no medication whatsoever. It remains an academic, if important, question as to whether this is a function of doctors failing to ask men about their pain or male patients failing to report it. The essential point is that *all patients should be regularly asked about their levels of pain.*

Patient education about pain has been recommended by the American Cancer Society as a way of encouraging patients to monitor (e.g. using a daily pain log) and report their pain.[144] In fact, it is seen as the cornerstone of effective pain management.[141] However, patient education is not simply providing patients with information so much as finding out what patients understand about pain. If patients have low expectations about pain control, they are more likely to be satisfied with inadequate pain management.[137] If patients believe that effective analgesia may mask their pain, rendering them unable to gauge whether their disease is progressing, they may be less willing to take it.

Healthcare staff should therefore sensitively but consistently…

- ask their patients about the quality and level of their pain;
- offer appropriate analgesic treatment (e.g. adhering to guidelines such as the WHO analgesic ladder);
- teach patients and their families about their medication and how best to manage their pain and any side-effects arising from the analgesia (e.g. constipation);
- encourage patients and families to monitor and continue to report levels of pain, making it clear throughout that treating the patient's pain is a vitally important goal;
- address all of the misconceptions about strong analgesia listed above;
- encourage patients and relatives to balance their focus on particular symptoms with a wider view, which acknowledges what is going well, and specific accomplishments of the patient (e.g. taking some exercise);
- encourage patients to take some level of control over their pain management (*see* Multidimensional Pain).

Assessing pain

Pain is a subjective state that cannot be measured objectively; patients' expressions of pain therefore should always be believed.[145] The interpretation and understanding of the pain may require a long process of assessment. Often a number of psychosocial factors contributing to the pain will subsequently emerge. The fact that a patient can sleep does not mean they are not in pain. The fact that a patient is quiet or uncomplaining does not mean they are not in pain—it may reflect their withdrawal and helplessness in response to their pain. And the fact that patients are reluctant to tell healthcare staff about their pain means that professionals must be vigorous and proactive in encouraging patients to talk about their pain.

Pain assessments should include:

- a careful history so that the time course of the pain is understood within the context of the patient's cancer and social concerns;[145]
- the site and qualitative features of the pain (dull, sharp, burning; acute, chronic, intermittent), and any circumstances that increase or decrease pain should be recorded. A number of features of pain should be repeatedly assessed so that the effects of any pain intervention can be monitored over time. These include: pain intensity, distress caused, interference with enjoyment of life, and satisfaction with current pain relief;[129]
- response to previous interventions;
- the patient's psychosocial context (their mood, level of anxiety, concurrent stresses, availability of social support, etc.);
- physical and neurological examination;
- sensitivity to ethnic differences in the way pain is perceived (e.g. expectations) and described.

Although a number of excellent scales exist for measuring pain (e.g. Brief Pain Inventory,[146] the McGill Pain Questionnaire, see Appendix 1), they may not always be ideal for use in clinical practice either because they are too difficult or take too long for patients to complete, or are too burdensome for clinicians to analyse and interpret.[129] Adjective-categorical scales (e.g. no pain/mild/moderate/severe/unbearable pain) should be generally avoided because they are too crude, leading people to assume mistakenly that there is equidistance between the labelled points.[147] Visual analogue scales (e.g. a ten-centimetre line with end-points labelled 'no pain' and 'worst possible pain') are preferable, though one should make it clear what one is assessing (average pain, worst pain, etc.) and the period of time in question (current pain, the past 24 hours, the past week, etc.) The shorter the time-frame the more reliable the measure is likely to be.

Monitoring pain intensity alone, however, may inadvertently lead the patient to focus on their pain and become more sensitized to it. Rather, it is important to distinguish between pain intensity, pain distress, pain interference, and pain tolerability. The patient should be encouraged to see that the aim of pain management is not always to extinguish all pain but to control it to a tolerable level, enabling the patient to continue with their everyday life, to concentrate, communicate, and to sleep and rest.[148]

Multidimensional pain

Psychological management of pain should be seen as an essential adjunct to comprehensive pain management. It is important to stress that psychological factors do not 'cause' cancer pain directly but can exacerbate a person's perception, and alter their experience of it.[149] Unless this distinction is understood, there may be a danger of dismissing genuine pain as 'just psychological'. Some clinicians have noted that patients who described their pain as 'severe' are more likely to be regarded by staff as having a psychological component to their pain; indeed, it may be difficult for healthcare staff to empathize with a patient's pain once it has exceeded a certain level of intensity, and consequently their judgements become unreliable.[128]

Pain and distress have an intimate relationship. Muscle tension, autonomic arousal, and psychological distress can exacerbate pain, while the experience of pain can lead to further muscle tension, arousal, and distress. Once again, people's beliefs and expectations are fundamental in shaping how they perceive experiences and react to them. Cultural and ethnic beliefs influence how people behave in response to pain and the meaning they ascribe to it.[134] People who believe that the presence of pain inevitably means that the disease is progressing are more likely to become distressed and anxious, more focused on their pain, and less likely to engage in other more pleasant and distracting activities. Women with metastatic breast cancer have been shown to report more pain if they believed the pain represented disease progression.[150] People who believe that one should *always* respond to pain by resting and avoiding physical activity may inadvertently withdraw from rewarding activities with the result that they lose their confidence and self-esteem in the process. It is not surprising therefore that pain is associated with depression in cancer patients, regardless of whether they have had depression in the past.[151]

A number of psychological strategies have been shown to be of help to people with chronic pain and, increasingly, people with cancer with advanced disease. The aim of these interventions is largely to help patients relinquish a passive, helpless relationship to their pain in favour of assuming a more active, self-managing role.[149]

Psychological strategies in pain management

Psychological support   Short-term psychotherapy,[152] either individually or in groups,[150] provides emotional support, information, continuity of care, and various ways of coping with pain and other symptoms. Cancer patients who receive active psychological support report less pain.[126] Patients (and their families) can be helped to communicate about their pain more effectively, express their distress and fears for the future, and find ways of maximizing their quality of life. Psychological support can enable the individual to describe the story of their pain within the broader context of their lives, thus clarifying the meaning of the pain while allowing other resources and qualities of the person to emerge.

Distraction   Distraction enables people to focus their mental energies on something other than their pain. This is not the same as denial and avoidance but rather an active approach to managing pain. Engaging in meaningful and stimulating activities seems to reduce the awareness of pain while giving the patient something different to think and talk about. Listening to music, watching films, talking to friends, creative activities (writing, art, playing music) can all lead to a sense of achievement and personal control.[126]

Relaxation and imagery   Anxiety heightens sympathetic nervous system activity which can lead to increased pain sensitivity. Both laboratory and clinical research over the past 40 years has shown that heightened anxiety can lead to higher pain and increased need for analgesia.[149] Relaxation combined with guided imagery or self-hypnosis training can reduce autonomic arousal and, indirectly, pain, although, as yet, few controlled clinical trials have tested these interventions with cancer patients. One of the few that has been conducted found that training in relaxation and imagery were significantly more effective than treatment-as-usual or therapist support in reducing the pain associated with bone marrow transplant (BMT) mucositis.[153] The authors concluded that the guided imagery component was especially powerful (e.g. imagining descending a staircase into deeper levels of relaxation).

Cognitive-behavioural approaches   How people think about their pain, and the assumptions and expectations they bring to pain, will affect the way they experience it (Fig. 5.1). For example, most cancer patients expect to have pain but this expectation, along with other assumptions about cancer, can lead to mental 'catastrophizing' and increased anxiety ('*I will now have this pain till I die*'). Similarly, believing that one is unable to exert control over pain can lead to helplessness and passivity in response to it. Moreover, when people have too much time on their hands, and lack mental stimulation, they are inclined to become preoccupied with their symptoms.

Cognitive-behavioural approaches to pain attempt to draw out the patient's underlying assumptions and expectations. Through examining, evaluating, and challenging these beliefs, the patient is encouraged to find more productive alternatives ('*This pain doesn't necessarily mean my cancer is any worse; it may help if I try to relax and distract*

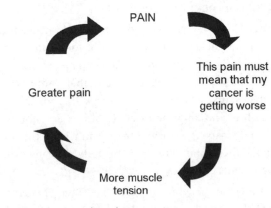

Fig. 5.1 Faulty assumptions can make pain worse.

myself by doing something useful'). There is often a strong problem-solving element to this approach. The behavioural component involves the patient setting graded tasks and goals for themselves to achieve; the achievement of even modest goals can lead people away from a sense of helplessness in the face of pain.

Control Finally, giving patients control over their analgesia may lead them to need less of it. One study has shown that BMT patients who were given control over their morphine infusion used 53% less morphine than those who were given the standard treatment, a continuous infusion.[154] Patients who were able to control their analgesia reported similar levels of pain and morphine side-effects but, unlike the continuous infusion group whose morphine dosage increased, they did not develop tolerance.

Depression

Clinical depression is thought to affect roughly 25% of people with cancer, with the prevalence rising as the disease progresses.[155] However, prevalence estimates ultimately depend on the methods of measurement used and some studies have found considerably lower rates.[156] More importantly, several investigations have found that oncologists are poor at recognizing clinical depression in their patients, and seem to rely heavily on whether or not the patient is sad, tearful, or irritable.[13] In a large study of nearly 2300 patients, oncologists accurately identified less than 30% of those who scored highly on a self-report questionnaire measuring psychological distress (GHQ-12).[157] However, communication courses appear to improve oncologists' use of psychological probing and thus improve their detection rates of psychological problems[158] and concerns.[15]

Depression is not inevitable in cancer and can usually be alleviated if it is detected. However, depression can result from a large number of causes so, rather than treat it merely symptomatically, these causes should be thoroughly explored. For example, is the patient suffering from a recurrence of a previous history of depression, the cumulative emotional exhaustion of cancer and its treatment, an appropriate reaction to loss, helplessness in the face of multiple social stresses, the biological effects of the cancer and its treatment, and so on? In short, depressed feelings should not always be interpreted as pathological but understood in the context within which they occur. For example, it is appropriate to mourn the loss of independence, one's physical capability or a body part. Tears are a normal expression of such feelings, just as they can be a release of tension or anger during periods when people are adjusting to significant change in their lives.

Clinical depression, however, involves persistently low mood which leaves people unable to enjoy anything in their lives and hopeless about the future. Severe depression can lead to delusions and agitation and such patients should always be referred for psychiatric assessment. The physical symptoms (e.g. appetite, concentration, and sleep problems) normally used for assessing depression can be features of the disease or its treatment, so are of limited value in the context of cancer. One must rely more heavily on psychological features of depression to assess its severity (for assessment and treatment of depression see Chapter 6—Working with Someone Clinically Depressed or Suicidal).

Table 5.4 Medical factors associated with the development of depression in people with cancer

---

Uncontrolled pain

Whole brain irradiation

Metabolic abnormalities

    Hypercalcaemia

    Sodium–potassium imbalance

    Anaemia

    Vitamin B12 or folate deficiency

Endocrinological abnormalities

    Hyper- or hypothyroidism

    Adrenal insufficiency

Medicine

    Steroids

    Interferon and interleukin 2

    Methyldopa

    Reserpine

    Barbiturates

    Propranalol

    Some antibiotics (amphotericin B)

    Some chemotherapy agents

Adapted from Massie MJ, Popkin MK. (1998) depressive Disorders. In: Holland JC. (ed.), *Psychooncology*, Oxford: Oxford University Press.

Chemotherapy and depression

A number of medical factors can directly or indirectly cause depression so these must be considered in any assessment of depression in cancer patients see Table 5.4.[159] However, the relationship between chemotherapy and depression works both ways. Those who receive particular chemotherapy agents are more likely to become depressed, and people who are depressed are less willing to accept a course of chemotherapy than those who are not depressed.[160] Corticosteroids, interferon, and some analgesics have been known to cause sudden changes of mood and behaviour. Prednisone is used as part of several treatment regimes, and intravenous dexamethasone, another steroid, is very commonly used with intravenous chemotherapy for its anti-emetic effects. It may also affect mood causing unexplained highs alternating with intense lows. The following chemotherapy and hormone agents are especially associated with the development of depression:[159]

    Corticosteroids

    Vinblastine

Vincristine
Interferon
Procarbazine
Asparaginase
Tamoxifen
Acetate

(For assessment and treatment options *see* Chapter 6—Working with Someone Clinically Depressed or Suicidal).

Intense fear

Cancer is a frightening disease because it involves numerous threats and uncertainties for the individual, and many changes imposed on the patient and family. Heightened anxiety among people with cancer is therefore common, especially around diagnostic interviews, at the start of new treatments and in the context of advanced disease.[161] However, generalized anxiety is often preventable if adequate support and information are available and healthcare staff are able to elicit and respond to the patient's concerns.[162] Cancer education is particularly effective at reducing anxiety when it is tailored to how patients understand the meaning of events.[163] Anxiety can also be alleviated by a number of psychological techniques such as relaxation training and cognitive-behaviour therapy. A meta-analysis of 25 controlled studies of psychological treatments designed to prevent anxiety in cancer patients revealed a moderate effect size of 0.42.[164]

Fear is a normal response to uncertainty and novelty, and most people harbour one or two long-standing phobias that they have successfully managed throughout their lives, usually by avoiding them. However, quite apart from cancer's mortal threat, there are a number of clinical contexts that are especially frightening to some patients because they either resonate with existing fears or, being unfamiliar, represent an overwhelming threat. High levels of anxiety during cancer treatment is not simply a horrible experience for the patient, it can sometimes prevent them from continuing with it. Examples of intense fear include:

Claustrophobia   This can occur during radiotherapy and/or diagnostic procedures (e.g. MRI), although will occasionally occur among patients in hospital isolation rooms. For example, radiotherapy to the head or neck usually requires fixing a customized plastic mould over the face. The mask ('jig') is then clipped to the radiotherapy table to ensure that the radiotherapy targets only the patient's tumour and not healthy tissue by keeping the head still. Some patients react with claustrophobia to confined diagnostic machines, especially closed Magnetic Resonance Imaging machines, while others can find even the radiotherapy room too small to be left alone in.

Needle phobia   A person's fear of needles is usually long-standing but can obviously interfere with blood tests and a number of treatments. Needle phobias can be related to a fear of the sight of blood, though often they result in a fall in blood pressure which is a form of shock reflex in response to a needle puncture.[165] Learning to recognize this vasovagal reflex and to respond by tensing up muscles in order to raise blood pressure, has been shown to be an effective treatment for such patients.[166] Other people, however, emphasize the pain sensation of their skin being punctured so an anaesthetizing cream can sometimes help to reduce this effect.

Panic attacks   Panic attacks are episodes of overwhelming anxiety which activate the autonomic nervous system, producing the 'fight-or-flight' response. The person concerned often feels an intense urge to escape but may be immobilized by their fear which, in itself, can be a terrifying experience. Though usually lasting only a few minutes, panic attacks are very intense experiences involving a racing heartbeat and hyperventilation that often lead the person to believe they are dying of a heart attack, going mad, or about to faint. Panic attacks also involve extreme muscular tension that can leave the individual feeling physically exhausted. Once a person has had a panic attack they understandably become fearful of having another one; thoughts and physical sensations of fear can mutually escalate out of control leading to self-fulfilling results. Although they are more common among patients with a history of anxiety or panic, panic attacks can occur for the first time during cancer treatment.

Treatment of intense fear

Although minor tranquillizers, such as short-acting benzodiazepine, may be helpful in acute situations (together with anti-depressants[167]), most patients will already be taking some form of medication and may be reluctant to take yet more. In contrast to pharmacological treatment, a more satisfactory and arguably more permanent approach is to help the patient to overcome their fear by learning practical and proven techniques for managing anxiety. This has the added advantage of enabling patients to feel more in control. The more recent the onset of the fear the more likely it will be amenable to a rapid intervention, though it would be misguided to assume that the anxiety is wholly to do with the cancer experience without exploring its broader associations. For example, in one case study, a woman who experienced a panic attack while undergoing radiotherapy for breast cancer later revealed that the treatment machine evoked memories of childhood sexual abuse.[168]

The most important measure in resolving intense fear is to conduct a careful assessment. Anxiety is often associated with depression in healthy people as it is among people with cancer, so an assessment of depression is advisable whenever someone reports anxiety.[163] In assessing intense fear, professionals should ask the patient:

- when and where the fear began;
- what bodily sensations they experienced;
- whether the fear predates the cancer;
- what the patient was aware of thinking and feeling when the fear started;

- what the patient identifies as the source of the threat (e.g. what do they imagine may happen? What do they associate with the threat?);
- how the patient feels they have managed since their cancer diagnosis;
- what additional concurrent stresses the patient is experiencing;
- how much support they receive;
- what memories or associations, if any, are evoked by the fearful experience.

Depending on the source of the anxiety, different treatment options can be considered. In any situation, enabling people to talk about their fears is often therapeutic in itself. Healthcare staff can help normalize the situation by reassuring patients that, given the situation they are in, fear is both common and understandable. This does not mean it cannot be ameliorated. Patients who are generally struggling with their illness and its treatment, and/or are poorly supported, may be best helped by access to ongoing emotional support and further assessment. Some people may be anxiously preoccupied with their disease and repeatedly checking their bodies for signs of disease progression. This type of constant worrying is discussed below (*see* Worry). Those patients whose anxiety has long predated the cancer, may require more specialist assessment and help from a clinical psychologist. On the other hand, some patients may have been poorly prepared for their treatment; thus, time spent clarifying information about aspects of their illness and treatment may provide the reassurance required.

Effective treatment of intense fear involves tackling the three main components of anxiety: bodily arousal, thinking, and behaviour (e.g. avoidance). Almost all patients who suffer intense fear will benefit from learning to relax because, whatever its source, anxiety involves the autonomic nervous system preparing the body to fight or run away (e.g. muscle tension, heart palpitations, shortness of breath, etc). Even among people with far advanced cancer, learning the skills of relaxation can help to reduce pain and increase a sense of tranquillity.[169]

Patients whose anxiety began as a result of a specific incident (e.g. needle, radiotherapy, etc.) will often benefit from a more focused cognitive-behavioural approach in which the patient's thoughts surrounding the threat are explored and challenged (*see* Cognitive-behaviour Therapy). As the assumptions underlying the fear are exposed and modified, the patient is also encouraged to confront their fears in gentle graded steps while maintaining a state of physiological relaxation. In this way, the patient gradually learns how to feel calm, safe, and in control when confronting their fears.

Although the techniques of cognitive-behaviour therapy usually require more extensive skill and training, the methods of systematic desensitization are more easily acquired and can be safely practised by nursing and radiotherapy staff. They are, in principle, the same as those used in overcoming anticipatory nausea and vomiting (see page 245). Thus, for example, the radiotherapy patient who feels claustrophobic wearing a face mask may benefit from the following graded steps:

- temporarily remove the patient from the object or place causing the distress. Slow everything down by dispelling any worries about the urgent need to continue immediately with treatment.

- normalize the patient's response to this far-from-normal situation. Many people feel they have failed, let themselves down, or are causing a nuisance to staff. Reassure them that their feelings are normal and that they are not alone in having them.

- assess the nature of the fear (as above). Explain clearly what you are proposing to do to help the patient manage the current difficulty.

- respond to the concerns of the patient with further information if required and appropriate (e.g. remind the patient that the mask is only loosely fixed to the radiotherapy table and that, if absolutely necessary, they could lift their head at any time—this provides a sense of safety by reassuring people that they are not trapped but have 'exit strategies').

- encourage the patient to relax their muscles and slow their breathing.

- once the patient is calm, hand them the mask and encourage them to touch and look at it.

- when the patient is ready, ask them to lie on a bed and relax. Ask them to imagine they are back in the treatment room while keeping their muscles relaxed.

- when they are fully relaxed ask the patient to place the mask over their face. Enabling people to feel that they are in control over what is happening, including the speed at which it is happening, is an essential element of treatment.

- once the patient is comfortable with this stage, explain that this time *you* will be placing the mask over their face. Remind them to keep as physically relaxed as possible and to continue to tell you what they are thinking and feeling. Let them know that you will stop whenever they want you to.

- when the patient has managed this stage, which may take some time, repeat it in the radiotherapy room with you present (i.e. a simulation of actual treatment). Emphasize that the patient can exercise control over the situation and the fact that they are safe, and, again, focus on thoughts and maintaining physical relaxation until the patient feels confident to resume treatment.

Worry

Worry is one of those mental activities that is so common that it can be easily overlooked, yet it can be a torturous, intrusive experience, causing great distress. One survey of over 600 cancer patients in remission found that the most common cancer-related problem they faced was fear or uncertainty about the future.[170] Worry is prevalent among people newly diagnosed, still undergoing treatment or facing limited survival.

Concern about physical symptoms and fears of recurrence are almost universal.[171] It is therefore worth exploring how worry works.

Worry is a chain of unpleasant thoughts or images which intrude on mental activity and demand attention. It is a highly adaptive feature of the human mind to be able to anticipate and plan for future scenarios.[172] People use their assumptions about the world to predict possible futures. If you can predict what may happen in the future, you may be able to solve any potential problems, rehearse how you would respond (e.g. to possible bad news), or even calculate a way to avoid the event altogether. Worry can therefore be a normal, helpful response to the possibility of future threat; in other words, it is a form of vigilance.

It is tempting to think that the best way to resolve a patient's worries is to reassure them. Not only is this unrealistic and potentially unethical, simple reassurance can paradoxically serve to raise anxiety levels.[163] Reassurance, of course, has its place when definitive answers can be given, and ensuring the patient has adequate information can often prevent many worries. But for those who seek repeated reassurances, or who tend to interpret every ache and pain as a sign of recurrence or disease progression, reassurance alone can be counter-productive. The immediate reduction in anxiety that reassurance gives is rewarding, albeit short-lived; however, before long, the act of seeking reassurance can become the automatic response to worrying thoughts. In short, it does not work. Moreover, before long, very dependent relationships can develop.

Experimental research has shown that, once worry has begun, it directs our attention to the threat and maintains a preoccupation with it.[173] Difficulties start when the threat cannot be resolved by worrying about it, which is often the case in cancer, a disease pervaded by uncertainty. Instead, worry accentuates the uncertainty and raises anxiety levels. In short, uncertainty promotes vigilance (through activation of the amygdala[174]) and worry is simply the mental (cognitive) component of heightened vigilance.

Persistent uncontrolled worrying is a key feature of 'generalized anxiety disorder', a condition which can be successfully treated with cognitive-behavioural therapy.[175] Cognitive-behavioural approaches work by (a) drawing out the hidden assumptions and thinking that underlie people's fears (*thoughts*), (b) teaching people to relax which enables them to control some of the autonomic arousal associated with their worrying (*physiological*) as they (c) gradually confront situations which have become avoided (*behavioural*). For example, the cognitive technique of de-catastrophizing aims to help people worry 'more productively'.

De-catastrophizing

Not all worrying is unrealistic. Many fears about the future may be entirely realistic. But many concern events which are highly unlikely. The possible becomes confused with the probable. For example, people frequently worry about the worst possible moment in their imagination, as if it were the only outcome. They fail to remember that whatever their imagined snapshot of the future, however realistic, the moment will always pass with time. And it is always only one of the several possible outcomes.

Worrying often produces so much distress and anxiety that people interrupt their own train of thought with something more benign (distracting themselves, thinking about something different, etc.). The events leading up to and including the imagined catastrophe are conjured up in vivid detail, but the individual breaks off their thinking when the image becomes too distressing. In some ways, therefore, the adaptive element of worry is never completed. The individual never gets to consider what is likely to happen, or how they and others would respond, if the catastrophe actually did come to pass.

By helping people think *through* their worries, and consider more realistically their 'worst case scenarios' and how they would manage them, the threat posed by the images and thoughts is diminished. Once the sting has been taken out of worrying thoughts, they are less likely to intrude on consciousness. For example, someone who constantly worries about a recurrence may not think beyond the point of the bad news interview, and they may fail to consider that, in fact, the healthcare team would have further goals to aim for and would not abandon them.

This form of intervention, while simple in principle, is not trivial. Because it often involves people articulating their worst fears, it is essential that the nature of the intervention is explained beforehand and the patient understands and agrees to it. No one should be pressured to talk about their fears unless they are willing and, if so, sufficient time, support, and privacy must be available because this kind of intervention can elicit strong emotions (for a clinical example of de-catastrophization *see* Chapter 3—Worrying about Children).

Insomnia

Roughly a third of cancer patients report sleeping difficulties that interfere with their daytime lives.[176] Problems usually involve either getting off to sleep or waking in the night followed by difficulty returning to sleep. Early morning wakening appears to be less common so may represent a useful clue that the individual is clinically depressed (though depression should be considered with any form of sleep disruption). Pre-existing sleep difficulties are often made worse by cancer.

Sleep disturbances in cancer patients can have a number of causes and the relationship between them is still far from clear.[177] Pain, increased frequency of nighttime urination, fatigue, worry, anxiety, depression, loss of daytime activity, and circadian rhythm disturbance can all contribute to insomnia. The picture can therefore be complex. For example, both insomnia and excessive REM sleep can cause increased fatigue and depression,[113] while increased fatigue causes patients to take daytime naps, which can lead to insomnia at night. Pain may create difficulties with sleeping while poor sleep may lead to difficulty managing pain.[177] Moreover, insomnia is not a simple function of treatments such as chemotherapy and radiotherapy, although it is often associated with them. A study of breast cancer patients who had not yet begun treatment revealed that nearly 90% reported insomnia although, interestingly, this was not confined to those who rated themselves as highly anxious.[178]

Assessing sleep disturbance must depend on the patient's own perception of their sleep, which is notoriously unreliable. For example, many people believe that they need eight hours a night, yet humans vary in their need for sleep. (There is, in fact, epidemiological evidence to suggest that risk of mortality among the general population is lowest among people who have seven hours of sleep nightly.)[179] People who claim to suffer with insomnia often under-report the amount of sleep they objectively get, though in one study lung cancer patients actually over-reported the amount of sleep they had had.[180] Sleep assessments should always include obvious factors like when and what the patient eats and drinks during the evening since people may be consuming stimulants (tea, coffee, cocoa) or excessive alcohol[1] without appreciating their effects on sleep.

Among the psychological causes of insomnia, worry, and anxiety are obvious candidates. Many researchers in the field have concluded that insomnia is often the result of an inability to switch off intrusive worrying thoughts and images at bedtime.[181] Undoubtedly people with cancer have a huge number of changes and uncertainties to worry about, so where worrying appears to be keeping people from sleeping, these concerns should be elicited and explored (see Worry) using cognitive-behavioural therapy techniques. For example, people with advanced disease may worry about dying in their sleep or have nightmares about dying. Encouraging patients to talk about these experiences enables the underlying fears to be isolated and addressed. Once insomnia has started, people frequently develop a worry about the insomnia itself, producing the self-fulfilling effect of being kept awake by trying too hard to get to sleep (e.g. in the belief that it is healthy to get a full eight hours sleep). It can remove some of the anxiety and urgency simply to reassure the patient that insomnia is not harmful in itself and that bedtime should be approached as an opportunity to enjoy some rest, rather than acquiring a particular number of hours of sleep. Paradoxical methods, such as asking the patient to try to stay awake as long as possible, can enable them to feel more in control and therefore less anxious about being awake.

Although benzodiazepines are frequently prescribed for insomnia, their long-term use is not advised, especially among older people where they have been associated with impaired cognitive function, falls and fractures, motor accidents, and even insomnia itself.[182] Prolonged use is also associated with problems of tolerance, dose escalation, and addiction.[183] Indeed, a recent comparison of benzodiazepines and behavioural treatment found that those treated with non-pharmacological methods sustained their improvements over two years follow-up, while those on drug therapies did not.[184]

A recent review of 48 studies, including two meta-analyses, found that non-pharmacological therapies produce reliable and durable benefits for between 70% and 80% of chronic insomnia sufferers.[185] These approaches included progressive muscle relaxation and paradoxical intention strategies (i.e. 'Try to stay awake'), and

---

[1]Alcohol is sedative at higher doses and a stimulant at lower doses. As alcohol is metabolised during the night the dose drops to stimulant levels, and may cause the person to wake.

stimulus-control (going to bed only when sleepy and not before normal bedtime, leaving the bedroom if unable to sleep after 20 minutes and returning only when sleepy, and using the bed only for sleeping, not for eating, television, etc.). There is good evidence that even simply training people to relax their muscles (progressive muscle relaxation) can lead to lasting sleep-onset improvements in people with cancer.[186]

An allied approach to sleep problems is to consider whether the effects of the stress and treatment of cancer have led to a disruption of the individual's sleep–wake schedule of activity. More rest and less physical activity during the day may lead to poor sleep at night with subsequent sleepiness the next day, leading to a cycle of deterioration.[177] In this regard, gentle daytime exercise (i.e. a walk) has been shown to decrease fatigue, emotional distress, and sleeping difficulties among breast cancer patients undergoing radiotherapy, possibly as a result of resynchronizing their rest–activity rhythms to coincide with the night–day cycle.[187]

Rehabilitation

With improved survival rates, cancer is progressively becoming regarded as a chronic illness. A period of recovery and convalescence is to be expected after any serious illness, but many cancer patients are left with enormous residual difficulties, requiring continued supportive care in its broadest sense. It is therefore increasingly necessary for cancer services to provide comprehensive programmes of rehabilitation to enable people with cancer to manage and resolve any enduring problems following their treatment. Although the effects of cancer and/or its treatment can result in significant residual problems that appear to be predominantly physical in nature, all have a strong psychological component. The section above on *Common Treatment Difficulties* lists a number of complications that people with cancer regularly face as they emerge from active treatment. These problems can be as much the focus of rehabilitation efforts as the difficulties that are mentioned below. Despite a surge of interest in cancer rehabilitation in the late 1970s and early 1980s, there has been a relative dearth of research or clinical attention to this topic since this time.[188]

Cancer rehabilitation involves helping people with cancer maximize their physical, social, psychological, and occupational functioning within the limits imposed by the disease and its treatment. The focus is on restoring quality of life that is equivalent to and preferably exceeding the individual's quality of life before the cancer. As such, its goals should always be defined by the patient in negotiation with the rehabilitation team. Several types of rehabilitation have been described:[189]

- **Preventive:** when a disability can be foreseen and prior training can reduce its severity (e.g. planning a mobility programme to prevent muscle weakness due to prolonged bed rest).
- **Restorative:** when a temporary disability is overcome (e.g. setting attainable goals to restore premorbid functioning).

- **Supportive:** when there is permanent loss of function, the goal of rehabilitation is to maximize quality of life and help the patient adjust to their loss (e.g. helping patients with disfigurements re-engage with the social world).

- **Palliative:** when advanced disease precludes the restoration of normal activities of daily life and where the aim is to minimize dependency and maximize quality of life (e.g. helping patients and families manage cognitive impairments).

Mobility

It has been estimated that muscle strength decreases by about 1% per day of bed rest, and this loss of strength is particularly apparent in lower weight-bearing muscles (e.g. quadriceps) and postural muscles (e.g. hip and lower-back muscles).[190] Bed rest and/or the effect of central nervous system disease can result in weakened, deconditioned muscles, as well as contribute to the problems of fatigue and insomnia. A programme of graded exercise can help restore weakened muscles and, for those who can tolerate it, aerobic exercises and activities are helpful in increasing endurance.[191] Rehabilitation efforts must progress from the patient's current level of functioning with due regard to their general medical condition (*see* CNS Tumours, page 223). Where the patient is bed-ridden, mobility training may start with changing position in the bed (which also prevents bed sores). Other people may require help in learning to walk, sit upright, or use a wheelchair and in learning to transfer to and from the wheelchair. Various prostheses help to maintain limb position and enhance mobility.

A number of different cancers frequently metastasize to the bones. Because there are currently only very inaccurate methods of predicting the risk of fracture in patients with bone metastases, rehabilitation professionals are wary about treating patients with bone secondaries. However, a recent review concluded that the risks of producing pathological fractures in cancer patients by increasing mobility and function are low.[192] Particular success has been achieved in the rehabilitation of patients who have had recent surgical repair of pathological or impending fractures. In some cases of breast cancer, bone secondaries may be the only site of cancer for many years. In some, they may never progress beyond bone; keeping the patient mobile and out of a wheel chair is then the main aim.

New drugs (bisphosphonates such as sodium clodronate and zoledronic acid) have been found to improve survival as well as prevent disability. Anticipating the risk of fracture by preventative strengthening of a weakened area, such as the neck of femur, or spinal cord or nerve root damage by elective spinal surgery is increasingly important. Patients appear to be at greater risk of fracture the more sites of bone metastases they have, and also if they have already had more than one fracture.[193] These crude indications may be of limited value in assessing the individual patient, and many patients, moreover, prefer to risk the possibility of a fracture rather than face the alternative to rehabilitation: bed rest or immobility. These alternatives are often life-long and have their own complications (e.g. weakness, atrophy, pressure sores, pneumonia, etc.).

Activities of daily living

For many patients, the focus of rehabilitation is helping the individual reintegrate back into their home and community. This involves the individual learning to manage routine activities of daily life such as dressing, bathing, toileting, cooking, shopping, etc. Rehabilitation may involve the patient developing the strength to cope with such activities and/or learning new ways to perform old tasks with or without adaptations to their home and additional equipment. Help with pacing and prioritizing their activities can also enable patients to conserve their energy, especially where they are suffering from fatigue.

Psychosocial rehabilitation

There are many other difficulties that are amenable to rehabilitation but beyond the scope of this book. Swallowing disorders (dysphagias), disorders of language (dysphasias), breathing difficulties (dyspnoea),[93, 194] bladder and bowel disorders, significant weight loss (cachexia), and lymphoedema are all candidates for a comprehensive rehabilitation programme.[191] However, there are more general psychosocial concerns that should also be addressed under the rehabilitation umbrella, and one might argue that psychosocial specialists need to focus their efforts on helping people maximise their adjustment to life during and particularly after their treatment.

The psychosocial problems that afflict people as a result of their cancer do not evaporate at the end of treatment. For some they become worse or only become apparent after treatment has ended. The confrontation of 'normal daily life' once active treatment has finished often highlights the very changes that have occurred which the individual must now adjust to or overcome.

Rehabilitation programmes which have psychosocial care at their core ensure that people with cancer are able to negotiate the transition from the hospital into the community without feeling they have been abandoned by the healthcare team to 'get on with their lives'. Ending treatment can be a time when people are particularly vulnerable to depression. Psychosocial rehabilitation helps people reintegrate with the social context of their lives. As described in Chapters 2 and 3, cancer has widespread effects on the patient, their partner, family, and other people; the world to which the individual 'returns' is often as changed as the patient themselves.

Many people with cancer finish treatment with mixed feelings about resuming the lives they led before their illness. They may need support in making the changes they feel are necessary to their personal and social lives (see Chapter 2—Ending Treatment). There may be relationship or sexual problems that only become clear as the patient feels well again. Patients may be anxious about returning to work—unsure whether they can still perform their job and, fearing stigma or pity, uncertain how much to reveal to colleagues. They may need support in adjusting to permanent changes to their body: how they look, feel, and what they are capable of doing (see Chapter 2—The Body). They may be facing unemployment, poverty, or a fundamental change in living standards resulting from loss of income. They may be suffering with residual depression or anxiety, intrusive worrying about recurrence or disease progression, or social phobia (a fear of meeting people).

Structured group rehabilitation programmes have been shown to help people with cancer manage the after-effects of treatment, while providing social contact and peer support. In one programme, patients and their partners benefited from attending a six-week group in which they received information about coping with cancer, undertook a relaxation and exercise programme, and used the sessions to 'problem-solve' cancer-related concerns.[195]

Rehabilitation teams

Rehabilitation teams must be multidisciplinary, reflecting the physical, psychological, and social needs of patients ending the treatment. In the US, where cancer rehabilitation is most developed, teams are often co-ordinated by 'physiatrists' (doctors who are trained in physical medicine and rehabilitation). In the UK, physiotherapists acquired professional autonomy in 1977 and the British Society of Rehabilitation Medicine was formed in 1984, although doctors are still simply referred to as working in rehabilitation medicine. Physiotherapists tend to focus on gross motor function, while occupational therapists concentrate on the fine motor skills and cognitive and perceptual abilities required for activities of daily living.[191] Specialists in physical exercise and health can advise on programmes of exercise to develop body composition and stamina, reduce fatigue and nausea, and improve emotional well-being. A review of 36 studies has concluded that exercise can positively affect all these parameters.[196]

Speech and language therapists target speech, language, and swallowing difficulties, while physiotherapists, and often nurses, play an invaluable role in mobility problems and psychosocial support. Social workers are essential for the co-ordination of discharge planning by arranging appropriate support in the community, and the chaplaincy service may be called upon for emotional and spiritual support.[191] Psychologists and psychiatrists provide expertise in tackling more complex psychological and relationship problems, while ex-patients can present the authentic voice of experience which can be both reassuring and inspiring. Finally, advice from dietitians/nutritionists enables patients and families to feel confident about their dietary intake, while the involvement of art, writing, and music therapists can restore patients' sense of confidence and self-esteem.

Prior to discharge, every patient should be carefully assessed and their individual needs documented, preferably by the key worker assigned to co-ordinate their care. The more that objective measures of current functioning can be recorded the easier it will be for the patient to monitor their progress. Once the individual's psychosocial concerns and motivation for rehabilitation have been assessed, clear achievable goals can be set by the patient in negotiation with rehabilitation staff. Although goals will be tailor-made to the individual's needs, their attainment may entail group exercises (e.g. relaxation training, return-to-work support group, etc.) as well as one-to-one therapies. It helps to involve families at an early planning stage so that they can contribute to the rehabilitation programme, maintain the motivation of the patient and obtain support for themselves from the rest of the rehabilitation team. A number of strategies can be used to ensure that patients maintain sufficient motivation during what is often a long rehabilitation. Patients and families should be encouraged to maintain a log or journal so that they can monitor progress and record difficulties.[191] Setting modest attainable goals with clear end-points and even rewards (e.g. a special meal or other treat) ensures that patients are not discouraged by setbacks.

Recurrence

> Not only did the chest x-ray show that I have secondary cancers in my ribs, but a recent cervical smear I had taken was also showing abnormalities, and unusually these appeared to be secondary breast cancer. Strangely I feel relieved that the cancer isn't in my lungs which is what I had been particularly worried about. It's hard to take it all in and all the old feelings that I had when I first learned I had breast cancer three years ago have come to the surface – mainly that I'm frightened and don't want to face the prospect of leaving my family without me. It's also so hard telling family and friends what is happening but you have to, even though you are still struggling to come to terms with it yourself.

Cancer recurrence is a devastating time for patients and their loved ones. Prior hopes that one may have been cured are dashed and the spectre of death reappears, only larger and more discernible. In returning to active treatment, if it is offered, patients are no longer buffered by their own ignorance of what to expect. While there is little published research to guide us, an early study found that many patients had difficulty communicating with loved ones about their recurrence because of the intrinsically painful nature of the subject, and that existential concerns were predominant.[197] Indeed, recurrence is often a time when the deeply held assumption described in Chapter 1 are revisited in earnest: life trajectory, relationship with other people, self-worth and personal control, assumptions about the body, and spiritual concerns.

The disappointment of recurrence rarely leaves much room for optimism and often signals a dramatic surge of hopelessness although, for some, it can feel like the inevitable outcome that they have long been dreading. Almost 80% of patients in one study described their recurrence as more upsetting than their initial diagnosis, while only 8% found their initial diagnosis more upsetting.[198] Those patients who were 'completely surprised' had more symptoms of post-traumatic stress disorder (intrusive thoughts and avoidance) than those who 'knew it could happen' (who did best) or who were 'not at all surprised'. All but one patient experienced a 'collapse of hope' following recurrence. Clinical depression has also been found to be more common among those with metastases.[151]

Roughly half the sample were concerned that their physician might decide not to treat the recurrent disease, and almost one in five believed their families would be less supportive than after their first diagnosis.[198] Facing treatment the second time round can be much harder for both patients and family and it is little wonder that patients fear that this time their family might be less able to sustain their support. Every one of the patient's family and friends must once again confront the very real probability that they will lose someone they love. A family that was previously reliant on 'positive thinking at all costs' may find this defence begins to wear thin as people feel the need to speak more authentically about their fears for the future. Now, more than ever, there is a need for openness and honesty between family members.

Following a recurrence, patients and families may be especially vulnerable to the promise of 'miracle cures' from alternative medicine.[199] They may regret previous treatment decisions and look elsewhere for their salvation. In their desperate search for survival, patients are susceptible to believing people who may offer little more than anecdotal evidence to support their claims (*see* Chapter 7—Complementary Therapy and Alternative Medicine). Yet it may be the fact that alternative medicine offers time and a willingness to attend to the emotional and existential suffering of patients that also gives it appeal. It should be noted that in the study mentioned above[198] the patients facing a recurrence believed that healthcare staff were not as interested and were not providing as much support or information as they had when the patient was first diagnosed. This latter perception may well have been accurate—nurses have been shown to use more blocking tactics in their communication with patients facing a recurrence than with other cancer patients.[200]

Clearly, recurrence is not only a devastating crisis for patients and their families but also a difficult time for healthcare professionals who may feel they have failed the patient and may now be blamed. It is a testing and alarming time in which patients and their families face a decidedly uncertain future in which they will increasingly be looking for the strength and resolve of their professional carers to show them the way. It is essential therefore that healthcare staff demonstrate that they are not over-whelmed by the tragedy of the recurrence. Instead they must strike a balance between acknowledging the significance of the recurrence and its emotional impact on the patient, and offering a reassuring sense of leadership and direction towards goals that can yet be achieved. These are the principles of palliative care.

Palliative care

Up until the nineteenth century, medicine concentrated on palliating symptoms while the disease took its course towards recovery or death. For the past century, however, scientific medicine has shifted almost all its attention to the search for underlying causes and ultimately cures.[201] As a result of this shift, palliative interventions became denigrated as 'merely symptomatic' and, with this, the traditional art of caring lost its stature.

With the flowering of the hospice movement in Britain in the late 1960s, however, palliative care was reborn with a new confidence of purpose (even though palliative medicine was not established as a distinct specialism until 1987). These days the hospice movement continues to spread across the world, and the effectiveness of palliative care interventions is being increasingly demonstrated.[202] However, despite the fact that most people want to die at home, death is frequently medicalized in the West and hospitals continue to be seen as the most appropriate place to die.[203] In the UK over

90% of patients spend the majority of their final year at home though only about 26% of deaths occur at home[204] (*see* Chapter 3—Caring).

Palliative care shares many of the same philosophical goals as psychosocial care and offers a patient-centred model of healthcare for other areas of medicine to emulate. It emphasizes that medical care and treatment should always be sensitive to the broader context of patients' lives: their family and social lives, their individual needs, their cultural and spiritual beliefs, and their social circumstances. Palliative care interventions unashamedly focus on ameliorating the symptoms of suffering; their success is evaluated in terms of the individual's quality of life rather than tumour regression or survival time. Cicely Saunders, one of the founding figures of the hospice movement, has highlighted the aspirations of palliative care. The professional team is there ...

> to enable the dying person to live until he dies, at his own maximum potential, performing to the limit of his physical activity and mental capacity with control and independence wherever possible. If he is recognized as the unique person he is and helped to live as part of his family and in other relationships, he can still reach out to his hopes and expectations and to what has deepest meaning for him and end his life with a sense of completion.[205]

(Saunders 1998, viii)

Palliative care is not limited to cancer, or even to the terminal stages of illness, though here we focus on the psychological and social issues affecting people with cancer who are dying.

Psychosocial issues for people who are dying

The images and assumptions we hold about death shape our responses to it. Not all cultures share the same attitudes and beliefs about death, let alone how it should be faced (*see* Chapter 2—Expectations about Illness). Death among Hindus, for example, is not a private family affair but more of a communal public event; children are not shielded from witnessing the death or attending the funeral. In fact, it is considered holy for anyone who has known the deceased to attend the funeral; an invitation is not necessary. Only after a year of wandering through the kingdoms of Yama, Lord of death, does the deceased reach the temporary abode of their ancestors where Yama decides whether they will go to *svarga* (heaven) or *narka* (hell).[206] But for Hindus death does not mark the end of life but the beginning of a new one (reincarnation).

Like Christians and Jews, Muslims regard life as a preparation for the next life where one will be held accountable; death represents the individual returning to Allah. Consequently, the dying person will wish to be facing Mecca. After they have died the body is prepared in much the same way as the individual would have prepared themselves for prayer: the body is washed and lain out with the head in the direction of Mecca. Ideally only Muslims of the same sex as the deceased should handle the body, but if this is not possible non-Muslims should wear gloves as a sign of respect. According to Islamic belief, the soul leaves the body immediately upon death and the body should be buried within two of the five daily prayer periods of the death.[207]

Dying therefore conjures up many varied images depending on the cultural beliefs that have been absorbed by the individual, but it should not be automatically assumed that any individual fully subscribes to all the beliefs and practices associated with their particular ethnic or religious community. Individuals vary within cultures as much as cultures vary from one another. The fear of death, however, is biological and natural. Like any creature, human beings struggle to hold on to life whenever possible. For example, patients are prepared to accept a considerably lower chance of benefit from second-line palliative chemotherapy than healthy subjects, oncologists, GPs, and nurses when these latter groups are asked to imagine such circumstances.[208] Only when death appears the more attractive option, or they are too exhausted to continue, will people choose death over life.

Religion can offer the comfort of spiritual guidance, often the consolation of meaning, and even the hope of a future to one's existence. Nonetheless, for many people death remains the ultimate fear of the unknown—dust to dust, ashes to ashes. Even when others are present, everyone must experience death on their own. This stark fact is not something that is easy to look at and, not surprisingly, death is associated with considerable anxiety.

But, in fact, people who know their cancer is incurable are generally less afraid of death *per se*, than they are of the process of dying. Images and expectations of slowly wasting away, enduring unremitting pain, and watching the distress of their helpless loved ones are common. The reality is usually quite different, particularly where there is input from nurses and doctors who specialize in palliative care and can provide reassurance and support regarding pain and other symptom control. The symptomatic treatment of the physically distressing processes of dying has improved dramatically thanks to the progress of palliative care doctors and nurses. In particular, there have been significant gains in the treatment of cancer pain with opiates, even if fears of addiction continue to abound in many parts of the world. Although not all pain can be controlled all the time, there has been steady progress in its management over the past 25 years. In 1978, a study of terminally ill cancer patients at home found that 28% suffered severe, mostly unrelieved pain during their last days at home, despite the use of drugs.[209] By 1993, another study of a similar population found that only 4% had had no pain relief and, during the last week before death, 87% had had little or no pain. A major task in palliative care is therefore to educate, prepare, and often reassure patients, their families, and sometimes professionals, about what is likely to happen during the process of dying.

Cancer's image as a wasting disease is also something of a caricature. The fact that cancer rarely kills people quickly is seen as its curse, rather than one of its few advantages over some other fatal illnesses. People commonly hold the view that they would prefer to die suddenly, without warning. Heart attacks and strokes are seen to inflict mercifully little suffering on their victims compared with cancer, but the reality is that sudden deaths often leave the bereaved entirely unprepared and therefore more traumatized by the loss. By contrast, the vast majority of people who die of cancer are given considerable warning, permitting them time to prepare themselves and their family for their impending death and, indeed, for the family to celebrate their lives. However, this leads to the other prevailing emotion among people who know they are dying: loss. In facing their death, the individual prepares to relinquish the essential elements that make up their lives: their goals and dreams, their relationships, their sense of agency and control, and their existential self. What can help mitigate these losses is palliative care's focus on helping people to achieve goals and derive meaning from their lives right up until their end.

Communicating needs

Appropriate palliative care is defined by the patient's wishes and needs, rather than by 'objective' criteria. People who are facing their death have many needs that change over time and it is not only the patient's current symptoms that need to be taken into account. Their previous experiences of treatment also shape their expectations and wishes. The age and stage of life a person has reached will affect their needs and concerns. For example, the young single person whose life has hardly begun, the parent of small children, the elderly person being cared for by their family—may all have differing yet overlapping concerns. Each person's individual history and current family context will also affect their decisions about which, if any, medical treatments they would be prepared to undergo. (*See* Chapter 6—Discussing resuscitation.)

Not surprisingly, palliative care professionals require sophisticated communication skills. They must carefully negotiate with their patients to ensure that interventions offered meet the individual's unique and changing needs. Not all patients are prepared to learn that they are terminally ill. Some people prefer to keep this knowledge at bay at times, even referring to their palliative treatment as curative, while at other times they are able to talk openly about their impending death (*see* Chapter 2—Denial and Avoidance; Chapter 6—Working with Someone in Denial). Communication can be especially challenging when, for example, the patient's cultural background discourages full disclosure of the prognosis, or where the family's desire to explore active treatment 'at all costs' conflicts with the patient's wish to feel well enough to pursue other goals (such as time with the family).

But communication with terminally ill patients is much more than a discussion of the relative merits of physical interventions. Palliative care ideally embodies the holistic model of patient-centred care in which psychosocial and spiritual concerns hold equal weight with physical ones. In addition, the planning and preparation for a good death involves seeing the patient as part of a family unit. Whilst the wishes of the patient remain paramount, the participation of family members is essential in resolving certain issues (e.g. Does the patient wish to die at home? Are the family supportive of this? What practical resources does the family need? And which members of the family are especially vulnerable and may need further support?).

As far as possible, communication with the patient should include as many of the family members as the patient wishes with, as always, the patient defining whom they regard as 'family'. This prevents the situation in which family members are with-holding information from the patient or vice versa. Where necessary, relatives and patients should first be counselled independently so that they can explore their fears of open disclosure (*see* Other People below). Ultimately, if the patient wants informa-tion about their condition, healthcare professionals are ethically bound to provide it and family members are unable to forbid it. Above all, families appreciate information that can help them care more effectively for their sick member since often the burden of care is on the family (with the support of primary care professionals). The patient's admission to hospital can induce conflicting feelings of relief and guilt in family mem-bers for, while most terminally ill cancer patients would prefer to die at home,[210] in the UK only 36% actually die at home, or in a residential or nursing home.

Ending Life

If there has been a reasonable period of remission, some people may feel they have regained a degree of 'normality' in their lives in which the threat of cancer and death has receded to become more distant and abstract again. The devastating realization that this time the end may truly be in sight marks a new relationship with what may have been faced earlier in the illness. For those who are newly diagnosed but face a ter-minal illness there is the additional shock and trauma of a catastrophic event that is sudden and unexpected (*see* Chapter 1). The core concerns (life trajectory, other peo-ple, self-worth and control, the body, existential issues) faced by newly diagnosed patients with cancer are equally pertinent to people facing the end of their lives, albeit with different priorities and urgencies. These will be briefly reviewed.

Life trajectory

Feelings of depression among people facing a terminal illness are probably quite under-standable when one considers the fact that they may be surrendering many of their life-long goals and ambitions. 'The loss of tomorrow'[211] is perhaps impossible to contemplate until one is faced with it. A wished-for future not only provides hope, it also sustains motivation and a buoyancy of mood. Among 120 terminally ill cancer patients, 99% rated 'having a sense of hope' as extremely or very important.[212] Loss of purpose, motivation, and hopes are tantamount to feeling depressed and it is not surprising there-fore to find that depression is commonly found among people who are terminally ill. However, while such emotional suffering should always be addressed, it is arguable whether drug treatments alone are the most appropriate response to concerns which are so clearly psychosocial and spiritual. The individual may already be taking a great deal of medication and may resist the loss of control implied by taking yet another drug which, in any event, may take nearly two weeks before any effect is discernible. However, anti-depressants (both tricyclics and SSRIs) have their place even if evidence for their effec-tiveness is currently limited and they are often prescribed 'too little, too late'.[213]

'Working through' loss allows people to articulate and release their feelings at their own rate. By enabling people to express their understandable sorrow and loss we normalize it.[211] By offering people emotional support, we ease their grief. Crying, after all, is a perfectly normal way for people to express and release their pent-up emotions. It is by working through their grief and tears that people find a way of integrating their illness with all that has gone before in their lives. Out of the turmoil caused by an amputated future emerges the possibility of new goals and a different kind of hope. It is notable that in a study in Scandinavia of suicide among cancer patients, the highest incidence was found among those who were offered no further treatment and no further contact with the healthcare system.[48] Palliative care, by contrast, offers continuity of help and support throughout the process of dying, extending to bereavement support for loved ones. It emphasizes the value of patients and staff making achievable realistic targets to aim for in terms of rehabilitation and symptom relief. It offers the promise of empathic care with the aim of preserving dignity. It *never* abandons hope.

Practical concerns

As the individual looks to the future beyond their own death they consider the practical needs facing their family and loved ones. The most practical of these concerns is to do with the disposal and distribution of their estate and thus the writing of a will. The financial security of loved ones is especially important when other people are dependent on the dying person (children, parents, a disabled partner, etc). Developing realistic long-term plans for the future security of loved ones is the overarching priority for many patients and their families. Planning the funeral is another practical activity that can give patients satisfaction while easing the burden of their loved ones who otherwise will be forced to organize it.

In the shorter term, families must look to the financial burden of caring for their loved one at home as well as, in some countries, the cost of hospitalization. In addition, the physical and emotional strains of caring need to be addressed through appropriate nursing, medical, psychosocial, spiritual, and community support. Families often underestimate the physical burdens of care, focusing more on the distress of losing someone they love (*see* Chapter 3—Caring).

Other people

Saying goodbye to a loved one is a mutual loss that can be as frightening as it is sad. The people we care about not only give us pleasure through their love, they are also embedded in the world we know, a reference point which helps to make the world a secure and safe place. Death inevitably severs the bonds between people and exposes their dependence upon one another. It is one of the most inevitable and painful aspects of human suffering.

Some people wish to put the record straight by repairing past hurts and restoring broken relationships, completing the unfinished emotional business of their lives. However, the prospect of separation can be so unspeakably distressing that a conspiracy of silence sometimes develops between the dying person and their loved ones. Discussing death would make it real and cause needless distress. Better to 'stay positive' and put it off until one is forced to deal with it. Unfortunately, such a response leaves everyone feeling isolated and unable to express their fears and sadness to the very person whom they would normally be turning to for support in any other crisis.

Yet there is often much to be said:[212] love, regret, thanks, memories, plans for the survivors' future. Open expression of these emotions can ease the later pain of bereavement, but both patients and families sometimes worry that the most important things that need to be said should be kept for the end, at the deathbed. It may come as a relief to realize that this is not the case but, rather, it may be easier to express such poignant matters earlier, and then 'safely put them away again', rather than leave them as 'unfinished business'.

The imminent death is a crisis that every member of the family will be facing, so helping all members of the family to communicate and support one another is the first of the two key tasks. The other is arranging support for the most vulnerable members of the family, or for any patient without adequate support who would welcome it. Emotional support, after all, is central to how people manage difficult change (*see* Chapter 3—Other People.)

The care of people with advanced disease should ideally include the entire family so that all key family members are kept fully informed, and so the staff can present a model of open communication. The 'family' (as defined by the patient) is a dynamic system of relationships which almost inevitably will be in various levels of turmoil as a result of the impending death of one of its members. If the person with cancer is facing a recurrence, the family will obviously have deep concerns about the patient. They will be hungry for news. A few families are already exhausted and some even resentful at having their lives massively disrupted again. Regular meetings between professionals and families go a long way towards helping families orientate themselves to the challenges that lie ahead.

Where there is evidence of blocked communication within family relationships, healthcare professionals can facilitate openness between family members by enabling patients or their relatives to share their thoughts and feelings with the professional first. For example, a patient may want to talk about their impending death with their family, but they feel forced to avoid discussing the topic because of their family's conspiracy of silence. By rehearsing what they might like to say if others (e.g. partner and children) were present, patients can explore their fears of talking more openly.

It may be helpful to remind family members that although the patient is dying they may wish to feel as involved as ever in the family, perhaps even more so. If appropriate, both patients and family members can also be warned that if they mutually protect each other from the distress of difficult conversations they may also forfeit each other's heartfelt support and an opportunity to resolve 'unfinished business'.

The family as a whole may need particular support in managing the death. A family meeting should be offered at which all issues of concern can be aired and explored. Professionals should ensure that: every member of the family has sufficient support; the family is communicating effectively; children's developmental needs are being addressed; and the family is able to talk about their future following the imminent death of one of its members. (Chapter 3 considers the broader issues facing families and carers.)

Self-concept and control

(*see* Chapter 2, Impact on Self)
People's sense of their own value is derived from their contact with others. In other words, people derive a sense of their worth through the social roles they perform in life (parent, teacher, friend, colleague, partner, etc.). Some of these roles are inevitably curtailed as patients become more ill or disabled by their cancer. Although some people with cancer are able to sustain some level of employment until the illness is advanced, others may already be pining for their working life. In one study of people experiencing recurrent disease, 75% reported missing work.[198]

Healthcare staff should encourage patients to retain roles that enable them to feel normal and valued, while supporting them when they are forced to relinquish important roles. Questions to consider include: Does the person feel they are using their time in meaningful and useful ways? Do they still have social roles that enable them to feel valued and respected by others?

Increasing ill health and frailty often leads other people to assume responsibility and 'speak for' the patient. However, the ability to make choices and decisions and to retain control is fundamental to many patients' self-image and self-worth. To lose this capacity is tantamount to a regression to childhood. A person's self-esteem, their sense of competence and control protects them against depression.[214] People rarely welcome this loss of control so healthcare staff can assist by helping the patient to reflect on their wishes: Does the patient feel they have control over current events in their lives or do they feel other people are making decisions for them? How do they feel about this situation and what, if anything, would they like to change about it?

Similarly, patients commonly fear losing their dignity as their disease progresses and control over their bodily functions diminishes. While acknowledging this deeply important concern, it may help to remind the patient that, as professionals and as people, we respect and value their inherent human integrity (their character and individuality) regardless of the state of their body. Palliative care is very much about preserving the dignity of the individual to the last.

The body

The end of life invariably involves the patient having to deal with physical decline. The body's failing capacities and the physical discomfort caused by disease progression increasingly become prominent concerns. Deterioration in one's appearance, and the capacity to express oneself or care for oneself can be equally distressing for both patients and their families. The primary role of healthcare in this respect is more obvious and concrete: palliation of physical symptoms. This is rightly the core concern of palliative medicine because pain and other physical symptoms are the source of much avoidable suffering and distress. Although a discussion of the palliation of physical symptoms (breathing difficulties, loss of strength, dysphagia, mucositis, etc.) is well beyond the scope of this book, we have discussed psychosocial aspects of pain and several other symptoms in earlier sections of this chapter. We also described rehabilitation interventions that are often equally applicable to patients with incurable illness as they are to patients emerging from a first encounter with cancer.

It is worth emphasizing, however, that physical difficulties experienced by patients also have a significant impact on their carers. Healthcare professionals should therefore provide carers with clear guidelines and practical advice regarding the care of their loved ones. This will allow them to feel symbolically included in the wider healthcare team (*see* General Practice). Maintaining open communication between the family and healthcare team also enables the needs of family members to be identified and addressed.

Furthermore, palliative interventions must always take account of the carer's needs. For example, loss of appetite and weight can cause anguish to both patients and carers alike. The giving and receiving of food is not only a literal means of sustaining life, but is symbolically embedded in the caring relationship. Carers may find it intolerable being unable to nurture their loved ones through giving them food. So although there is little objective evidence that appetite stimulants, like megastrol acetate, improve quality of life, there's good evidence that they do improve appetite,[215] and this is likely to have a beneficial effect on the carer's capacity to care.

Existential/spiritual

For many people in the world, formal religions provide an important source of guidance, reassurance, and meaning to people facing their death. The frequency of personal prayer has been found to be an important influence on people's psychological well-being.[216] Furthermore, the social cohesion of many religious communities is also an important source of support, not only spiritual but practical and emotional support as well. Nonetheless, spiritual doubts and questions occur, and in one ethnically diverse American sample, as many as 40% of patients reported wanting help with these difficulties.[217] Among a sample of 120 terminally ill cancer patients, over 90% rated their spiritual concerns as being either 'very' or 'extremely' important to them.[212] Healthcare staff frequently underestimate the importance of these questions to their patients,[218] and should therefore routinely ask patients whether they would like the support of their religious leader or would like to talk through these issues with a counsellor. Some people regain their faith at the very end of their lives.

The human search for meaning and purpose is not limited to the spiritual beliefs embodied in formal religions (see Existential Beliefs in Chapter 2). Everyone has core beliefs about the nature of existence and these are not always framed with reference to a god. Often they appear to be more concerned with constructing a moral summary or overview of one's existence in the world. Like other life transitions, such as adolescence and 'mid-life crises', the end of life can be a time to reflect on the past before reorienting oneself to the future. In this regard, the principles of a 'life review' are relevant.

Life review

Conducting a 'life review' is a recognized therapeutic intervention in the care of older people[219] and is considered helpful in enabling developmental change. In simple terms, it involves the patient telling the story of their lives so that 'unfinished business' from the past (regrets, conflicts, anger, missed opportunities, etc.) can be better understood and integrated into a more coherent life narrative. This process reminds the individual of the richness and value of their life and relationships, so that death can be faced with the 'sense of completion' to which Cicely Saunders refers.

Life reviews, whether written or described orally, can help family members and professionals become more aware of the past, present, and future concerns of the dying patient and, in the process, these caregivers may become more understanding and supportive of the individual's needs.[220] The person is seen afresh in the full context of their life story. One of the positive aspects of a life review is that it can involve the caregiver or family member as much as the patient, and can be an activity that spans many days with the potential use of diverse media (photographs, letters, family trees, etc.). Life reviews are designed to be affirming of people's lives. Where there is a risk that the individual may ultimately view their life as a failure or a waste, it is best avoided unless conducted by someone experienced in such techniques.

Communication at the end of life

Doctors often underestimate what a patient already knows or suspects about their illness, and sometimes fail to inform them adequately. However, as in other areas of cancer care, honest communication about the patient's prognosis must be tempered by the patient's desire to know. Although 85% of a sample of 1032 UK palliative care patients stated that they wanted 'as much information as possible, good and bad', nearly 8% did not want to know any details, preferring to 'leave it up to the doctor'.[221] Finding out how much the patient wants to know is therefore always the first step in communicating difficult news; denial or avoidance are valid psychological defence mechanisms which should be respected and worked with. They are often merely temporary sanctuaries.

There is never a need for brutal honesty; if the patient wants a full disclosure then this should be given alongside the clear message that, despite the incurability of the disease or the patient's impending death, the medical team values the individual and will never abandon them. Communication should serve to reduce uncertainty, while giving the patient and family a sense of direction and a goal to work towards.[203] (see Chapter 6—Breaking Bad News).

In most circumstances it is difficult for doctors to estimate accurately a patient's length of survival and it is doubtful that giving firm 'deadlines' is useful, beyond very rough parameters, because they can become the focus of intense worry. In one American study, over 80% of palliative care patients rated their chances of living more than six months as much higher than their doctors' estimation.[222] These patients were also twice as likely to receive life-extending treatments as those patients who accepted the possibility that they would not survive six months. In fact, the longer and better the doctor knows the patient, the more the doctor overestimates their patients' survival time.[223] Hope somehow sustains our will.

As death approaches, it is helpful to warn family members about what the process of death may be like (noisy, rattling, increasingly intermittent breathing, cold extremities, skin mottling, etc.) so that family members can begin to prepare themselves for the physical changes that will occur as their loved one dies. Reassurance should also be given about steps the medical team may need to take and an explanation given regarding any medication used (e.g. morphine) and its action. Whenever possible, patients should continue to be asked for their permission before interventions are offered, and their questions should be answered honestly and supportively. Giving family members tasks to perform allows them to feel involved and useful during what can be a protracted and painful period of waiting. It also helps to ask family members about cultural or religious customs and practices that should be observed before and after the death; one should never make assumptions about these because there can be enormous diversity within any cultural or religious group.

The waiting period is not only emotionally exhausting, it can also evoke unexpected feelings and thoughts in loved ones which can be alarming (e.g. emotional numbness, wishing it were all over, 'selfish' thoughts concerning the future, etc.). Loved ones can be helped by normalizing their feelings, acknowledging their efforts at caring, and reassuring them that they are coping with a situation that they have never faced before or ever been taught to deal with. Encourage loved ones to take breaks from the patient's bedside and to attend to their own needs and those of others, which may have become overlooked. Family members often feel that they ought to be present at the actual time of death, though if they choose not to be present they should not be made to feel guilty. Following the death, the family should be given as much time as they need with the deceased and all cultural and religious customs should be sensitively observed. All families should be given opportunities to discuss the death with the patient's doctor at a specified time. Ideally well before the death, health-care staff should try to assess the extent to which relatives may be vulnerable to a difficult or complicated bereavement. This is especially the case among those who are socially isolated or lack support in the period immediately following the death. A clear offer of follow-up bereavement support should be made to those who are particularly vulnerable.

Bereavement care

Unlike hospices, where bereavement support is usually an integral part of the care of families, hospital-based cancer services rarely offer much help to the newly bereaved. Most bereavement services in the UK, for example, tend to be provided by volunteers within the charitable/voluntary sector. This situation prevails in spite of research evidence, collected over the past forty years, which shows that bereavement has serious health consequences. This conclusion is based both on epidemiological studies, as well as on psychobiological research that has documented significant effects of bereavement on the cardiovascular, endocrine, and immunological systems.[224, 225]

Bereavement care isn't glamorous and its lack of funding is probably due to people seeing bereavement, rightly, as a natural event in almost anyone's life. Its neglect though belies its significance. The death of a spouse has been rated as one of the most stressful life events that people can face. The epidemiological evidence is particularly alarming in terms of the effects of grief on physical health, psychological health, and mortality among survivors. In one study, clinical depression was found in 47% of older widows during the first year after bereavement.[226] Another study found that four times as many bereaved as non-bereaved people had spent part of the preceding year in hospital;[227] the cost implications of this finding to healthcare services are significant. In an earlier study, there was a sevenfold increase in risk of mortality among the bereaved, compared with controls, in the first year following bereavement.[228] And lastly there is evidence of increased suicide among single men losing a parent[229] and among widowed people,[230] especially men.

In the absence of hospital-based bereavement services, the healthcare team who have cared for the deceased should ensure that the bereaved have sufficient emotional or 'confiding' support in their community. It is helpful to assess this before the death and to consider what resources should be activated for those in need of additional support: primary care team, community bereavement support, a voluntary bereavement organization, the relative's church or school, etc. General practitioners can play an important role in preparing families for an imminent death and offering support after it has occurred. All relatives should be provided with information about bereavement support within their local community, and healthcare staff should convey the clear message that obtaining bereavement support is in no sense a sign of failure or weakness. Talking about one's grief is usually the most therapeutic strategy for anyone, though cultures vary in terms of prescribed customs and timescales associated with the period of mourning.

Relatives should always be given opportunities to discuss the death with the medical team at a later date if they wish; after a protracted illness, relatives are often exhausted and their emotional reserves at a low ebb. Written information about practical steps that need to be taken after a death (funeral, registering the death, etc.) as well as the emotional aspects of bereavement can be particularly valuable. Healthcare teams may also wish to send a card of condolence a month to six weeks after the death; this is often the time when the wider community support that was present at the funeral has diminished, and normal daily routines have returned, revealing the bleak reality of life without the deceased. The other side of the condolence card might also remind the bereaved about local bereavement resources.

Essentially the task of bereavement is one of adjusting to a world in which the deceased is no longer present.[231] In the same way that adjusting to a cancer diagnosis can involve a re-examination of deeply held assumptions about one's life, so too does profound loss present bereaved people with fundamental challenges to their mental maps of the world. For example, the life trajectory of the bereaved person is irrevocably altered. For some people, a world without the deceased is one that has lost all meaning and purpose so the future may seem empty and futile. For others, especially when the death is unexpected, living without the deceased may represent an unimaginably frightening prospect full of uncertainty. People often resort to a temporary denial of the death, before gradually absorbing its reality and implications. For the majority, however, mourning is a mixture of emotional pain, pining, anxiety and sadness, exhaustion, and moving on. Mourning, like cancer, is a stressful psychosocial transition.[232]

The process of grief is as varied as it is long. It is shaped by the cultural and religious rituals associated with bereavement as well as the meaning that the death has for the individual in the context of their prevailing culture. Historically, for example, child mortality used to be so high that 'it was sometimes said that you were not a woman until you had lost your first child[233]' (Parkes 2002, p. 19). As Colin Murray Parkes has noted, the reflective French philosopher Montaigne put in writing that he had lost 'two or three children in their infancy, not without regret, but without great sorrow.[234]' Today there are widely varied cultural expectations regarding the course of people's bereavement.

Alarm and grief pangs

In the very early stages of mourning there may be denial, disbelief, or dreamlike dissociated feelings. Alarm and uncertainty about the future soon follow, together with intense pangs of grief and yearning for the deceased. Here is how C.S. Lewis described his spasms of grief for his beloved wife: '*I've plenty of what are called "resources". People get over these things. Come, I shan't do so badly. One is ashamed to listen to this voice but it seems for a little to be making out a good case. Then comes a sudden jab of red-hot memory and all this "commonsense" vanishes like an ant in the mouth of a furnace.*'[235]

(Lewis 1961, pp. 5–6).

Mitigation

An estimated 40% of bereaved people experience what has been termed a 'mitigation' of their grief, a vague or sometimes striking sense that the dead person has been 'found' again. It may even be the beginnings of a form of resolution or recovery. Occasionally the bereaved person believes they have seen, heard, or smelled their loved one again, though other people experience it more in terms of a spiritual presence. C.S. Lewis again: '*I suppose I am recovering from a good deal of mere exhaustion... suddenly at the very moment when, so far, I mourned H. the least, I remembered her best. Indeed it was something (almost) better than memory; an instantaneous, unanswerable impression. To say it was like a meeting would be going too far. Yet there was that in it which tempts one to use those words. It was as if the lifting of the sorrow removed a barrier*'. (p. 39)

Anger, guilt, and sadness

The wish to attribute blame, or at least a reason, in the face of painful loss is as common as it is understandable, yet anger can sometimes turn inwards causing the bereaved person to blame themselves. Anger may be focused on healthcare staff for not having done more, towards God, or even towards the deceased for having abandoned the living. Guilt may be to do with not having said important things to the deceased (love, thanks, apologies), for having neglected their needs in some way, or it may even be derived from feelings of relief or liberation associated with the death.

The protracted turmoil caused by the many emotions described above can lead to emotional exhaustion and feelings of despair and depression. The bereaved, especially those who have lost a partner, often feel lonely and alone in managing their loss and in facing the future. It can feel disloyal to reinvest emotional energy in new relationships and new goals, and it takes time to realize that laughing and enjoying oneself again is not a betrayal of the deceased.

Reviewing a bereavement

Bereavement is an inescapable fact of life which the vast majority of people negotiate without professional aid, but nonetheless professionals can help people in mourning by listening to their concerns, helping them to consider their options, and providing reassurance regarding their progress. When reviewing someone's grief, it is helpful to consider the following factors that can influence the course of the bereavement[231] and possibly lead to complicated bereavement reactions:

- **What was the nature of the relationship with the deceased?** Consider the strength of the attachment, dependency on or by the deceased, the security provided by the deceased, ambivalent feelings caused by the death, etc.

- **What was nature of the death?** Was it expected or a shock? Was it 'age-appropriate'?— The death of a young person is usually perceived as more 'wrong'. Did the dying person suffer physical, emotional, or spiritual distress? Was the deceased able to make plans in anticipation of their death?

- **What losses has the bereaved person experienced in the past?** A history of multiple losses, childhood loss, depression, or other mental health problems is likely to resonate with the current loss. Have there been problems grieving in the past?

- **Does the bereaved person feel comfortable about expressing their grief to others?** People's cultural background, their social context, their age, sex, and personality can all influence the individual's readiness to engage in the work of grief that needs to be done.

- **Is there sufficient support available to the bereaved?** Does the bereaved person have good emotional supports around them or are they isolated? Does the rest of the relative's family live locally or far away? Does the bereaved person have other people to support and therefore may be neglecting their own need to grieve?

- **How much concurrent stress is the person facing?** e.g. unemployment, retirement, financial difficulties, menopause, children leaving home, social dislocation, etc.

Complicated grief

People vary enormously in both the form and the duration of their mourning, and it is unwise to be prescriptive regarding 'the normal course', even within a particular culture. However, in reviewing someone's bereavement, one should be concerned about people who use defences early on and fail to relinquish them (see model of adjustment–Chapter 1). As in cancer generally, denial can be helpful in the short term but can be counter-productive if sustained too long. Idealizing the dead person is common but becomes unhelpful when it leads the bereaved to enshrine aspects of their home or lives, preventing them from rebuilding a productive and fulfilling life for themselves. Rationalizing, intellectualizing, or rapidly resuming the busyness of life as if nothing has happened are unhelpful if these reactions prevent the bereaved person from confronting their real feelings of loss. Finally, drugs and alcohol are a more obvious way of keeping painful thoughts and feelings at bay, although, sadly, prescribed psychotropic medications are also sometimes used in this way.

There are occasions therefore when people become stuck in their grief, and the natural processes of adjustment falter or remain unfinished. It helps to be aware of these complicated bereavements so that help can be offered sooner rather than later. There are three main forms of complicated grief to be aware of:[231]

Chronic grief   In chronic grief the individual becomes stuck and unable to reinvest emotional energy in new goals and new relationships. The bereaved person withdraws into their grief as if it were a safe haven in its own right. Two years is sometimes used as a rule-of-thumb or yardstick for determining whether someone is stuck. Queen Victoria famously never resolved her grief for her adored Albert who died in 1861; she enshrined his memory all over London yet she rarely appeared in public thereafter, despite reigning until 1901.

Delayed grief   Here the individual may have had an emotional reaction at the time of the death but it was insufficient to the loss. Often a later event, usually another loss of some sort, precipitates a powerful grief reaction that the individual may be aware is out of proportion to the current situation. Occasionally, the reason for a delayed grief reaction is that the individual is overwhelmed by more than one loss or highly stressful event, leading them to put their grief 'on hold' as they attempt to resolve these other issues.

Masked grief   In masked grief a delayed grief reaction manifests itself as some other form of problem. For example, physical symptoms (often similar to those from which the deceased died) or psychological problems (such as depression or a phobia) sometimes mask an underlying bereavement that has not been adequately resolved.

'Recovery' from bereavement

Mourning is an exhausting time of adapting to change and processing emotions, during which the individual must forge a new identity from the ashes of their loss. As with most personal transitions people benefit from expressing their thoughts and feelings in words so as to make better sense of them and integrate their loss within the unfolding story of their lives. People swing between intense despair and resigned acceptance, between pining for what has been lost and a sense that they are beginning to re-engage with their changed world; rarely is there linear progress.

Healthy grief, according to Dutch scientists,[236] therefore involves an oscillation or swinging between thinking about and missing the deceased ('loss orientation'), and working practically to rebuild one's life ('restoration orientation'). If only one form of grief is pursued, then complicated grief reactions are likely to occur. Intriguingly, some research has indicated that widowed men benefit more from an 'emotionally-focused' intervention, while widowed women benefit more from a 'problem-focused' intervention.[237] This suggests that interventions that teach people *new* methods of resolving problems, rather than their normally preferred methods, may be of more use to them than interventions that offer more of their habitual methods of resolving problems.

It is difficult to know what constitutes a 'recovery' from bereavement. Is it even appropriate to think in terms of recovery? Does a parent ever fully recover from the death of a child? Somehow one has to rebuild a life in which there is a place for the memory of the dead person without that memory remaining an obstacle. Sometimes the maintenance of a continuing bond with the deceased can serve to deny the reality of their passing, and sometimes it can be an expression of the positive impact of the loved one carried forward into the new life of the bereaved.[238] Robert Weiss[239] has suggested five criteria that may indicate successful recovery:

(i) **Ability to give energy to everyday life** as opposed to being emotionally preoccupied with the loss.

(ii) **Psychological comfort** and freedom from intense emotional distress.

(iii) **Ability to experience pleasure** rather than feel guilty, for example, that one is dishonouring the dead.

(iv) **Investment in the future**, having things to look forward to and achieve.

(v) **Ability to function in social roles** as spouse, parent, etc., and member of the community.

References

1. Salmon P. (2000). *Psychology of medicine and surgery: a guide for psychologists, counsellors, nurses and doctors.* Chichester: Wiley.
2. Lee E. (1995). *A good death: a guide for patients and carers facing terminal illness at home.* London: Rosendale Press.
3. Robinson L and Stacey R. (1994). Palliative care in the community: setting practice guidelines for primary care teams. *British Journal of General Practice* **44**:461–4.
4. Northouse L. (1989). The impact of breast cancer on patients and husbands. *Cancer Nursing* **12**:276–84.
5. Harcourt D, Rumsey N, and Ambler N. (1999). Same-day diagnosis of symptomatic breast problems: psychological impact and coping strategies. *Psychology, Health and Medicine* **4**:57–71.
6. Poole K. (1997). The emergence of the 'waiting game': a critical examination of the psychosocial issues in diagnosing breast cancer. *Journal of Advanced Nursing* **25**:273–81.
7. Poole K, Hood K, Davis BD, Monypenny IJ, Sweetland H, Webster DJ, *et al.* (1999). Psychological distress associated with waiting for results of diagnostic investigations for breast disease. *The Breast* **8**:334–8.

8. Thomas C. (2001). *What are the psychosocial needs of cancer patients and their main carers? A study of user experience of cancer services with particular reference to psychosocial need.* Lancaster: Institute for Health Research, Lancaster University.

9. Ambler N, Rumsey N, Harcourt D, Khan F, Cawthorn S, and Barker J. (1999). Specialist nurse counsellor interventions at the time of diagnosis of breast cancer: comparing 'advocacy' with a conventional approach. *Journal of Advanced Nursing* **29**:445–53.

10. Parle M, Jones B, and Maguire P. (1996). Maladaptive coping and affective disorders among cancer patients. *Psychological Medicine* **26**:735–44.

11. Maguire P. (1999). Improving communication with cancer patients. *European Journal of Cancer* **35**:1415–22.

12. Söllner W, DeVries A, Steixner E, Lukas P, Sprinzi G, Rumpold G, *et al.* (2001). How successful are oncologists in identifying patient distress, perceived social support, and need for psychosocial counselling? *British Journal of Cancer* **84**:179–85.

13. Passik SD, Dugan W, McDonald MV, Rosenfeld B, Theobald DE, and Edgerton S. (1998). Oncologists' recognition of depression in their patients with cancer. *Journal of Clinical Oncology* **16**:1594–600.

14. Maguire P. (1985). Barriers to the care of the dying. *British Medical Journal* **291**:1711–13.

15. Maguire P, Booth K, Elliott C, and Jones B. (1996). Helping health professionals in cancer care acquire key communication skills – the impact of workshops. *European Journal of Cancer Care* **32a**:1486–9.

16. Fallowfield L, Lipkin M, and Hall A. (1998). Teaching senior oncologists communication skills: results from phase I of a comprehensive longitudinal program in the United Kingdom. *Journal of Clinical Oncology* **16**:1961–8.

17. Jacobsen PB, Roth AJ, and Holland JC. (1998). Surgery. In: JC Holland (ed.), *Psychooncology*, Oxford: Oxford University Press.

18. Volicer BJ, Isenberg MA, and Burns MW. (1977). Medical surgical differences in hospital stress factors. *Journal of Human Stress* **3**:3–13; Cited in Salmon P. (2000). *Psychology of medicine and surgery: a guide for psychologists, counsellors, nurses and doctors.* Chichester: Wiley.

19. Johnston M. (1982). Recognition of patients' worries by nurses and other patients. *British Journal of Clinical Psychology* **21**:255–61.

20. Salmon P and Manyande A. (1996). Good patients cope with their pain: postoperative analgesia and nurses' perceptions of their patients' pain. *Pain* **68**:63–8.

21. Ward SE, Goldberg N, Miller-McCauley V, Mueller C, Nolan A, Pawlik-Plank D, *et al.* (1993). Patient-related barriers to management of cancer pain. *Pain*, **52**:319–24.

22. Maguire P. (1992). Improving the recognition and treatment of affective disorders in cancer patients. In: K Granville-Grossman (ed.), *Recent advances in clinical psychiatry*, Edinburgh: Churchill Livingstone.

23. Johnston M and Vogele C. (1993). Benefits of psychological preparation for surgery: a meta-analysis. *Annals of Behavioral Medicine* **15**:245–56.

24. Devine EC and Cook TD. (1986). Clinical and cost-saving effects of psychoeducational interventions with surgical patients: a meta-analysis. *Research in Nursing and Health* **9**:89–105.

25. Auerbach SM, Meredith J, Alexander JM, Mercuri LG, and Brophy C. (1984). Psychological factors in adjustment to orthognathic surgery. *Journal of Oral Maxillofacial Surgery* **42**:435–40.

26. Blanchard CG, Ruckdeschel JC, Labrecque MS, Frisch S, and Blanchard EB. (1987). The impact of a designated cancer unit on house staff behaviors toward patients. *Cancer* **60**:2348–54.

27. McArdle JM, George WD, McCardle CS, Smoth DC, Moodie AR, Highson AV, *et al.* (1996). Psychological support for patients undergoing breast cancer surgery: a randomised study. *British Medical Journal* **312**:813–17.

28. Northouse LL and Northouse PG. (1996). Interpersonal communication systems. In: R McCorkle, M Grant, M Frank-Stromberg, and S Baird (ed.), *Cancer nursing: a comprehensive textbook*, 2nd edn, pp. 1211–22. Philadelphia: W.B. Saunders Co.

29. Cancer Research UK. (2003). http://www.cancerresearchuk.org/aboutcancer/specificcancers/breastcancer

30. Cancer Facts and Figures. (2003). American Cancer Society.

31. Meyerowitz BE. (1980). Psychosocial correlates of breast cancer and its treatment. *Psychological Bulletin* **87**:108.

32. Rowland JH and Massie MJ. (1998). Breast cancer. In: JC Holland (ed.), *Psychooncology*, Oxford: Oxford University Press.

33. Polinsky ML. (1994). Functional status of long-term breast cancer survivors: demonstrating chronicity. *Health and Social Work* **19**:165–73.

34. France L, Michie S, Barrett-Lee P, Brain K, Harper P, and Gray J. (2000). Male cancer: a qualitative study of male breast cancer. *The Breast* **9**:343–8.

35. Schunemann H and Willich N. (1998). Lymphoedema of the arm after primary treatment of breast cancer. *Anticancer Research* **18**:2235–6; Cited in Pain SJ, Purushotham AD. (2000). Lymphoedema following surgery for breast cancer. *British Journal of Surgery* **87**:1128–41.

36. Schover LR (1991). The impact of breast cancer on sexuality, body image, and intimate relationships. *CA: A Cancer Journal for Clinicians* **41**:112–20.

37. Dr Elisabeth Whipp – Personal communication.

38. Roberts R and Fallowfield L. (1990). Who supports the cancer counsellors? *Nursing Times* **86**:32–4.

39. Ambler N, Rumsey N, Harcourt D, Khan F, Cawthorn S, and Barker J. (1999). Specialist nurse counsellor interventions at the time of diagnosis of breast cancer: comparing 'advocacy' with a conventional approach. *Journal of Advanced Nursing* **29**:445–53.

40. Ganz PA, Shag AC, Lee JJ, Polinsky ML, and Tan SJ. (1992). Breast conservation versus mastectomy: is there a difference in psychological adjustment or quality of life in year after surgery? *Cancer* **69**:1729–38.

41. Margolis G, Goodman RL, and Rubin A. (1990). Psychological effects of breast-conserving treatment and mastectomy. *Psychosomatics* **31**:33–9.

42. Fallowfield LJ, Baum M, and Maguire GP. (1986). Effects of breast conservation on psychological morbidity associated with diagnosis and treatment of early breast cancer. *British Medical Journal* **293**:1331–4.

43. Moyer A. (1997). Psychosocial outcomes of breast-conserving surgery versus mastectomy: a meta-analytic review. *Health Psychology* **16**:284–98.

44. Harcourt D and Rumsey N. (2001). Psychological aspects of breast reconstruction: a review of the literature. *Journal of Advanced Nursing* **35**:477–87.

45. Rowland JH, Holland JC, Chaglassian T, and Kinne D. (1993). Psychological response to breast reconstruction. Expectations for and impact on postmastectomy functioning. *Psychosomatics* **34**:241.

46. Al-Ghazal SK, Fallowfield L, and Blamey RW. (2000). Comparison of psychological aspects and patient satisfaction following breast conserving surgery, simple mastectomy and breast reconstruction. *European Journal of Cancer* **36**:1938–43.

47. Moadel AB, Ostroff JS, and Schantz SP. (1998). Head and neck cancer. In: JC Holland (ed.), *Psychooncology*, Oxford: Oxford University Press.

48. Bolund C. (1985). Suicide and cancer: II. Medical and care factors in suicides by cancer patients in Sweden:1973–1976. *Journal of Psychosocial Oncology* **3**:31–52; Cited in Breitbart W, Chochinov HM, and Passik S. (1998). Psychiatric aspects of palliative care. In: D Doyle, GWC Hanks, N MacDonald (ed.), *Oxford textbook of palliative medicine*, 2nd edn, Oxford: Oxford University Press.

49. Bjordal K and Kaasa S. (1995). Psychological distress in head and neck cancer patients 7–11 years after curative treatment. *British Journal of Cancer* **71**:592–7.

50. Charlton R, Rumsey N, Partridge J, Barlow J, and Saul K. (2003). Disfigurement – neglected in primary care? *British Journal of General Practice* **53**:6–8.

51. Robinson E, Rumsey N, and Partridge J. (1996). An evaluation of the impact of social interaction skills training for facially disfigured people. *British Journal of Plastic Surgery* **49**:281–9.

52. Madden TC and Jehu D. (1987). Psychological effects of stomas – I. Psychosocial morbidity one year after surgery. *Journal of Psychosomatic Research* **31**:311–6.

53. White CA and Unwin JC. (1998). Post-operative adjustment to surgery resulting in a stoma: the importance of stoma-related cognitions. *British Journal of Health Psychology* **3**:85–93.

54. Bernhard J and Hürney C. (1998). Gastrointestinal cancer. In: JC Holland (ed.), *Psychooncology*, Oxford: Oxford University Press.

55. Passik SD and Ricketts PL. (1998). Central nervous system tumors. In: JC Holland (ed.), *Psychooncology*, Oxford: Oxford University Press.

56. Rees GJG. (1989). *Clinical oncology*. Tunbridge Wells: Castle House Publications.

57. Kirschblum S, O'Dell M, Ho C, and Barr K. (2001). Rehabilitation of persons with central nervous system tumours. *Cancer* **92**:1029–38.

58. Bakker M, Weug D, Crommelin M, and Lybeert M. (1999). Information for the radiotherapy patient. *Radiography* **5**:99–106.

59. Buick DL, Petrie KJ, Booth R, Probert J, Benjamin C, and Harvey V. (2000). Emotional and functional impact of radiotherapy and chemotherapy on patients with primary breast cancer. *Journal of Psychosocial Oncology* **18**:39–62.

60. Watson M. (1991). Breast cancer. In: M Watson (ed.), *Cancer patient care: psychosocial treatment methods*, Cambridge: BPS Books and Cambridge University Press.

61. Decker TW, Cline-Elsen, and Gallagher M. (1992). Relaxation therapy as an adjunct in radiation oncology. *Journal of Clinical Psychology* **48**:388–93.

62. Mose S, Budischewski KM, Rahn AN, Zander-Heinz AC, Bormeth S, and Bottcher HD. (2001). *International Journal of Radiation Oncology*Biology*Physics* **51**:1328–35.

63. Hammick M, Featherstone C, and Benrud-Larson L. (2001). Information giving procedures for patients having radiotherapy: a national perspective of practice in the United Kingdom. *Radiography* **7**:181–6.

64. Eardley A. (1988). Patients' worries about radiotherapy: evaluation of a preparatory booklet. *Psychology and Health* **2**:79–89.

65. Rainey L. (1985). Effects of preparatory patient information for radiation oncology patients. *Cancer* **56**:1056–61.

66. Thomas R, Dalya M, Perryman C, and Stockton D. (2000). Forewarned is forearmed – benefits of preparatory information on video cassette for patients receiving chemotherapy or radiotherapy – a randomised controlled trial. *European Journal of Cancer* **36**:1536–43.

67. Montgomery C, Lydon A, and Lloyd K. (1999). Psychological distress among cancer patients and informed consent. *Journal of Psychosomatic Research* **46**:241–5.

68. Cross A and Salmon P. (2000). Physical side-effects experienced by women with breast cancer: the women's perspective. *Journal of Radiotherapy in Practice* **1**:213–9.

69. Greenberg DB. (1998). Radiotherapy. In: JC Holland (ed.), *Psychooncology*, Oxford: Oxford University Press.

70. Auchincloss SS and McCartney CF. (1998). Gynaecologic cancers. In: JC Holland (ed.), *Psychooncology*, Oxford: Oxford University Press.

71. Knobf MT, Pasacreta JV, Valentine A, and McCorkle R. (1998). Chemotherapy, hormonal therapy and immunotherapy. In: JC Holland (ed.), *Psychooncology*, Oxford: Oxford University Press.

72. Slevin ML, Stubbs L, Plant HJ, Wilson P, Gregory WM, Armes PJ, *et al.* (1990). Attitudes to chemotherapy: comparing views of patients with cancer with those of doctors, nurses, and general public. *British Medical Journal* **300**:1458–60.

73. Kiebert GM, Stiggelbout AM, Klevit SB, Leer JW, van de Velde CJ, and de Haes HJ. (1994). Choices in oncology: factors that influence patients' treatment preference. *Quality of Life Research* **3**:175–82.

74. Fallowfield LJ. (1992). Behavioural interventions and psychological aspects of care during chemotherapy. *European Journal of Cancer* **28A**:S39–S41.

75. Luebbert K, Dahme B, and Hasenbring M. (2001). The effectiveness of relaxation training in reducing treatment-related symptoms and improving emotional adjustment in acute non-surgical cancer treatment: a meta-analytic review. *Psycho-Oncology* **10**:490–502.

76. Burish TG, Snyder SL, and Jenkins RA. (1991). Preparing patients for cancer chemotherapy: effect of coping preparation and relaxation interventions. *Journal of Consulting and Clinical Psychology* **59**:518–25.

77. Jacobsen PB, Hann DM, Azzarello LM, Horton J, Balducci L, and Lyman GH. (1999). Fatigue in women receiving adjuvant chemotherapy for breast cancer: characteristics, course, and correlates. *Journal of Pain and Symptom Management* **18**:233–42.

78. Frumkin LR. (1996). Weight gain in women receiving adjuvant chemotherapy for breast cancer. *Journal of the American Medical Association* **276**:855.

79. Fugh-Berman A and Epstein S. (1992). Tamoxifen: disease prevention or disease substitution? *The Lancet* **340**:1143–5.

80. Turken S, Siris E, Seldon D. (1989). Effects of tamoxifen on spinal bone density in women with breast cancer. *Journal of the National Cancer Institute* **81**:1086–9.

81. Dr Elisabeth Whipp – personal communication.

82. Roth AJ and Scher HI. (1998). Genito-urinary malignancies. In: JC Holland (ed.), *Psychooncology*, Oxford: Oxford University Press.

83. Andrykowski MA and McQuellon RP. (1998). Bone marrow transplantation. In: JC Holland (ed.), *Psychooncology*, Oxford: Oxford University Press.

84. Marks DI, Friedman SH, Delli Carpini LD, Nezu CM, and Nezu AM. (1997). A prospective study of the effects of high-dose chemo and bone marrow transplantation on sexual function in the first year after transplant. *Bone Marrow Transplantation* **19**:819–22.

85. Alby N. (1991). Leukaemia: bone marrow transplantation. In: Watson M (ed.), *Cancer patient care: psychosocial treatment methods*, Leicester: BPS Books.

86. Ball AB, Baum M, Breach NM, Shepherd JH, Shearer RJ, Thomas JM, *et al.* (1998). Surgical palliation. In: D Doyle, GWC Hanks, and N MacDonald (ed.), *Oxford textbook of palliative medicine*, 2nd edn, Oxford: Oxford University Press.

87. Jemal A, Murray T, Samuels A, Ghafoor A, Ward E, and Thun MJ. (2003). Cancer statistics, 2003. *CA: A Cancer Journal for Clinicians* **53**:5–26.

88. Sarna L. (1998). Lung cancer. In: JC Holland (ed.), *Psychooncology*. Oxford: Oxford University Press.

89. Walker A, O'Brien M, Traynor J, Fox K, Goddard E, and Foster K. (2002). *Living in Britain: results from the 2001 general household survey*. London: HMSO.

90. Hill KM, Muers MF, Connolly CK, and Round CE. (2003). Do newly diagnosed lung cancer patients feel their concerns are being met? *European Journal of Cancer Care* **12**:35–45.

91. Chemotherapy and non-small-cell lung cancer. *Drug and therapeutics bulletin* **40**:9–11.

92. Cox P and Kennelly GM. (1980). The role of curative radiotherapy in the treatment of lung cancer. *Cancer* **45**:678–702; Cited in Brown ML, Carrierei V, Janson-Bjerklie S, and Dodd MJ. (1986). Lung cancer and dyspnea: the patient's perception. *Oncology Nursing Forum* **5**:19–24.

93. Gallo-Silver L and Pollack B. (2000). Behavioral interventions for lung cancer-related breathlessness. *Cancer Practice* **8**:268–73.

94. American Cancer Society (2001). *Cancer facts and figures, 2001*. Atlanta, Georgia: ACS. Cited in Eton DT and Lepore SJ. (2002). Prostate cancer and health-related quality of life: a review of the literature. *Psycho-Oncology* **11**:307–26.

95. Pirl WF, Siegel GI, Goode MJ, and Smith MR. (2002). Depression in men receiving androgen deprivation therapy for prostate cancer: a pilot study. *Psycho-Oncology* **11**:518–23.

96. Anderson BL and Cyranowski JM. (1994). Women's sexual self-schema. *Journal of Personality and Social Psychology* **67**:1079–100.

97. Steginga SK, Occhipinti S, Dunn J, Gardiner RA, Heathcote P, and Yaxley J. (2001). The supportive care needs of men with prostate cancer. *Psycho-Oncology* **10**:66–7.

98. Airey C, Becher H, Erens B, and Fuller E. (2002). *Cancer national overview 1999/2000*. London: UK Department of Health.

99. Helgason ÁR, Dickman PW, Adolfsson J, and Steineck G. (2001). Emotional isolation: prevalence and the effect on well-being among 50–80-year-old prostate cancer patients. *Scandanavian Journal of Urology and Nephrology* **35**:97–101.

100. Mock V. (2001). Fatigue management: evidence and guidelines for practice. *Cancer* **92**: 1699–707.

101. Escalante CP, Grover T, Johnson BA, Harle M, Guo H, Mendoza TR, *et al*. (2001). A fatigue clinic in a comprehensive cancer centre – design and experiences. *Cancer* **92**:1708–13.

102. Winningham ML, Nail LM, Burke MB, Brophy L, Cimprich B, Jones LS, *et al*. (1994). Fatigue and the cancer experience; the state of the knowledge. *Oncology Nursing Forum* **21**:23–36.

103. Graydon JE. (1994). Women with breast cancer: their quality of life following a course of radiation therapy. *Journal of Advanced Nursing* **19**:617–22.

104. King KB, Nail LM, Kreamer K, Strohl RA, and Johnson JE. (1985). Patients' descriptions of the experience of receiving radiation therapy. *Oncology Nursing Forum* **12**:55–61.

105. Andrykowski MA, Curran SL, and Lightner R. (1998). Off-treatment fatigue in breast cancer survivors: a controlled comparison. *Journal of Behavioral Medicine* **21**:1–18.

106. Wharton RH. (2002). Sleeping with the enemy: treatment of fatigue in individuals with cancer. *The Oncologist* **7**:96–9.

107. Curt GA, Breitbart W, Cella D, Groopman JE, Horning SJ, Itri LM, *et al*. (2000). Impact of cancer-related fatigue on the lives of patients: new findings from the fatigue coalition. *The Oncologist* **5**:353–60.

108. Valentine AD and Meyers CA. (2001). Cognitive and mood disturbance as causes and symptoms of fatigue in cancer patients. *Cancer* **92**:1694–8.

109. Cella D, Lai JS, Chang CH, Peterman A, and Slavin M. (2002). Fatigue in cancer patients compared with fatigue in the general United States population. *Cancer* **94**:528–38.

110. Greenberg DB. (1998). Fatigue. In: JC Holland (ed.), *Psychooncology*, Oxford: Oxford University Press.

111. Greenberg DB, Sawicka J, Eisenthal S, and Ross D. (1992). Fatigue syndrome due to localized radiation. *Journal of Pain and Symptom Management* **7**:38–45.

112. Haylock PJ and Hart LK. (1979). Fatigue in patients receiving localized radiation. *Cancer Nursing* **2**:461–7.

113. Winningham ML. (2001). Strategies for managing cancer-related fatigue syndrome. *Cancer* **92**:988–97.

114. Suzanne Cowderoy – Personal communication.

115. Morrow GR and Hickok JT. (1993). Behavioral treatment of chemotherapy-induced nausea and vomiting. *Oncology* **7** (Supplement):83–9.

116. Morrow GR, Roscoe JA, Hickok JT, Andrews PR, and Matteson S. (2002). Nausea and emesis: evidence for a biobehavioral perspective. *Supportive Care in Cancer* **10**:96–105.

117. Carey MP and Burish TG. (1988). Etiology and treatment of the psychological side-effects associated with cancer chemotherapy. *Psychological Bulletin* **104**:307–25.

118. Burish TG and Jenkins RA. (1992). Effectiveness of biofeedback and relaxation training in reducing the side-effects of cancer chemotherapy. *Health Psychology* **11**:17–23.

119. Lyles JN, Burish TG, Krozely MG, and Oldham RK. (1982). Efficacy of relaxation training and guided imagery in reducing the aversiveness of cancer chemotherapy. *Journal of Consulting and Clinical Psychology* **50**:509–24.

120. Redd WH, Dadds MR, Futterman AD, Taylor KL, and Bovbjerg DH. (1993). Nausea induced by mental images of chemotherapy. *Cancer* **72**:629–36.

121. Jacobson PB and Schwartz MD. (1993). Food aversions during cancer therapy: incidence, etiology, and prevention. *Oncology* **7**:139–43.

122. Montgomery GH and Bovbjerg DH. (2000). Pre-infusion expectations predict post-treatment nausea during repeated adjuvant chemotherapy infusions for breast cancer. *British Journal of Health Psychology* **5**:105–19.

123. Watson M, Meyer L, Thomson A, and Osofsky S. (1998). Psychological factors predicting nausea and vomiting in breast cancer patients on chemotherapy. *European Journal of Cancer* **34**:831–7.

124. Walker LG. (1992). Hypnosis with cancer patients. *American Journal of Preventive Psychiatry and Neurology* **3**:42–9.

125. Alden P. (1997). Using hypnosis with patients undergoing chemotherapy. *Contemporary Hypnosis* **14**:87–93.

126. Syrjala KL and Abrams J. (1999). Cancer pain. In: RJ Gatchel and DC Turk (ed.), *Psychosocial factors in pain: critical perspectives*, London: The Guildford Press.

127. Yates PM, Edwards HE, Nash RE, Walsh AM, Fentiman BJ, Skerman HM, *et al.* (2002). Barriers to effective pain management. *Journal of Pain and Symptom Management* **23**:393–405.

128. Breitbart W and Payne DK. (1998). Pain. In: JC Holland (ed.), *Psychooncology*. Oxford: Oxford University Press.

129. Twycross R, Harcourt J, and Bergl S. (1996). A survey of patients in pain with advanced cancer. *Journal of Pain and Symptom Management* **12**:273–82.

130. Portenoy RK. (1990). Pain and quality of life: clinical issues and implications for research. *Oncology* **4**:95–101.

131. Bolund C. (1985). Suicide and cancer: I. Demographic and social characteristics of cancer patients who committed suicide in Sweden:1973–1976. *Journal of Psychosocial Oncology* **3**:17–30. Cited in Breitbart W, Chochinov HM, and Passik S. (1998). *Psychiatric aspects of palliative care.* In: D Doyle, GWC Hanks, and N MacDonald (ed.), *Oxford textbook of palliative medicine*, 2nd edn, Oxford: Oxford University Press.

132. Lyne ME, Coyne PJ, and Watson AC. (2002). Pain management issues for cancer survivors. *Cancer Practice* **10** (supplement), S27–S32.

133. Larsen MM (1996). Unscheduled cancer pain admissions costly: close to $5 million a year at M.D. Anderson. Abstract presented at 8th world congress on pain. Cited in *Oncology News International* **5**(10).

134. Lasch KE. (2002). Culture and pain. *Pain: Clinical Updates* 10(5).

135. Yanes G, Kittleson J, Smock T, and Obbens E. (1993). Pain incidence and analgesic use in outpatients seen by radiation oncologists. Poster presented at the 7th World Congress on Pain.

136. Brennan JH and Leach C. (1996). Pain prevalence, analgesic use and psychological distress in patients attending a U.K. oncology centre. Poster presented at the 10th world congress on pain, Vancouver, Canada.

137. Dawson R, Jablonski ES, and Sellers DE. (2002). Probing the paradox of patients' satisfaction with inadequate pain management. *Journal of Pain and Symptom Management* 23:211–20.

138. Foley KM. (1985). Treatment of cancer pain. *New England Journal of Medicine* 313:84–95.

139. Miaskowski C, Dodd MJ, West C, Paul S, Tripathy D, Koo P, *et al.* Lack of adherence with the analgesic regimen: a significant barrier to effective cancer pain management. *Journal of Clinical Oncology* 19:4275–9.

140. Larue F, Colleau SM, Fontaine A, and Brasseur L. (1995). Oncologists and primary care physicians' attitudes towards pain control and morphine prescribing in France. *Cancer* 76:2181–5.

141. Ferrell BR, and Juarez G. (2002). Cancer pain education for patients and the public. *Journal of Pain and Symptom Management* 23:329–36.

142. Fife BL. (1993). A comparative study of the attitudes of physicians and nurses toward the management of cancer pain. *Journal of Pain and Symptom Management* 8:132–9.

143. Sloman R, Ahern M, Wright A, and Brown L. (2001). Nurses' knowledge of pain in the elderly. *Journal of Pain and Symptom Management* 21:317–22.

144. American Cancer Society (2001). National comprehensive cancer network. *Cancer pain treatment guidelines, version 1.* American Cancer Society. Cited in Ferrell BR, and Juarez G. (2002). Cancer pain education for patients and the public. *Journal of Pain and Symptom Management* 23:329–36.

145. Foley KM. (1998). Pain assessment and cancer pain syndromes. In D Doyle, GWC Hanks, and N MacDonald (ed.), *Oxford textbook of palliative medicine*, 2nd edn, Oxford: Oxford University Press.

146. Daut RL, Cleeland CS, and Flanery RC. (1983). Development of the Wisconsin Brief Pain Questionnaire to assess pain in cancer and other diseases. *Pain* 17:197–210.

147. Williams A. (1994). Assessment of the chronic pain patient. *Clinical Psychology Forum*, (September 1994), British Psychological Society.

148. Dr Nick Ambler – personal communication

149. Turk DC and Feldman CS. (1992). Noninvasive approaches to pain control in terminal illness: the contribution of psychological variables. In: DC Turk and CS Feldman (ed.), *Noninvasive approaches to pain management in the terminally ill*, New York: Haworth Press.

150. Spiegel D and Bloom JR. (1983). Pain in metastatic breast cancer. *Cancer* 52:341–5.

151. Ciaramella A and Poli P. (2001). Assessment of depression among cancer patients: the role of pain, cancer type and treatment. *Psycho-Oncology* 10:156–65.

152. Breitbart W, Passik S, and Payne D. (1998). Psychological and psychiatric interventions in pain control. In: D Doyle, GWC Hanks, and N MacDonald (ed.), *Oxford textbook of palliative medicine*, 2nd edn, Oxford: Oxford University Press.

153. Syrjala KL, Donaldson GW, Davis MW, Kippes ME, and Carr JE. (1995). Relaxation and imagery and cognitive-behavioral training reduce pain during cancer treatment: a controlled trial. *Pain* 63:189–98.

154. Hill HF, Chapman CR, Kornell JA, Sullivan KM, Saeger LC, and Benedetti C. (1990). Self-administration of morphine in bone marrow transplant patients reduces drug requirement. *Pain* 40:121–9.

155. Maguire P. (2000). The use of antidepressants in patients with advanced cancer. *Supportive Care in Cancer* **8**:265–7.

156. Lansky SB, List MA, Hermann CA, Ets-Hokin EG, DasGupta TK, Wilbanks GD, *et al.* (1985). Absence of major depressive disorder in female cancer patients. *Journal of Clinical Oncology* **3**:1553–60.

157. Fallowfield L, Ratcliffe D, and Saul J. (2001). Psychiatric morbidity and its recognition by doctors in patients with cancer. *British Journal of Cancer* **84**:1011–5.

158. Jenkins V, Nicholls K, and Fallowfield L. (2002). Communication courses improve clinicians' ability to detect distress in patients during cancer consultations. Poster presented at the 19th annual conference of the British Psychosocial Oncology Society, Harrogate, UK.

159. Massie MJ and Popkin MK. (1998). Depressive disorders. In: Holland JC (ed.), *Psychooncology*, Oxford: Oxford University Press.

160. Colleoni M, Mandala M, Peruzzotti G, Robertson C, Bredart A, and Goldhirsch A. (2000) Depression and degree of acceptance of adjuvant cytotoxic drugs. *The Lancet* **356**:1326.

161. Noyes R, Holt CS, and Massie MJ. (1998). Anxiety disorders. In: JC Holland (ed.), *Psychooncology* Oxford: Oxford University Press.

162. Maguire P, Faulkner A, and Regnard C. (1993). Eliciting the current problems of the patient with cancer. *Palliative Medicine* **7**:63–8.

163. Stark GPH and House A. (2000). Anxiety in cancer patients. *British Journal of Cancer*, **83**:1261–7.

164. Sheard T and Maguire P. (1999). The effect of psychological interventions on anxiety and depression in cancer patients: results of two meta-analyses. *British Journal of Cancer* **80**:1770–80.

165. Hamilton JG. (1995). Needle phobia: a neglected diagnosis. *Journal of Family Practice* **41**:169–75.

166. Ost LG, Sterner U, and Fellenius J. (1989). Applied tension, applied relaxation and the combination in treatment of blood phobia. *Behaviour Research and Therapy* **27**:109–21.

167. Slaughter JR, Jain A, Holmes S, Reid JC, Bobo W, and Sherrod NB. (2000). Panic disorder in hospitalized cancer patients. *Psycho-Oncology* **9**:253–8.

168. Brennan JH. (2000). Changing tack: the importance of the therapeutic relationship. *Primary Care and Cancer*, **20**:31–4.

169. Fleming U. (1985). Relaxation for far-advanced cancer. *The Practitioner* **229**:471–5.

170. Dunkel-Schetter C, Feinstein L, Taylor SE, and Falke RL. (1992). Patterns of coping with cancer. *Health Psychology* **11**:79–87.

171. Somerfield MR, Stefanek ME, Smith TJ, and Padberg JJ. (1999). A systems model for adaptation to somatic distress among cancer survivors. *Psycho-Oncology* **8**:334–43.

172. Eysenck MW. (1992). *Anxiety: the cognitive perspective.* Hove, UK: Lawrence Erlbaum Associates Ltd.

173. Aldrich S, Eccleston C, and Crombez G. (2000). Worrying about chronic pain: vigilance to threat and misdirected problem solving. *Behaviour Research and Therapy* **38**:457–70.

174. Davis M and Whalen PJ. (2001). The amygdala: vigilance and emotion. *Molecular Psychiatry* **6**:13–34.

175. Durham RC and Allan T. (1993). Psychological treatment of generalised anxiety disorder: a review of the clinical significance in outcome studies since 1980. *British Journal of Psychiatry* **163**:19–26.

176. Davidson JR, Waisberg JL, Brundage MD, and Maclean AW. (2001). Nonpharmacological group treatment of insomnia: a preliminary study with cancer survivors. *Psycho-Oncology* **10**:389–97.

177. Ancoli-Israel S, Moore PJ, and Jones V. (2001). The relationship between fatigue and sleep in cancer patients: a review. *European Journal of Cancer Care* **10**:245–55.

178. Cimprich B. (1999). Pretreatment symptom distress in women newly diagnosed with breast cancer. *Cancer Nursing* **22**:185–94.

179. Kripke DF, Garfinkel L, Wingard DL, Klauber MR, and Marler MR. (2002). Mortality associated with sleep duration and insomnia. *Archives of General Psychiatry* **59**:131–6.

180. Silberfarb PM, Hauri PJ, Oxman TE, and Schnurr P. (1993). Assessment of sleep in patients with lung cancer and breast cancer. *Journal of Clinical Oncology* **11**:997–1004.

181. Borkovec TD, Robinson E, Pruzinsky T, and DePree JA. (1983). Preliminary exploration of worry: some characteristics and processes. *Behaviour Research and Therapy* **21**:9–16.

182. Endeshaw Y. (2000). Commentary on Holbrook AM, Crowther R, Lotter A, Cheng C, and King D. The role of benzodiazepines in the treatment of insomnia. *Canadian Medical Association Journal*, 2000 162:225–33. Cited in *Journal of the American Geriatrics Society* **49**:824–6.

183. Hirst A and Sloan R. (2003). Benzodiazepines and related drugs for insomnia in palliative care (Cochrane Review). In: *The Cochrane Library (Issue 1)*. Oxford: Update Software.

184. Morin CM, Colecchi C, Stone J, Sood R, and Brink D. (1999). Behavioral and pharmacological therapies for late-life insomnia: a randomized controlled trial. *Journal of the American Medical Association* **281**:991–9.

185. Morin CM, Hauri PJ, Espie CA, Spielman AJ, Buysse DJ, and Bootzin RR. (1999). Nonpharmacologic treatment of chronic insomnia. An American academy of sleep medicine review. *Sleep* **22**:1134–56.

186. Cannici J, Malcolm R, and Peek LA. (1983). Treatment of insomnia in cancer patients using muscle relaxation training. *Journal of Behaviour Therapy and Experimental Psychiatry* **14**:251–6.

187. Mock V, Dow KH, Meares CJ, Grimm PM, Dienemann JA, Haisfield-Wolfe ME, *et al.*(1997). *Effects of exercise on fatigue, physical functioning and emotional distress during radiation therapy for breast cancer*. Oncology Nursing Forum **24**:991–1000.

188. DeLisa JA. (2001). A history of cancer rehabilitation. *Cancer* **92**:970–4.

189. Dietz JH. (1981). *Rehabilitation oncology*. New York: Wiley.

190. Gillis TA and Donovan ES. (2001). Rehabilitation following bone marrow transplant. *Cancer* **92**:998–1007.

191. Tunkel R and Passik SD. (1998). Rehabilitation. In: JC Holland (ed.), *Psychooncology*, Oxford: Oxford University Press.

192. Bunting RW and Shea B. (2001). Bone metastasis and rehabilitation. *Cancer* **92**:1020–8.

193. Dr Elisabeth Whipp – personal communication.

194. Corner J. (1996). Non-pharmacological intervention for breathlessness in lung cancer. *Palliative Medicine* **10**:299–305.

195. Heinrich RL and Schag CC. (1985). Stress and activity management: group treatment for c patients and spouses. *Journal of Consulting and Clinical Psychology* **53**:439–46.

196. Courneya KS, Mackey JR, and Jones LW. (2000). Coping with cancer. Can exercise help? *The Physician and Sports Medicine* **28**:49–73.

197. Weisman A and Worden J. (1985). The emotional impact of recurrent cancer. *Journal of Psychosocial Oncology* **3**:5–16.

198. Cella DF, Mahon SM and Donovan MI. (1990). Cancer recurrence as a traumatic event. *Behavioral Medicine* **13**:15–22.

199. Mahon SM. (1991). Managing the psychosocial consequences of cancer recurrence: implications for nurses. *Oncology Nursing Forum* **18**:577–83.

200. Wilkinson S. (1991). Factors which influence how nurses communicate with cancer patients. *Journal of Advanced Nursing* **16**:677–88.

201. Wall PD. (1986). Editorial – 25 volumes of pain. *Pain* **25**:1–4. Cited in Saunders C. (1998). Foreword. In: D Doyle, GWC Hanks, and N MacDonald (ed.), *Oxford textbook of palliative medicine*, 2nd edn, Oxford: Oxford University Press.

202. Hanks GW, Robbins M, Sharp D, Frobes K, Done K, Peters TJ, *et al.* (2002). The imPaCT study: a randomised controlled trial to evaluate a hospital palliative care team. *British Journal of Cancer* **87**:733–9.

203. Jeffrey D. (1998). Communication skills in palliative care. In: C Faull, Y Carter, and R Woof (ed.), *Handbook of palliative care*, Oxford: Oxford University Press.

204. Seale C and Cartwright A. (1994). *The year before death.* Avebury: Aldershot. Cited in Payne S and Ellis-Hill C. (2001). Being a carer. In: S Payne and C Ellis-Hill (ed.), *Chronic and terminal illness: new perspectives on caring and carers*, Oxford: Oxford University Press.

205. Saunders C. (1998). Foreword. In: D Doyle, GWC Hanks, and N MacDonald (ed.), *Oxford textbook of palliative medicine*, 2nd edn, Oxford: Oxford University Press.

206. Laungani P. (2002). Hindu spirituality in life, death, and bereavement. In: JD Morgan, and P Laungani (ed.), *Death and bereavement around the world. Volume I: major religious traditions*, Amityville, NY: Baywood Publishing.

207. Morgan JD. (2002). Islam. In: JD Morgan, and P Laungani (ed.), *Death and bereavement around the world. Volume I: major religious traditions*, Amityville, NY: Baywood Publishing.

208. Balmer CE, Thomas P, and Osborne RJ. (2001). Who wants second-line, palliative chemotherapy? *Psycho-Oncology* **10**:410–8.

209. Parkes CM. (1978). Home or hospital? Terminal care as seen by surviving spouses. *Journal of the Royal College of General Practitioners* **28**:19–30.

210. Townsend J, Frank A, Fermont D, Dyer S, Karran O, andWalgrave A, *et al.* (1990). Terminal care and patients' preferences for place of death: a prospective study. *British Medical Journal* **301**:415–7.

211. Bolund C. (1993). Loss, mourning and growth in the process of dying. *Palliative Medicine* **7**:17–25.

212. Greisinger AJ, Lorimor RJ, Aday LA, Winn RJ, and Baile WF. (1997). Terminally ill cancer patients: their most important concerns. *Cancer Practice* **5**:147–54.

213. Lan Yi K, Chidgey J, Addington-Hall J, and Hotopf M. (2002). Depression in palliative care: a systematic review. Part 2. *Treatment. Palliative Medicine* **16**:279–84.

214. Seligman ME. (1975). *Helplessness: on depression, development and death.* New York: WH Freeman.

215. Jatoi A, Kumar S, Sloan JA, and Nguyen P. (2000). On appetite and its loss. *Journal of Clinical Oncology* **18**:2930–2.

216. Maltby J, Lewis CA, and Day L. (1999). Religious orientation and psychological well-being: the role of the frequency of personal prayer. *British Journal of Health Psychology* **4**:363–78.

217. Moadel A, Morgan C, Fatone A, Grennan J, Carter J, Laruffa G, *et al.* (1999). Seeking meaning and hope: self-reported spiritual and existential needs among an ethnically-diverse cancer patient population. *Psycho-oncology* **8**:378–85.

218. Koenig HG, Bearon LB, Hover M, and Travis JL 3rd. (1991). Religious perspectives of doctors, nurses, patients and families. *Journal of Pastoral Care* **45**:254–67.

219. Knight B. (1986). *Psychotherapy with older adults.* London: Sage.

220. Pickrel J. (1989). "Tell me your story": using life review in counselling the terminally ill. *Death Studies* **13**:127–35.

221. Fallowfield LJ, Jenkins VA, and Beveridge HA. (2002). Truth may hurt but deceit hurts more: communication in palliative care. *Palliative Medicine* **16**:297–303.

222. Weeks JC, Cook EF, O'Day SJ, Peterson LM, Wenger N, Reding D, *et al.* (1998). Relationship between cancer patients' prediction of prognosis and their treatment preferences. *Journal of the American Medical Association* **279**:1709–14.

223. Christakis NA and Lamont EB. (2000). Extent and determinants of error in doctors' prognoses in terminally ill patients: prospective cohort study. *British Medical Journal* **320**:469–72.

224. Parkes CM (1990). Risk factors in bereavement: implications for the prevention and treatment of pathologic grief. *Psychiatric Annals* **20**:308–13.

225. Irwin M, Daniels M, and Weiner H. (1987). Immune and neuroendocrine changes during bereavement. *Psychiatric Clinics of North America* **10**:501–11. Cited In: J Holland, Rowland J (ed.), *Handbook of psychooncology*, Oxford: Oxford University Press, 1990.

226. Parkes (1972). Bereavement: studies of grief in adult life. Madison, Conn.: International Universities Press.

227. Clayton P, Halikas I, and Maurice W. (1972). The depression of widowhood. *British Journal of Psychiatry* **120**:71–78.

228. Rees WD and Lutkins SG. (1967). Mortality of bereavement. *British Medical Journal* **4**:13–16.

229. Bunch J, Barraclough B, Nelson B, and Sainsbury P. (1971). Suicide following the death of parents. *Social Psychiatry* **6**:193–9.

230. Duberstein P, Conwell Y, and Cox C. (1998). Suicide in widowed persons: a psychological autopsy comparison of recently and remotely bereaved older subjects. *American Journal of Geriatric Psychiatry* **6**:328–34.

231. Worden JW. (1991). Grief counselling and grief therapy, 2nd edn. London: Routledge.

232. Parkes CM. (1971). Psycho-social transitions: a field for study. *Social Science and Medicine* **5**:101–15.

233. Parkes CM. (2002). Grief: lessons from the past, visions for the future. *Bereavement care* **21**:19–23.

234. Michel Eyguem de Montaigne (1533–1592). Cited in Parkes CM. (2002). Grief: lessons from the past, visions for the future. *Bereavement Care* **21**:19–23.

235. Lewis CS. (1961). *A grief observed.* London: Faber and Faber.

236. Stroebe MS and Schut H. (1999). The dual process model of coping with bereavement: rationale and description. *Death Studies* **23**:197–224.

237. Schut HA, Stroebe MS, and van den Bout J. (1997). Intervention for the bereaved: gender differences in the efficacy of two counselling programmes. *British Journal of Clinical Psychology* **36**:63–72.

238. Gal-Oz E and Field NP. (2002). Do continuing bonds always help with adjustment to loss? *Bereavement Care* **21**:42–3.

239. Weiss R. (1993). Loss and recovery. In: MS Stroebe, W Stroebe, and RO Hansson (ed.), *Handbook of bereavement: theory, research and intervention.* Cambridge: Cambridge University Press.

Chapter 6

Communication

Communication and ethics..298
  Disclosure of diagnostic information 298
  Consent, collaboration, and choice 299
Information 302
  Information supply and demand 302
  Written information 305
  Video 307
  Audiotapes...307
  Internet and computer-based information 308
  Information and support centres 308
Staff–patient relationships 309
  What do healthcare professionals want in their patients?.........................309
  What is appropriate professional distance?.....................................311
  What are patients looking for in the professionals who care for them?................313
Patient-centred communication 315
  Cultural assumptions and differences 316
  Working through interpreters 318
  Language..319
Eliciting concerns..320
  Assessing the whole person 321
  Conducting a patient-centred clinical interview 323
  Problem-solving..328
  Clarifying and challenging assumptions 329
Specific communication issues 330
  Giving bad news 330
  Discussing resuscitation..335
  Identifying vulnerability 336
  Working with people with special needs.......................................338
  Working with someone clinically depressed or suicidal...........................342
  Working with denial and avoidance 346
  Anxiety, worry, and uncertainty 348
  Working with someone acutely confused or cognitively impaired 350
  Angry, difficult, or disliked patients 351
Professional issues in communication 353
  Communication between professionals..353
  Healthcare teams and patient confidentiality 354
  Communication training 355
References 355

> The nurses are kind, gentle and caring – but nurses cannot get involved with patients or the pain would destroy them. The radiographers are gentle, meticulous and efficient – but they have an enormous workload, and they cannot get involved. The doctors are caring, careful, informative and distant – but their job is to preserve my life and they too cannot get involved. And always there are 'no guarantees'. It has been such a long, hard year.

The quality of healthcare is intimately tied to the quality of communication between professionals and their patients and families. Communication is not simply information flow between people, but also involves messages of support and concern. It is often these 'non-specifics' of healthcare that make all the difference. Patients and professionals have valuable information that the other person can helpfully use, so this chapter is about *what* needs to be communicated and *how* people can best communicate with one another.

As if it were not obvious, there is growing evidence that healthcare staff can help prevent physical, psychological, and social suffering by providing a supportive environment in which patients' wider concerns are acknowledged and addressed. It is the build up of these concerns that has been found to predict high levels of distress (e.g. more severe anxiety and depression).[1] Where healthcare professionals can help patients to identify and describe their concerns, distress can be prevented or minimized. For example, a study of 60 women with breast cancer found that women who saw their doctors as being more caring and emotionally supportive during their cancer diagnosis tended to have fewer cancer-related post-traumatic stress symptoms, less depression, and less distress.[2]

This chapter is not advocating that healthcare professionals should deal with all the diverse needs of their patients, let alone the emotional care of those who are most vulnerable. Doctors and nurses do not have to become psychotherapists to recognize that people with cancer have complicated lives and are not only concerned about their bodies and their illness but have other concerns too. In the context of the fear, uncertainty, and turmoil that cancer often unleashes, patients and families expect professionals to be kind and supportive guides throughout their ordeal. As Alan Radley has noted, 'the psychological effectiveness of the doctor is not some spin-off from clinical practice; *it is intrinsic to the role of the physician as healer*'[3] (Radley 1994, p. 97). The same could be said of any member of the healthcare team.

One problem, though, is that people with cancer rarely discuss their psychosocial or even their physical concerns (e.g. pain) with a healthcare professional unless prompted, and healthcare staff are generally poor at eliciting and recognizing the worries and difficulties of their patients. These communication challenges are at the heart of this chapter.

There are more than enough sound reasons to strive for better communication in healthcare. Among other things, high quality communication ...

- improves the accuracy and efficiency of medical care;
- improves the relationship between patient and healthcare professional;

- enhances the patient's participation in their care and their satisfaction with it;
- encourages patient 'compliance' with treatment regimens;
- reduces the distress of patients and families and improves their quality of life;
- enables healthcare staff to respond to the patient's current symptoms (pain, depression, etc.);
- elicits personal and social concerns before they become entrenched and more severe;
- reduces complaints and litigation.

In the end professionals cannot know what their patients need (e.g. pain relief, psychosocial support) unless there is effective communication between them and, since patients often fail to voice their concerns, it is the responsibility of healthcare staff to elicit them. But no one has to do it all. Acknowledging the patient's concerns and responding to them by drawing in appropriate other members of the healthcare team is good supportive care.

Efficiently drawing out and addressing patients' needs and concerns is a skill that, like any other clinical skill, can be learned. Doing it thoughtfully and supportively, however, takes time.

Time to care

Interviews with 577 people who had had cancer in the previous six years found that satisfaction with their initial diagnostic interview was related to the amount of time spent with their doctor.[4] In both qualitative and quantitative studies, lack of time in consultations with doctors is the most common source of patient dissatisfaction, (even though admittedly patients' perception of the length of an interview seems to be influenced by their satisfaction with its quality).[5] But, far from being given more time, many healthcare staff feel they have less time than ever to share information, let alone time to draw out the physical and psychosocial needs of their patients.

> Patients are often afforded more privacy, thought, and time during a meeting with a bank manager, accountant, or veterinary surgeon than with a doctor.[6]

> (Fallowfield 1993, p. 476)

In today's climate of managed care and waiting-list medicine, doctors are sometimes penalized for taking the time to provide a caring service that attends to the broader needs of their patients. In the under-funded National Health Service, UK oncologists see dramatically more new patients per year than their European counterparts with consequently less time for each patient. In the United States, market forces such as health maintenance organizations have such a grip on the provision of healthcare that doctors schedule ever-shorter consultations so as to be able to see more patients. Ironically, it is largely due to the increasing cost of ever more successful medical interventions that has led doctors to spend less and less time with their patients. How does this affect the relationship between patient and doctor? What should the public realistically expect of doctors and nurses in the context of healthcare that emphasizes throughput at the expense of quality of care? A report of the Royal College of Physicians of London puts it baldly:

> Careful communication will be the first thing to go when the doctor is under time pressures. When emphasis is placed on 'patient through-put', time spent talking to patients is time taken from activities that can be 'counted': half-an-hour explaining the implications of an illness to a patient does not register on any performance indicators. Time spent on one patient is time taken away from others.[7]

(Royal College of Physicians of London 1997, p. 8)

The power of the therapeutic relationship between doctor and patient is not some historical artefact but remains central to the art of medicine. Society still expects doctors to communicate effectively and sensitively with their patients about their illnesses, and to accurately assess their diverse needs. We expect medical 'wisdom', care, and honesty. We expect doctors to be clear where the best resources exist for further care and support if required and, where these resources do not exist, we expect doctors and other healthcare staff to campaign alongside their patients for better services. Increasingly, the missing resource is adequate time, so there is all the more reason for using it well.

Communication and ethics

The public are increasingly well informed about illness and disease, and there is an unprecedented amount of information in the public domain about prevention, early detection, and treatment of major diseases such as cancer. Information that was once the preserve of the few is now available through mass media: press, radio, television, and especially the Internet. Alongside this deluge of information there has been growing consumer activism with an emphasis on consumer rights. The right to information about any part of one's personal history, for example, is a core ethical principle of 'Western' individualism. So it would be hard to argue that information about the body should be one of the rare exceptions to the public's access to information.

From an ethical point of view therefore, people have a *right* to information about their bodies. This includes information about their diagnosis, all treatments being proposed, and their likely prognosis. Accordingly, healthcare staff have an ethical *duty* to provide this information to the best of their abilities, provided patients show a desire for it. However once again, establishing how much patients want to know, and conveying it sensitively, takes time. And, because they are usually the leaders of clinical teams, it usually falls upon doctors to convey the most important information.

Disclosure of diagnostic information

More patients than ever in the West want to have a full explanation of their diagnosis. In the USA and the UK, for example, about 90% of people with cancer want to know their diagnosis, their treatment and likely side-effects,[8, 9] with recent studies suggesting as many as 98% wanting to know whether the illness is cancer.[10] In France, almost 90% of patients in one study wanted direct communication about their illness and use of the word 'cancer', and most people wanted more information that they were given[11] On the whole, younger, better educated, and female patients are inclined to request and be offered more information from their doctors than older, less well-educated, and male, though one must always be wary about this kind of generalization.

Despite this cultural drift in many parts of the West towards ever-greater openness about diagnosis and prognosis, not all cultures share this enthusiasm for full information and patient autonomy in decision making.[13] In fact, the prominent view that truthful disclosure is a prerequisite for ethical practice can obscure cultural and individual differences even *within* the West. In many cultures, including the West until fairly recently, the full disclosure of a cancer diagnosis is seen as potentially harmful, causing unnecessary psychological suffering for patients and families alike. In one Japanese survey, for example, only a third of the sample thought that people in general should be informed of their cancer diagnosis, and fewer still said they would want a family member informed.[14] The emphasis on modesty and non-verbal behaviour in Japanese culture means that 'sensing what has been politely and respectfully left unsaid is a well-used skill'.[13]

No matter what the statistics may suggest with regard to the disclosure of diagnostic information, the preferences of every patient must be sought before diagnostic tests are carried out[13] and probably at every key consultation. How much information does the patient want? How involved does the patient want the family (or others) to be in the disclosure process? These preferences should then be recorded and shared with the entire healthcare team.

Consent, collaboration, and choice

Cultural changes in the West over the past few decades, as well as medical progress in the treatment of many cancers, has led to a greater emphasis on the rights of the consumer and a concern for individual autonomy.[15, 16] This has been reflected in medical practice in many countries by the increasing provision of both information to patients and shared clinical decision making. Nonetheless, in a UK national survey of 65 000 cancer patients in 2000, 11% reported that they would like to have been more involved in decisions regarding their care and treatment.[17]

Cancer treatments require healthcare staff to make choices in the best interests of their patients with their informed consent. Consent is the patient's agreement for a health professional to provide a particular package of healthcare. Without consent one only has paternalism.[18] For the patient's consent to be valid, the patient must be competent to make the specific decision, have received sufficient information on which to base their decision, and not be acting under pressure from others. However, procedures for obtaining informed consent are not always designed primarily to meet the needs of patients, so much as to protect clinicians from medico-legal challenges. Informed consent regarding treatment is often sought after the patient has already committed themselves to a medical intervention (e.g. surgical patients are often asked to sign their consent after they have been admitted to hospital and while waiting for their surgery).[19]

How risks and options are described in the consent process will influence the patient's decision—for example, whether outcomes are described in terms of chances of survival or chances of death, percentages rather than probabilities, etc. People reason in very different ways. One cannot assume that logical, systematic, deductive reasoning is the public's preferred method of reaching decisions. Another method is known as the 'naturalistic model of decision making'[20] in which people construct a mental image of the option that seems optimal, based on 'rules of thumb' drawn from past experience. They then use the image to simulate whether the option would work for them in the current context.

Occasionally, treatment choices are sufficiently balanced to warrant the involvement of the patient in making the decision; the anticipated quality of life of the individual sometimes becomes the most important deciding factor. The most celebrated choice in cancer care is between having a mastectomy and breast conserving surgery (that is, among patients for whom it is clinically advisable to be given this choice). In advanced cancer there may be a choice between having an anti-cancer treatment versus symptomatic care, between having treatment now or having it later, or trying an experimental treatment versus a conventional one.[21]

One 1994 study found that the treatment policy of surgeons had an impact on women's risk of becoming anxious and depressed.[22] Women treated by surgeons who, whenever clinically possible, encouraged their patients to choose between having a lumpectomy or mastectomy were compared with women treated by surgeons who favoured mastectomies or favoured lumpectomies. The study found that women treated by surgeons who offered choice, whether or not the woman was ultimately able to exercise a choice (due to the clinical situation), were subsequently less depressed and anxious three years later. The authors suggested that the critical variables were the communication style of the surgeons and the fact that they provided adequate information to their patients.

Of course, to make a choice one must understand the options and be free to choose. Informed consent, whether to a clinical treatment or a research trial, requires that patients be made fully aware of the clinical implications of their disease and the proposed treatment, its risks and possible benefits. But how much information constitutes being made 'fully aware', or even adequately informed? In the case of clinical trials, detailed information reveals the state of medical ignorance that has led to a randomized trial.[23] Some authors regard the practice of obtaining full written informed consent to be unnecessarily cruel and argue that the procedure for obtaining it should be as humane for the individual patient as all other aspects of clinical care.[24] Others have similarly warned that providing choice, even where real choices exist, may place an unfair burden of responsibility on patients and that informing them about medical uncertainties can undermine their confidence in their doctor.[21] If people are provided with adequate information so that they can make a truly informed choice, there is a concern that it could undermine or short-circuit the protective function of denial and avoidance. The evidence on this last point, however, suggests that making detailed information available does not undermine patients' ability to use denial and avoidance.[8]

It also turns out that although many people in the West want information, control, and choice, they rarely want to carry sole responsibility for treatment decisions. In fact, the evidence to date suggests, for example, that many people do not want active participation in clinical decisions but prefer to leave these decisions to their doctors. Of the 62 women in the 1994 study who were offered choice of a mastectomy or a lumpectomy, 23 found it difficult to make a decision, and eight refused to choose.[22] Asked how they felt about being offered choice, 26 expressed positive reactions, 13 were unable to say, and 10 were 'unenthusiastic'. The authors concluded that people have a right to decline to participate in decision making. Another British study found that of 150 women with recently diagnosed breast cancer, 20% wanted an active role in deciding their treatment, 28% preferred to share decision making, and 52% wanted the surgeon to decide.[25]

An earlier study from Canada used card sort methodology to examine the degree of participation preferred by 436 cancer patients. This showed that only 12% wanted 'active collaboration' with their physician, while 59% chose to adopt a less active role, preferring their physicians to make clinical decisions on their behalf.[26] More recently, among a sample of 1012 women with breast cancer, 22% wanted active collaboration, 34% wanted the doctor to be responsible for decisions, and 44% wanted to share decisions.[27] None of these snapshot surveys measured whether people's preferences for information or control over their treatment changed over time. It is well established that decision making is impaired by high anxiety levels[28] and it seems likely that the closer the patient is to their diagnosis the more they are inclined to delegate the responsibility for decision making to their doctor.[15]

In summary, medical culture is moving towards the provision of more choice and more shared decision making with patients. Patients have a *right* to information about their bodies, and medical staff have an ethical *duty* to provide it, but patients are not *obliged* to exercise that right. Although the situation continues to change, at present some patients seem to want active participation in their treatment while many clearly do not. For those patients and families who do not want the responsibility of deciding between treatment options (due to an understandable fear of later regret) the medical team may be required to make the decision on their behalf. After all, it is quite reasonable for a patient to ask their doctor: *'If you were in my position, what would you decide to do?'* The apparent safety of a doctor's firm recommendation may be the very thing some patients are looking for. Their clinical opinion is what many people expect from an expert.

No matter what level of control over their treatment people want to assume, the problem remains as to how the healthcare professional or clinical researcher can convey complex medical information to the patient while still allowing them control over the depth and speed of the information presented. There is frequently a mismatch between the information people are offered by their doctors and nurses and the information they require,[29] and many patients report that their need for information changes during the course of their illness and its treatment.[30] The challenge for healthcare staff, especially doctors, is to be flexible in response to how much information, choice, or control a patient wants at any particular time.

Information

In this section we consider methods of conveying information about cancer and its treatment beyond face-to-face contacts. Although much of this information flows from professionals to patients, it should be remembered that people with cancer regularly learn about cancer from friends, family members, and especially other patients. Indeed, the experiences of other patients who have had a particular cancer or treatment can be an invaluable source of information for some people.

Information can be conveyed through many media and no single medium is ideal for every context or individual. The diversity of people's needs must be met with a diversity of media. People with learning disabilities or those with cognitive impairments, for example, may benefit from information that is presented in pictorial form or through audio and videotape, rather than through words alone. Consulting rooms where diagnostic information is given should therefore routinely contain pictorial representations of the body so as to aid explanations.

It should not be assumed that even a leaflet or video with apparently high face validity is necessarily interpreted the way it was designed to be understood.[31] It is therefore usually a poor substitute for direct contact. The advantage of face-to-face communication is precisely to do with the corrective feedback that is possible when information is exchanged *between* two people.

Information supply and demand

The thirst for information among people with cancer cannot be overstated. Making information available whenever it is needed is critical to quality cancer care.[32] For example, in 2001 the Cancer Council Victoria in Melbourne, Australia received over 49 000 phone calls for information and support.[33] The state of Victoria has a population of just 4.6 million. In 2003, the free UK national telephone information service Cancer BACUP was receiving 60 000 visits to their Internet website per month, and in the year 2000 BACUP distributed over a quarter of a million booklets or fact sheets to UK residents.

The desire for information is apparent, but why is information so important? When Australian patients were asked this question,[34] the four strongest reasons were that information ...

- gives people a sense of control over the situation;
- reduces anxiety by reducing uncertainty;

- can be used to *do* something, thereby actively contributing to one's recovery;
- enables people to predict and plan the future.

Providing information, however, is no simple matter. During medical consultations, between half and three quarters of medical patients who want more information simply do not ask for it.[35] For the patient and family, clinical appointments are often a time of high stress and uncertainty, making them a poor environment in which to understand and remember complex information. Cancer patients commonly complain that they are given either too much or too little information by their doctors. They frequently feel uncomfortable asking further questions at a later date[36] yet their need for information obviously changes during the course of their illness and its treatment.[30] Moreover, people with less formal education have more misconceptions about cancer than well-educated people, yet they are also less likely to request information directly.[37] There is therefore an important role for information that is simple and clearly presented.

While 95% of patients in one study ranked their hospital consultant as the primary source of information about cancer, and GPs were ranked as the second most important source, doctors were not rated highly in terms of quality of the information they provided.[38] The specialist nurse was ranked as providing the best quality of information and GPs in particular scored poorly. Patients do not always feel comfortable about using their doctors as a source of information. When asked about their attitudes towards information, patients in another study described a combination of (a) *faith* in their doctors ('doctor knows best' and good patients do not ask), (b) a need to maintain *hope* by avoiding potentially 'dangerous' information, and (c) an awareness of the plight of less fortunate patients (what the authors labelled *charity*), leading to a reluctance to make demands on the limited resources of information.[39]

Doctors, meanwhile, often complain that they have insufficient time to assess carefully how much information a patient actually wants, and they sometimes lack the communication skills required to conduct an interview that effectively and sensitively elicits the concerns of the patient.[40] The reality of busy clinics is that doctors often lack the time to provide information in an unhurried way that is sensitive to the patient's capacity to absorb it. Consequently, information delivery becomes rationed by the professional rather than being under the control of the patient, and doctors often end up relegating and delegating information delivery to other staff. Yet information delivery is vitally important to doctors if they wish their patients to comply with their treatment plan and the medical advice given.

Information can reduce the threat and uncertainty embedded in the word 'cancer'. The adequacy of information about diagnosis and treatment has been found to predict whether or not a patient develops a psychological disorder,[41] and there is no evidence that making detailed information available undermines patients' ability to use denial and avoidance.[8] People will take in what they are ready to take in, but the healthcare professional should always be vigilant about providing more information than is welcome.

Factual information (about the disease, its treatment, its likely course, etc.) can lessen the traumatic impact of the diagnosis by correcting mistaken beliefs about the disease and its prognosis, and increasing the patient's sense of control, safety and predictability (i.e. preparing the patient for what is to follow).[42]

Rarely, however, do cancer services offer advice to patients about what they can do to help themselves manage their illness, actively contribute to their own treatment, and minimize the risk of the cancer returning,[43] despite the popularity and helpfulness of such information. The only repository of such ideas, albeit with limited evidence to support them, often seems to be within complementary therapy and alternative medicine (which may explain in part the current popularity of such treatments).

Providing the optimal level of information at the point of *diagnosis* is more complex still; it seems that both too much and too little information can lead to later psychological problems.[44] One study of breast cancer patients indicated that although patients who felt well informed about their diagnosis and treatment experienced less anxiety and depression a year later than those who felt inadequately informed, most women acknowledged that they had been too shocked on hearing the word 'cancer' to absorb much of the rest of the interview.[45]

A review of the information needs of cancer patients[46] concluded that most patients' primary areas of concern are:

- the extent of the disease;
- the prognosis and likelihood of cure;
- the available treatment options;
- side-effects of treatment and their likely impact on the patient's normal life;
- how the patient can care for themselves and resume a normal lifestyle.

Over the course of their illness and its treatment people with cancer report that their need for information changes.[30] It is therefore important that patients and their families are told how to access further information whenever they need it. The use of information and support centres in cancer facilities is an obvious solution to general information needs, though only professional staff are able to answer detailed questions about the patient's specific medical condition and care. People may feel embarrassed asking the same question twice, so if there seems doubt, the information should be freely offered again without leaving the patient feeling either patronized or foolish. Some people continue to doubt the veracity of what they have been told, fearing that professionals may be withholding bad news. All questions should be answered, whether direct or indirect, no matter how trivial they may seem, while at the same time healthcare professionals must be sensitive to how much the patient is ready to hear and what they are interested in learning.

Please let me know if you have any questions about your illness or its treatment and I will always be happy to answer them. You might like to write down some questions before our appointments together. If you ask me a direct question I will, of course, try to answer it as truthfully as I can, though not everybody wants to hear every detail about their illness, so it would be helpful if you could think about how much information you want from me. There is a lot of information to take in, so please don't be shy about asking the same question more than once.

Written information

Written information in the form of booklets and leaflets is a common form of information delivery in cancer care and can be particularly effective in preparing people for imminent treatments.[47] It may be a poor substitute for face-to-face communication but can be helpful when it bolsters what has been discussed. In the UK some excellent booklets on specific cancer sites and specific treatments have been produced by national charities such as Cancer BACUP and Cancerlink, though many cancer hospitals also produce their own information booklets or sheets. However, despite the availability of quality information, a 2000 national survey of UK 65 000 cancer patients found for example that only 24% of women with ovarian cancer reported that they had received written information at the time of their diagnosis.[17]

Appendix 2 provides an example of a psychosocial booklet that was designed to normalize people's emotional reactions and experiences as a result of having cancer. It is drawn from many of the key themes described in this book and has been rated as highly helpful by many people with cancer over the past few years.

One problem with printed information is that it tends to be either too superficial or too complex for many users; rarely does one find both simple and complex information in the same booklet. This means that people cannot easily access the information they are looking for without having to search through several booklets or coming across information that they may not wish to have read. However, more sensitive information, such as prognosis or risks of treatment, tends to be absent in these booklets in order to protect those who do not wish to know, or are not ready for such information.

Printed material has the advantage of being fairly easy and inexpensive to produce and distribute, until new information necessitates a reprint. However, it presents information in a static, linear way that does not readily engage the reader or easily allow them to explore the subject area to a level of complexity that satisfies their needs. Static information can be used interactively (e.g. in discussion of a booklet with a professional) and such methods are considered to enhance their effectiveness,[48] though the added benefits of discussion presumably hold true for any medium of information delivery.

Patient-held records offer an interesting model of sharing information between staff and patients and is well established in other areas of medicine, including child health and obstetrics. They enable patients to 'own' and review their treatment plan, diagnostic test results, medication, etc., as well as record their own diary of events. They also hold the promise of more consistent information sharing among the professionals caring for the patient. However, patient-held records currently represent additional work for staff and not all patients welcome it—in one study some patients found it burdensome and an 'unwelcome reminder' of their disease.[49] A randomized trial of patient-held records among people with advanced cancer found no evidence that it improved patient satisfaction with information provided by professionals.[50] The authors of this study concluded that, while often popular among patients, patient-held records need the support of the entire healthcare team, which is currently difficult to engender. More work to overcome these barriers is currently underway within Britain's National Health Service.[51]

Written material is not the ideal medium for everyone: literacy rates are lower than one might expect. For example, in the United States about 20% of the population is functionally illiterate.[52] Even among people who can read and write, reading can be perceived as difficult and tiring. Because nearly half the population read at a Grade 8 (13 or 14 years old) level or lower,[53] it must always be checked that information is at an appropriate reading level. It should also be translated into appropriate local languages. A number of readability formulae are available though Gunning's Fog Index, introduced in 1968, is one of the best known for calculating the number of years of education required to read the text. This paragraph, for example, requires at least a Grade 14 (i.e. post-secondary) education, according to the Fog Index.

Gunning's Fog Index

$$F = [(\text{number of words/number of sentences}) + \text{number of words greater than two syllables}] \times 0.4$$

In addition to readability, which these days can be automatically checked by word-processors, Philip Ley has suggested several other criteria to be considered when producing written information for patients.[54] Written information must be:

- **Noticed** It should be physically well-presented. If it is not attractive and lacks 'eye appeal', it is less likely to be read.

- **Legible** Elderly patients may have difficulty reading small print or poor layout.

- **Read** Use words that are familiar to the target reader, use short words and sentences and avoid negatives. All these are likely to improve the chances that something is read. Helping people to prioritize the written material they have been given is also helpful when there is a lot available.

- **Understood** Information must be checked for clarity and readability. Text should preferably be written at the Grade 4 or 5 level (aged 9–11) or even lower. Technical terms should be clearly defined. Use active rather than passive sentences, and make all instructions explicit and specific.

- **Believed** Not all information is necessarily believed. It should be clear who is being targeted with the written material. Sources of the information should be cited and should preferably be perceived as credible, expert, and appealing to the intended readership. Any likely counter-propaganda should be confronted and addressed, and the acceptability of the material should be checked with a sample of the target audience.

- **Regularly checked**   Ensure that it is current and up-to-date.

Video

In 2000, 88% of British households possessed a video player, a proportion that appears to have been rising in a linear fashion by about 2–3% per year.[55] Videos, and increasingly DVDs, have the advantage of allowing patients and their families to review information in the comfort of their own home, in their own time. By weaving the personal testimonies and stories of patients with the advice of an 'expert', information can be conveyed in ways that allay rather than reinforce people's anxieties. Videos can also convey complex information by using simple diagrams and animations.

However, in spite of their enormous potential value, both in terms of information delivery as well as skill transmission, few formal evaluations have been undertaken of the many videos that have been produced. [56] Too often videos lack any underlying theoretical basis for behaviour change, and their authors rarely have a clear notion of what their video aims to achieve and thus what variables to measure when evaluating the video. Nonetheless videos designed to prepare patients for radiotherapy and chemotherapy have been evaluated and found to be helpful, reducing levels of anxiety and depression.[57] This approach has much potential.

Audiotapes

Audiotapes for transmitting general information have particular value for those unable to see or read. But they have further applications. Audiotapes of clinical consultations have the obvious advantage that they are tailor-made for the patient and therefore a source of highly relevant information which can be reviewed later with relatives. They also enable those for whom the consultation is not in their first language to review the contents at their leisure. The use of tape recordings of medical consultations appears to improve patient retention and recall of information and facilitates patients' requests for clarification[58] but does not appear to reduce psychological morbidity[59] or improve quality of life.[60]

One double-blind randomized study found that 75% of patients reviewed the tape of their initial post-diagnosis consultation, and those provided with a tape were more satisfied with the consultation as well as with their medical care in general.[60] This study was unable to replicate an earlier finding[59] that taped consultations lead to more psychological distress among poor-prognosis patients. Three months after the consultation, 98% of patients were positive about the use of audiotaped consultations and reported they would recommend it to other cancer patients. An Australian study found that those patients receiving bad news were more likely to want to listen to their tape than those who received neutral or good news though, significantly, one patient reported that having the consultation taped inhibited discussion.[61]

It seems therefore that most people would find it useful to receive a taped record of important consultations, such as those in which treatment options are being discussed. However, as always, the patient should be given the choice and no pressure should be exerted on them to listen to the tape.

Internet and computer-based information

Increasingly, people in the West are turning to the Internet as a largely free repository of information. In 2000 a third of British households had access to the Internet.[55] The breadth of information on the Internet is at once staggering and overwhelming; entering the term 'breast cancer' into a well-known search engine in 2003 yielded over 2.5 million web pages. The problem becomes one of discriminating what is good information from what is inaccurate, out-of-date, or irrelevant. Healthcare providers will be increasingly called upon to advise their patients on reputable up-to-date sites known for their accuracy. They will also be expected to provide web-based information about their own services to enable prospective patients to orientate themselves to the institution, its personnel, and the treatments offered.

Like the Internet, CD-ROMs offer the potential advantage of interactivity that is absent with linear media such as written material and videos. They can enable people to control the rate and depth of the information they receive. However, the rise of CD and DVD-ROM packages appears to have been largely eclipsed by the growing influence of the Internet.

Information and support centres

Information centres have the advantage of providing a wide range of current information whenever the patient (or family member) is ready to absorb it. However, new information can also provoke distress (e.g. when it reveals the uncertainty of the patient's condition). Information and support centres therefore ideally link these two components of supportive care to ensure that support is always at hand whenever sensitive information is made available. In practice, the seeking of information is simply the pretext used by many patients to obtain emotional support.

Many cancer information and support centres are attached to cancer treatment facilities and staffed by trained volunteers. Information centres can provide orientation information about local cancer services and personnel, access to information booklets, multimedia and internet-based information about cancer and its treatment, emotional support, practical and financial advice, as well as route to local and national support organizations. Despite their accessibility, a survey of UK information centres revealed that they are used considerably more by women than by men, and more by middle-aged people than older patients.[62]

Some centres have successfully deployed trained ex-patient volunteers whose mere presence can provide a source of hope for newly diagnosed patients.[63] They also bring the authentic voice of experience which, when tempered by training in listening skills, can deliver much needed empathic support. All volunteers, however, whether ex-patients or not, require vetting, regular support, and clinical supervision. They must be trained to recognize and refer more complex psychological and social issues that are beyond their level of competence. (*see* Chapter 7—Voluntary Support)

Staff–patient relationships

People are only 'patients' to healthcare professionals. To everyone else they are parents, children, siblings, relations, friends, colleagues. For those newly diagnosed with cancer the role of 'patient' and the relationships they form with healthcare staff must be learned through experience.

Hospital wards and treatment clinics are seen by patients to be owned by the staff who work in them. Patients can feel like they are temporary guests. When people are guests they try to fit in with the way their hosts do things. Most of the ways hospital wards and clinics work, however, amounts to unwritten rules that are taken for granted by the staff, but which have to be surmized and learned by patients. Clear written information about ward and clinic routines, and what the patient is allowed and not allowed to do, can therefore be helpful in reducing stressful ambiguity. A ward clerk or hospital volunteer should be deployed to welcome and orientate both patients and visiting relatives to the ward environment. Patients from minority ethnic communities often face the added stress of trying to maintain their cultural practices (e.g. diet, prayer, etc.) in the face of healthcare staff who may seem unsupportive and insensitive to these needs.

But developing an adequate understanding of their patients is challenging for most healthcare professionals when they lack adequate 'clinical' time. Often they also struggle to provide continuity of care. Patients who see a different doctor every time they attend a hospital clinic are unlikely to feel guided and supported through the ordeal they are going through. One of the few studies that has examined the number of doctors seen by patients found that, among a group of Scottish palliative care patients, those with an illness of less than one year had seen an average of 28 doctors.[64] One patient had met 73 doctors in little more than two years.

It can be unsettling and potentially distressing when people's expectations are not met. So it therefore may be helpful to consider some of the many expectations held by staff and patients.

What do healthcare professionals want in their patients?

Healthcare professionals want patients who can articulate clearly the nature and history of their symptoms and, more importantly, what they understand by them. They need their patients to tell them about any pain, side-effects of treatment, and broader 'psychosocial' concerns, so they can respond appropriately and relieve unnecessary suffering. The patient's most important concerns may not always be about their illness.

The reality is that patients do not always tell their professional carers everything consistently and may, in fact, tell members of the healthcare team different things depending on the interest shown by healthcare staff in the past.[65] Patients may not have the concerns that healthcare staff imagine them to have and their needs can change from day to day, from hour to hour. They may want no information one day, detailed information the next. They may want to talk one moment, be silent the next. Understanding what a person needs sometimes takes time and patience.

Patients rarely know what is expected of them. So orientating patients to unfamiliar medical settings, and explaining different ways in which they can help staff deliver their care, is time well spent. For example, encouraging patients to make a list of questions prior to their consultations not only saves everyone time, but leads to a consultation in which the patient's concerns are more likely to be addressed.[66] Let people know that you want to hear about their concerns.

Healthcare professionals are constantly meeting patients who have different needs and who harbour different expectations of professionals. In the face of so much that is new and frightening, patients understandably depend on professionals for their safety. As Radley has noted, 'there is a need for doctors to conduct their clinical practice without displacing (or disrupting) *the integrity of the patient as person*'[3] (Radley 1994, p. 106). This is no simple matter for it requires the professional to be receptive and responsive to the patient's initial dependency, while gradually handing back control to the patient, in as much as the patient wants to assume it.

> At the root of the healing relationship everywhere is the client's (and family's) wish for the reassurance that all is well or can be redeemed; and its reciprocal is the healer's hope, if not expectation, that he can indeed reassure and cure. Included in this relationship is the realistic impossibility of certainty. What, in fact, are legitimate expectations and false hopes? It is often at this point that fact and fantasy, reality and wish, collide.[67]
>
> (Stein 1985, p. 25)

Patients come to their doctors with the 'expectant faith'[68] that this person will resolve the medical problem and make the situation safe again. Doctors naturally want to meet this expectation but, in the context of cancer, they know that for many people this will not be possible. While harbouring their own uncertainties, they must work with people who earnestly want to return to a life without uncertainty. The pressure on professionals to provide good news is like a 'tractor beam' that must be sensitively navigated. Faced with their patients' yearning for a positive outcome, healthcare staff need to choose their words carefully, but they are also constantly exploring this tension between the patient's need to depend on them for their safety and their need to be in control over their lives again.

Faced with these complicated expectations and their patients' considerable distress, professionals may wish to maintain a safe 'professional distance' from their patients.

It may be less distressing for the healthcare professional to focus on physical symptoms like pain, rather than the *feelings* that the patient has about these symptoms (the fear, perhaps, that their cancer has spread). But too much professional distance can lead to remote impersonal care.

What is appropriate professional distance?

The first time I met Mr H. [surgeon], I felt absolutely relaxed and trusted him (I still do!) completely. He is an open, friendly and smiling person with a great charisma. Dr M. on other hand, from the very first time I met him, made me anxious and tense. He doesn't smile, no warmth radiates from him and he doesn't seem, or even make the effort to pretend to be interested in how I feel. I may well be over-sensitive, but I refuse to take the entire responsibility of my not feeling at ease with Dr M.

Healthcare staff need to establish a working alliance with their patients based on trust, balancing respect for the patient's dignity and privacy with kindness and concern. Patients often feel very supported and reassured when they see that their doctor is moved by their experience without being overwhelmed by it. It is reassuring to know that one's nurse or doctor really cares.[34]

But how much compassion should one show? Is there not a risk that by offering emotional support one may inadvertently cause the patient to become overly dependent? Might professionals become overwhelmed by the complicated emotional concerns of the patient and their family if they take an interest in them, and be unable to meet their needs? If we offer compassion, how long before we suffer 'compassion fatigue'[69] or emotional burnout? (*see* Chapter 7).

Historically, 'professional distance' is embodied in the uniforms and white coats that healthcare staff wear. These are symbols of professional disinterest and expert status, but they are also potential barriers to establishing a trusting and confiding relationship. There is no doubt that professional distance has its place as, for example, when doctors are required to examine 'private parts' of the body. During a physical examination, both the patient and doctor generally assume a disinterested, dispassionate dissociation from what is happening in order to manage the socially taboo situation (i.e. sexual overtones) of one person (the patient) allowing a relative stranger (the doctor) access to their body. 'The unflinching composure, and the holding of a middle-distance gaze, are things people do in the clinic to transform themselves into an object for medical examination'[3] (Radley 1994, p. 99). So one function of 'professional boundaries' is to confine both patients and professionals to their respective roles, so as to protect each of them from behaviour that would be inappropriate to these roles.

However, professional distance can also become an acute barrier to effective communication, such as the nurse who maintains a breezy surface brightness at all times that isolates the patient and keeps their distress at bay. Peter Maguire has shown that doctors and nurses often use 'distancing tactics' to block patients from disclosing or exploring their emotional concerns.[40]

Distancing tactics

Jollying along	'There's no need to be so glum …'
Normalization	'You are bound to be worried at this stage, it's quite normal …'
Offering reassurance	'I'm pretty confident you are going to be all right'.
Offering advice/fixing it	Giving advice without acknowledging the genuine concerns of the patients. Trying to fix the problem before properly acknowledging it.
False reassurance	Doctor avoids giving bad news in the face of a direct question but reassures instead.
Switching	Changing the topic, the person being discussed or the time-frame ('Yes, but how do you feel now?').
Selective attention[70]	Focusing on concerns which the professional feels confident addressing while ignoring the patient's concerns.
Passing the buck[71]	Although it may be appropriate to refer to the expertise of another person, it can also be used as a way of avoiding a distressing topic.
Using jargon[71]	Professionals, and increasingly patients, use medical terms that are not always well understood.

Maguire found that doctors and nurses used these distancing or blocking strategies because they were …

- afraid of unleashing strong emotions that they would be unable to contain;
- worried that eliciting their patients' emotions might be damaging to them (equating the expression of emotion in their patients with distress);
- concerned that by asking patients to talk about their concerns, they would be encouraging them to ask a difficult question (e.g. 'How long have I got?');
- anxious to avoid a conversation that would be emotionally distressing to the professional themselves.

However, healthcare professionals are more likely to communicate well with their patients if they …

- have sufficient time
- see it as a legitimate part of their role
- have been trained in communication skills
- set a high value on communicating well and see this as a priority[72]
- feel confident at handling distress and emotional concerns
- feel well supported (e.g. access to clinical supervision)
- are aware of further sources of psychosocial support for the patient.

In summary, professional boundaries are there to preserve a therapeutic function and should not undermine compassion based on the common experience of being human.[73] They are ethical and social constraints that are there to benefit and protect the patient, enabling them to feel safe to receive the care of professionals without the intrusion of normal social ambiguities (confidentiality, sexual interest, etc.). They are there to ensure that both the professional and the patient observe the implicit rules governing their respective roles. For example, the over-involvement of professionals can lead patients to worry about burdening their professional carers with their emotional concerns. Professional distance, however, can be used to overprotect the professional from the patient's distress, thereby blocking its expression, and is sometimes a sign that the professional is becoming emotionally drained and burned out (*see* Chapter 7). 'Appropriate' professional distance therefore depends on the people involved and the context they find themselves in, but it is invariably wiser to err on the side of 'being human' than retreat to the safety of professional indifference.

What are patients looking for in the professionals who care for them?

> Some nurses smiled or waved whenever they came to my end of the ward; to others I felt invisible. Sometimes the absence of a smile made me feel desolate, and I felt lonely and neglected when the nurses were busy elsewhere in the ward, even though I did not need anything and I knew that other patients had greater needs. I appreciated it when anyone found a few minutes to spend with me.

Patients invest their safety in the hands of their doctors, nurses, and radiographers. But it is usually doctors who represent figures of enormous importance in the eyes of patients. As David Spiegel has noted, 'patients rely on their doctors for their very lives, and they invest elaborate wishes and fears in them'.[32]

> I'm not quite sure that I trust him [*the surgeon*] to be wholly honest with me anymore, but I couldn't be bothered to pursue my questions today. I'll leave it all in his hands. I suddenly feel that he is no longer the centre of my universe as he has been for the last 3 months – quite a big step in my rehabilitation I think.

An Australian study[34] asked women with cancer what they regarded as important in their relationship with their specialist doctor in helping them to reach a decision about their treatment. Five themes emerged:

- the doctor cared for, understood, and respected them
- they could trust and have confidence in the doctor
- the doctor would give them enough time
- they would be listened to by their doctor
- the doctor would be open and honest

There is often a tension, however, between wanting one's doctor to be authoritative and certain (denoting safety and hope), and wanting them to be honest about the uncertainties. 'Although the mature part of us knows that all knowledge and treatment is *probabilistic*, the frightened child in patients and healers alike craves *absolute certainties*'[67] (Stein 1985, p. 25). Doctors in particular are constantly required to tolerate and work with this tension.

Patients want doctors:

- **Always to be honest** Trust is the basis of the doctor–patient relationship. False hope remains false and, likely or not, will be found out with damaging results for the relationship. Being honest, however, does not mean brutal honesty, nor imposing information where it is not wanted. It is also acceptable to say 'I don't know'. This response too is honest and will be respected more than a smoke-screen of mystifying technical language, though similarly it should not be used to get out of answering difficult questions.

- **To provide patients with a 'model' of the treatment plan** Provide a clear rationale for why the patient is having a particular treatment and explain how it works in a language that the patient is likely to understand. Such 'treatment models' are valuable and highly reassuring, but all too often absent. Patients are more likely to 'comply' with a treatment if they have a model for how it is thought to work. Giving patients a treatment model that they can understand is also an important element of informed consent. In one Australian study, a third of patients were unclear what their treatment plan was meant to achieve.[74]

- **To provide patients with a role in their own treatment** Patients are frequently keen to do something active to help their treatment and recovery and prevent recurrence, yet rarely are they given anything active to do. Encouraging people to discontinue unhealthy practices (e.g. smoking, fatty foods, sedentary lifestyle, etc.) and adopt healthier practices (stress reduction, gentle exercise, healthy diet, etc.) allows patients to feel more in control by doing all they can to maximize their health.

- **To provide a 'road map' for the future** Always communicate with the patient about what you are hoping to do next, and the steps you have agreed for the future. A clear plan establishes mutual goals that can be worked towards, thereby conveying hope. This reduces unnecessary worry and allows the patient and family to prepare themselves for what is to come. A coherent road map is as important for patients who cannot be cured as it is for those who can. People feel safer and more relaxed when they can anticipate clearly what is about to happen. For this they must be able to trust the healthcare professional.

I felt that I was being pushed down an endless dark tunnel – I could see no end and kept coming upon obstacles with no warning. I was always having to look out for myself. No one was guiding me. I was alone and helpless.

- **To be a source of leadership and guidance** Cancer patients value doctors who are authoritative with a clear sense of direction, but who are nonetheless responsive to their patients' views and needs. By adopting the role of patient, people permit doctors special access to their bodies, and in temporarily delegating this control to the doctor the patient enters into an implicit contract that the doctor will restore the patient's control over their own life.[67] Thus, doctors must always be ready to hand decision making control back to the patient as soon as, and as much as, the patient is ready to assume it.

- **To be a source of information and support**   All healthcare professionals can provide patients with the 'safety signals' they are looking for,[75] but doctors represent the ultimate medical authority and the source of the most definitive information about the patient. Patients therefore value doctors who share information openly and sensitively, and who are emotionally supportive.[76] It is singularly disconcerting to see a doctor who has forgotten one's clinical situation and treatment stage, just as it is to see a different doctor at each consultation.

- **To have sufficient time**   If doctors are to be supportive and informative, they need sufficient training and adequate time with their patients. A UK national survey of 65 000 cancer patients in 2001 revealed that 30% of patients had spent less than ten minutes with their doctor during their most recent outpatient appointment.[17]

Patient-centred communication

The word 'communication' includes the same root as community, common, and communism; in other words, to share. Communication occurs when information is shared rather than conveyed in one direction alone. Not surprisingly, therefore, communication training usually starts with teaching healthcare staff how to listen and pay attention to the concerns of their patients. This is known as patient-centred care.

Patient-centred care puts the concerns of individual patients at centre stage. It involves healthcare professionals showing respect for and sensitivity to the diversity of their patients' needs, while demonstrating both their professional expertize and their common humanity. It involves preparing people for what is to come (such as unfamiliar treatments) and helping them to make sense of what has already occurred (eliciting concerns).

Similarly, patient-centred communication occurs when the patient's perspective becomes the focus of what is discussed. In Chapter 1 we described how people with cancer can only make sense of information about their illness by fitting it into their existing knowledge and beliefs.[77] Whatever professionals need to communicate with patients, it must *fit* with what the patient currently understands about their illness. The difficulty is that people's understanding, beliefs, and attitudes are never fixed but continually evolving, so the only way to find out what a person understands (and wants to understand) is to listen to what the patient says. There must be a constant dialogue between healthcare providers and the patient (and family members) so that professionals can learn how the patient currently understands their situation, their illness, their treatment, and any concerns they may have. The extent to which the patient's wider family is involved must be determined by the patient, and local cultural practices will have a bearing on this.

There is also an expectation that staff communicate effectively with one another. It is deeply alarming to discover that the surgeon and the oncologist appear to be in conflict about one's treatment plan. The team must work to a consistent and co-ordinated plan that is agreed by everyone and openly available to the patient. This is particularly difficult when the patient is forced to communicate with different doctors at every clinical appointment; recall the study of palliative care patients in Scotland which found that, on average, patients had seen 28 doctors in the year since their diagnosis.[64]

Finally, the head of the clinical team should be ultimately responsible for telling the patient important news such as diagnostic and prognostic information. In addition, it helps the patient and the family to know that a particular professional has been appointed the 'key worker', a person who is well-informed and up-to-date about the patient's illness and treatment, to whom they can direct further concerns and questions.

Cultural assumptions and differences

Cultural differences are often more apparent than real. The emotional and social concerns of people confronted by a life-threatening illness appear to be broadly similar the world over.[71] Nonetheless, people make sense of all new information on the basis of what they know, and what they know is what they have learned from their social and cultural background. Equally, everyone, including professionals, conveys information using the terms and conventions they have learned from their own personal and professional background. So to the extent that people's social backgrounds—their values, assumptions, beliefs, and language—are different, there is room for miscommunication and misunderstanding.

For example, many people in the West believe that germs cause disease. Some cultures, however, are influenced by the traditional Chinese belief that a healthy body is in a state of balance, and that disease is the result of a lack of balance between *yang* (hot) and *yin* (cold).[78] Some cultures believe that illness is a consequence of the soul having left the body or been stolen, while others regard illness as a form of possession by powerful spirits which only an exorcism will remove. Disease is commonly seen as a punishment for a breach of taboo or sin. In Christianity this has sometimes been known as divine retribution; in Islam, Allah rewards the good and punishes the sinful. The only difference between these traditional beliefs and scientific medicine is that the latter is falsifiable and can be proven wrong.[78] The trust that the public have in their healing experts, however, is very similar the world over. These underlying belief systems about illness can affect the interpretation and comprehension of what healthcare personnel are both saying and proposing to do. It is therefore essential to understand the patient's cultural frame of reference when discussing their illness ('*What do you understand about these kinds of illness?*' '*What do you think caused this problem?*')

The way people communicate also varies enormously from culture to culture. Many Asians consider it disrespectful to look someone in the eye for it implies that one has the same or superior social standing. Some Asian patients may therefore avoid direct eye contact out of respect for the perceived superior status of healthcare professionals.[78] By contrast, many people from the Middle East perceive eye contact between a man and a woman as a 'sexual invitation'. Thus, healthcare staff should be aware that the eye contact they make with their patients may be interpreted in ways they did not intend.

Many non-Western cultures share a social hierarchy in which age carries authority and men are considered the head of the household. Often the behaviours of men and women are more clearly prescribed than in the West. Consequently, being medically examined by a member of the opposite sex may offend some patients' sense of modesty, depending on their culture. In the largely Islamic Middle East, for example, female nursing is a low-status profession because a nurse violates the laws of the Koran when she either looks at or touches the body of a male stranger. Consequently, there is a shortage of nurses and huge salaries are often paid to foreign nurses.

Patients in the West are reported to be increasingly assertive, expressive, open, and direct with healthcare staff, and expect to participate in their treatment. This is often not the case in other cultures, nor even among everyone in the West. Asian patients are more likely to regard the doctor and nurse as authority figures with high social standing. Western doctors may therefore find it more difficult interviewing someone who appears quiet, deferential, and passive, and who may understate their problems and rarely express their feelings.[79]

Likewise, the use of first names is considered friendly and egalitarian in America, though disrespectful in most other cultures, including many European ones.[78] To avoid any possible discourtesy, healthcare staff should therefore address adult patients by their titles (Mr, Mrs, Ms, etc.) unless invited to use their first names. And one should not assume that both members of a couple, or even their children, will share the same surname; in many societies this is not the norm.

Gestures, physical contact, diet, dress, the expression of emotion, pain, and modesty, quite apart from customs and ceremonies, can all differ from culture to culture. For example, nodding (as if to say 'Yes') does not always denote understanding or agreement; it may simply reflect embarrassment and a concern with loss of dignity at not having understood. Even the West's obsession with getting things done by a particular time is not shared by all cultures.[78] Finally, patients from any culture may be too embarrassed to discuss certain issues unless the healthcare professional shows sensitivity, concern, and patience.

Healthcare staff should:

- find out as much as possible about the minority ethnic patients in the community served by the service. Learn a word or two of greeting in the language of your patients;

- allow more time for interviews with patients whose first language is not English. Time pressures only intensify the stress of communication for both the professional and the patient;

- check that you are pronouncing the patient's name correctly;

- find out whether the patient has family and friends living in the general area and how much support they have. Any individual may feel cut off from natural sources of support but social and cultural isolation may be more of an issue for people from minority ethnic backgrounds;
- ask individual patients and families about their values and lifestyle and any particular needs that the healthcare service could helpfully respond to;
- learn how the patient and family understand cancer. What does it mean to them in terms of its cause and likely course? In some cultures the word cancer is taboo (*see* Control, Consent, Collaboration, and Choice);
- respect cultural differences without generalizing—there are always many variations within any one culture. Each person is unique and not everyone conforms to the supposed norms of their cultural and ethnic background;
- enquire as to what people mean when they use the words they do. Words have multiple meanings and euphemisms are common. Consider the ones used by healthcare staff in terms of possible ambiguities and potential for misunderstanding;
- learn to find something positive in every cultural difference. Respect each person's values, beliefs, and choices as you do your own;[80]
- remember that non-English-speaking patients are often quite lonely in hospital and may feel that staff avoid them. Think about whether you unwittingly avoid people with whom it is harder to communicate;
- if English is not the patient's first language, speak slowly and clearly but without raising your voice. Avoid idioms such as 'starting from scratch' or 'fed up'; in other words, any expression whose meaning cannot be inferred from the meanings of the words that make it up;[80]
- consider the use of an interpreter rather than using a member of the family to translate. Family members are likely to be emotionally involved and may choose to filter information between the patient and the professional.

Working through interpreters

- Appointments using interpreters usually take much longer than normal so always assign more time for the interview.
- Consider the ethnicity and dialect of the interpreter. Remember that there are many dialects within any language. For example, the Chinese dialects Cantonese, Hakka, and Fukien are all very different.[80]
- Check that the patient feels comfortable talking through the interpreter and that the interpreter is clear about confidentiality rules. Always use interpreters of the same sex as the patient, especially if there are intimate matters to be discussed.
- Meet the interpreter before the interview so as to build rapport and ensure that they feel comfortable with you. Discuss how you will manage the interview together and

invite the interpreter to tell you of any cultural misunderstandings that arise during the interview. Invite the interpreter to let you know if the interview is going too quickly or any difficulties the interpreter feels the patient may be having. The interpreter in this sense can act as the patient's advocate during the interview. They may be able to 'read' the patient's non-verbal behaviour more accurately than you.

• If one is forced to use a non-professional interpreter, make it clear that they must translate exactly what they hear and refrain from adding their own bias or opinion unless they make this explicit.

• However, do not be alarmed if interpreters talk more than you were expecting. They may be explaining a concept or term you have used, for which there is no direct translation.

• Allow time for introductions and for the patient and the interpreter to talk for a few minutes in their own tongue.

• Avoid jargon so as to make the interpreter's job easier. In some instances, where the patient's English is fair, the interpreter may be used only for instances where the patient does not understand.

• Do not allow the presence of the interpreter to obstruct your relationship with the patient more than is necessary. Sit facing the patient and speak to them rather than the interpreter. Listen and look at the patient when they are talking to the interpreter because you may still be able to pick up the emotional message from the patient's facial expressions and gestures.

• End the interview as you would normally by inviting the patient to ask you any questions, or tell you any concerns that they may be having. Allow the interpreter and the patient some time to discuss the interview and how it went and ask the interpreter afterwards for any feedback they wish to give. If there is to be a further meeting with the patient try to employ the same interpreter so as to ensure continuity.

Language

Not all miscommunication is caused by cultural difference. Some of it is caused by the language that people use to communicate. A UK national survey of 65 000 cancer patients in 2000 found that 16% could not understand all or even most of their doctors' answers to their questions.[17] In a 2001 survey of the British lay public's understanding of cancer terms, only about half the sample understood that 'the tumour is progressing' meant that the cancer had spread, while only a fifth of men were able to locate the prostate gland.[81]

Words are ultimately slippery vague things that mean different things to different people, and even different things to the same person in different contexts. The most effective way of knowing one's message has been received is to ask for it back. Healthcare staff seldom check that their remarks and explanations have been understood. It is often helpful to ask the patient and their family to summarize their understanding so that one can confirm or gently amend it.

- Adapt your vocabulary to that of the patient while explaining terms that they are likely to encounter in the future. Be prepared to explain the same information on several occasions.

- Avoid euphemisms and long words. Try instead to use words that the patient has already used or is likely to know. For example, do not use the word 'utilize' when the word 'use' will do. Say 'chemotherapy drug' rather than 'chemotherapy agent'.

- Patients should be respected as intelligent adults but do not expect even well-educated patients to understand medical jargon. Jargon mystifies and intimidates. If you choose to use words like prognosis, metastases, biopsy, etc., always check first that the patient fully understands them. The majority of the population do not understand these words.[82]

- Keep your sentences short and simple. English can be expressed in many convoluted ways. Give instructions in a clear logical order and preferably write them down: 'First you will have your operation. Then you will have the chemotherapy we talked about'. Do not say 'Before your chemotherapy starts you'll have your operation.'

- From time to time ask the patient in a gentle and supportive way to tell you *what* they have understood, not *if* they have understood. This will enable you to clarify any misunderstandings that have occurred. If you simply ask 'Do you understand?' you are likely to receive the answer 'Yes.' This may simply mean 'Yes, I'm listening but actually I don't understand'.[80] Better to ask *what* they understand.

- Judge how much people are likely to remember, given the context and the likely impact of what you have said. When people are very anxious they find it hard to retain a great deal of information. A written summary (or tape recording) of what you have talked about can be enormously helpful for patients and families to refer to later.

Eliciting concerns

Why do I hide my feeling from professional people? Fear of being classed a case of nerves? Not a coper? Labelled? Who knows?

In this section we consider how healthcare professionals can assess their patients' physical and psychosocial concerns in the context of routine clinical interviews. This is a vitally important component of supportive care. Before describing the normal course of clinical interviews and the kind of questions that can help elicit these concerns, we briefly look at why this is rarely as simple as it sounds.

The more concerns people have the more they are likely to be distressed,[83] yet rarely are these concerns expressed by patients or identified by healthcare staff.[1] It seems that, whether their concerns are physical,[84] psychosocial,[29] or spiritual[85] many patients are reluctant to complain about them due to commonly held expectations and assumptions.

Common assumptions which deter patients from revealing their physical, spiritual, or psychosocial concerns

- Raising difficulties is seen as the responsibility of doctors, not patients.[12]
- Patients and relatives sometimes lack the confidence, social skills, or language to ask questions to healthcare professionals, or express their feelings.
- Healthcare professionals are seen as too busy and important to be burdened with the patient's concerns.
- Patients feel constrained by the common social pressure to 'think positively' at all times.
- Patients may feel shame at admitting they have particular difficulties (e.g. sexual, financial, literacy, etc.).
- Those harbouring guilt about their previous lifestyle (e.g. smoking) may be more reluctant to voice their concerns.[71]
- 'Complaining' about side-effects may lead staff to view the patient as not coping, a nuisance, or ungrateful. It may even risk treatment being stopped.[71]
- Emotional and even physical distress is often seen as inevitable and untreatable.

Similarly, healthcare staff are generally poor at detecting even severe levels of distress in their patients,[86, 87] and oncologists tend to leave it to their patients to raise concerns if they have them[12] or simply block patients' attempts to communicate their concerns (see What is Appropriate Professional Distance?). The resulting impasse amounts to a failure of communication.

The onus is therefore on healthcare professionals to draw out and attend to these concerns wherever possible, in so far as the patient wishes to talk about them.

Assessing the whole person

Incorporating a psychosocial assessment into key clinical interviews (e.g. those around diagnosis, treatment, end of treatment, follow-up appointments, etc.) can have therapeutic merit in its own right, yet does not need to be excessively lengthy or drawn out. By acknowledging the patient's own unique feelings and concerns, healthcare professionals can assist their patients' psychosocial adjustment (described in Chapter 1). Furthermore, by enabling people to identify their concerns, professionals can help patients prioritize them into more manageable chunks and, in doing so, the professional becomes a natural part of the patient's extended support network.

Asking about issues of importance to the patient does not mean that the professional has to deal with them all. It is vital, however, that all healthcare staff are aware of what further resources exist and how they can be accessed—for example, information about palliative care specialists, social workers, clinical psychologists, counsellors, relaxation training courses, voluntary and self-help groups, information centres, and other more general community resources.

The following open-ended questions merely provide a starting point for eliciting the patient's concerns. From here the professional should funnel the interview to elicit the specific concerns that require attention.

- *You have had to face a lot of change in your life recently. How do you feel you are managing at the moment? Do you have any particular concerns that we have not perhaps discussed?*

- *How do you feel your treatment is going? Are there any physical problems you are having that you may not have mentioned to me? For example, any pain or discomfort? (What do you think may be causing that?)*

- *What sort of support do you have? (Are you able to talk to them openly?) How is your [family, partner ...] dealing with your illness? Do you feel they are well supported? Is there anyone you are particularly worried about? How do you feel you and your [family, partner ...] are getting on with one another?*

- *How are your spirits, your general mood? (How long do the low spells last? How low do you get? Do you have times when you can enjoy yourself? Do you ever have thoughts that it would be easier not to go on? How far have you taken these thoughts?)*

- *Do you have any particular worries or things you are especially anxious about?*

- *How are you spending your time? Have you got things to look forward to and things to achieve? Do you feel you are still involved in things you have always enjoyed?*

- *Do you have any practical worries: financial concerns, accommodation, the need for equipment at home (commodes, incontinence pads, special mattresses, etc.), or domestic support (help with shopping, preparing meals, cleaning, and laundry)?*

- *How are you feeling about yourself these days? How do you feel you have changed since you learned you were ill? Do you feel you have lost confidence in yourself in any areas of your life?*

- *Do you feel your illness has changed the way you look at your life or left you with big (existential/spiritual) questions? (Do you feel it would be helpful to discuss these questions with someone? Would you say that you have a faith? Do you practise your faith?)*

- *Have you managed to talk to anyone about these changes? (Would you find it helpful to talk to someone about some of these concerns?)*

- *Is there anything we have not discussed that you would like to ask me about?*

Having identified the patient's concerns, the professional should summarize them clearly and work with the patient to consider what sources of support and information are required to resolve the concerns.

- Some concerns may be resolved immediately (e.g. providing further information) or through a further consultation with the professional at a later date.

- Some concerns may be resolved through the patient taking action (becoming more socially active again, obtaining information, attending a support group, taking more physical activity, etc.).

• Some concerns may require a referral to another service (other medical specialist, social worker, spiritual leader, clinical psychologist, counsellors, etc.). It is essential that the professional conducting the interview is aware of specialist resources that are locally available as well as their referral criteria. In discussing a possible referral to a 'mental health professional', such as a psychologist or psychiatrist, it is important to reassure the patient that such referrals are commonplace and in no sense a sign of failure, shame, or 'weakness'.

Conducting a patient-centred clinical interview

Relationships between healthcare professionals and patients usually begin with an interview of some kind, whether at the bedside or in a clinic. It has been estimated that during a 40-year career an oncologist will conduct about 200 000 clinical interviews.[88] In any relationship far more time is spent clearing up communication mistakes than it would have taken to communicate effectively in the first place, so learning to conduct a clinical interview effectively is an essential clinical skill for all healthcare professionals.

Clinical interviews are the main medium through which information is exchanged and occur at different points and in different contexts throughout the patient's medical care. They are key opportunities for staff to learn about the patient's symptoms and concerns and for patients to be updated, in as far as they wish to be, about their condition and its treatment. From this dialogue shared new goals can emerge.

Setting—introductions—purpose of meeting—establishing rapport

A few conditions should always be observed wherever possible:

1. Interviews should be conducted with as much privacy as possible and with no interruptions. If interruptions do occur, an apology to the patient should be made, their permission sought and, after the interruption has been dealt with, the clinician should summarize what has occurred thus far in the interview. Ensure you have sufficient time so as to avoid any impression that you are in a hurry.

2. Wherever possible, patients should be fully clothed and seated rather than lying down. During bedside interviews, the professional should sit next to the patient so that they are not looking down on the patient from above. Also avoid talking across a desk.

3. Use the patient's name and title, introduce yourself with a smile and explain your role within the healthcare team. A little small talk at this point allows patients to feel comfortable with their surroundings and clearer about people's names and roles. Above all, convey your interest and concern. By demonstrating openness and kindness you will encourage the patient and their family to express themselves freely. It may seem obvious that smiling and eye contact often express far more than words when building rapport, yet both can be easily overlooked (see Cultural Differences).

4. Share your mutual expectations of the meeting with the patient so that you establish a common understanding about why you are meeting. There is a common tendency for clinical interviews to begin abruptly, after perfunctory introductions, without the purpose and context of the meeting first being established. Declaring expectations can mean that neither of you leaves the meeting feeling empty-handed. Of course, whatever the initial expectations, neither of you is obliged to stick rigidly to the agenda—the door always needs to be left open for new information, questions and concerns raised by the patient or their family.

Building rapport—the tone of communication

Every healthcare professional knows that the start of a new relationship with a patient is critical to how that relationship develops. 'Establishing rapport', as it is sometimes known, sets the tone of what people expect of one another. Showing respect and courtesy to a patient, for example, not only conveys good manners but also facilitates a collaborative working relationship.

The tone of a relationship often has less to do with what is said than the non-verbal style and attitude of the people present. Unfortunately, it is the nebulous human qualities of respect, kindness, and warmth that tend to evaporate when overstressed professionals lose sight of the person within the patient. One adage, however, has lost none of its truth: 'Treat the person in front of you in the way you would wish your mother (father, sibling, child) to be treated.'

Establishing and maintaining therapeutic tone to a relationship is about doing one's best to 'tune in' to the patient's frame of reference so as to understand what the patient is experiencing. Indeed, this musical metaphor can be extended by noting the three main elements of communication:[89]

Pitch Are you communicating in a way that the patient can understand? Are you on the same level? Are you in tune with their current concerns?

Pace Are you going at the patient's speed? Have they understood what you have said and taken it in, or do they need more time to absorb this before further issues are discussed?

Pulse Are you in tune with the emotional state of the patient? Do you have a sense of what they are feeling at this moment, given what you know about what they have gone through recently and what you are discussing? Are you communicating with the patient in a way that resonates with what they are currently feeling?

Communication skills

Following the introductions, the interview proceeds with the business of the meeting, as agreed at its start. What distinguishes patient-centred interviewing from the more traditional focus on the professional's agenda is that the entire interview is conducted from the patient's frame of reference, starting and ending with their understanding and concerns. This style of communication is certainly much preferred by patients, relatives, and friends to traditional styles.[90] The professional's agenda must be fulfilled, of course, but with reference to the patient's story—their perceptions and understanding, the impact of the illness on their lives, and their concerns, fears, and questions. However, even at post-treatment follow-up consultations, doctors often organize the interview around clinical investigations rather than widen its scope to include new or residual symptoms the patient may be having, let alone address broader psychosocial concerns and the impact the disease has had on the patient's quality of life.

There is a common tendency for healthcare professionals to be over-directive in their style of interviewing, to interrupt patients and ask closed rather than open-ended questions. These styles usually inhibit patients from disclosing the concerns they have and might wish to express; they denote a professional who is hurried, stressed, or unconcerned. It can be sobering to ask a patient's permission to make an audio recording of your clinical interview with them, and then listen to how much you use, or fail to use, the following skills.

Active listening   Listening effectively is the core element of effective communication and the most challenging skill for most people to acquire. Healthcare professionals must learn to hear not only the words the patient is using, but also the thoughts and feelings behind the words and, most importantly, the patient must *feel* that the professional is listening, concerned, and interested. Active listening is mostly achieved and conveyed through non-verbal behaviour.

Rather than focusing solely on the facts of what the patient is telling you, try to notice the way they are feeling: their tone of voice, their eye-contact, posture, and other physical cues. Notice and respond to the patient's references to their feelings. Sometimes 'throwaway' or seemingly trivial remarks may reflect a more widespread feeling. For example, someone using the phrase 'There's probably no point' is conveying a feeling or attitude that may reflect more general feelings of hopelessness. Similarly, an apparent lack of feeling within a patient who is discussing something that one might expect to be emotionally charged *may* indicate depressive withdrawal (or 'flattening of affect').

As the interview progresses, think about how the patient seems to be making sense of what you are discussing. How has their mood changed during the course of the interview? Consider your own feelings too; these can be a valuable source of information about what the patient may be feeling. By acknowledging the feelings that lie behind what the patient is saying, and by maintaining a posture of interest and concern, the professional enables the patient to feel safe, supported, and more inclined to reveal their genuine concerns.

Open and closed questions   Open questions do not confine people to tight answers, but encourage them to speak more broadly. The closed question '*Are you still in pain?*' may well produce a yes-or-no type answer—useful, but not very informative. The more open question '*Can you tell me about any pain you are still having?*' is likely to produce a more detailed and helpful answer. Open questions are particularly useful at the start of an interview when the professional is trying to develop a general picture of the patient's experience and interpretation of their symptoms. From this general overview the interviewer can funnel down with more closed questions to tease out specific issues of concern.

The use of closed questions is unavoidable when professionals are gathering clinical assessment information, but they should never be used exclusively unless the patient has difficulty communicating. They are equivalent to using a clinical checklist and, by their nature, they limit the information obtained. If a sequence of checklist-type questions is to be asked, the professional should preface it by saying something like: *'I would now like to ask you a few questions about … Will that be all right with you?'*

Clarification   As the interview progresses, any ambiguities in what the patient has said can be clarified with more direct questions: *'You mentioned a "funny feeling" in your stomach. Can you try to describe this a bit more?' 'I'm not sure I understand the last bit you were talking about. You mentioned … Can you go over that again for me?'*

Facilitation   Some people can find it difficult to talk openly and may need encouragement. Reflecting back and summarizing a little of what the patient has said encourages them to develop their thoughts. Showing interest through eye contact, nodding, and saying short affirming words or sounds like *'Yes … Mmm … Okay … Go on … Right'* are gentle but important ways of facilitating. *'Is there anything more you would like to say about this?'* is a more explicit invitation to expand on a subject, or close it.

Acknowledging   Feelings can sometimes be overwhelming to the person having them. They may feel ashamed or embarrassed by them, or be reluctant to disclose them to loved ones. Professionals have the advantage of detachment and experience and are therefore sometimes seen as safer to talk to. It therefore helps if professionals feel comfortable asking about the feelings that underlie what is being discussed. However, professionals are often reluctant to acknowledge strong feelings such as anger or despair, lest they provoke yet stronger emotions that become difficult to contain. This is perhaps due to lack of training and possibly a fear of the unknown. Unfortunately it leads professional staff to use 'distancing behaviours' to block patients from expressing their feelings (*see* What is Appropriate Professional Distance?).

In reality, the release of intense emotion is usually short-lived (and often tiring to the person concerned). If strong emotions are provoked, the professional should always be prepared to remain with the feelings, and acknowledge them (*'That seems like a real worry for you'*) until the patient is ready to move on, rather than attempt to change the subject (a typical blocking tactic). The relief that emotional expression offers can be enormous, provided it does not leave the person concerned feeling embarrassed or ashamed. Professionals must therefore show that they are comfortable with the patient's feelings and are not judgemental about them.

Support   Like facilitation, support is conveyed through the quality or tone of the relationship and much of this is non-verbal. Healthcare staff are generally trained to be active, practical, and problem-solving, so the temptation to assume this active, busy role can be strong. Yet not all problems *can* be resolved easily. There are moments in clinical interviews when it is more helpful and supportive simply to listen and acknowledge the patient's feelings.

Showing that one is moved by what the patient is saying can be conveyed by facial expression, silence, taking the patient's hand (if this is culturally appropriate), or using words, e.g. *'That sounds very difficult'*. However, unless the expression of support is natural and genuine ('authentic'), the professional will be dismissed as insincere.

A revealing source of information about what is emotionally going on within the patient is often what the professional is feeling within themselves. One of the most powerful and sophisticated skills in clinical interviewing is learning to observe one's relationship with the patient, and notice how one's own feelings have changed over the course of the interview.[91]

Summarizing and structuring the interview　After a topic has been fully discussed, the professional should summarize what has been said and what plans, if any, have been agreed. Summarizing at regular intervals throughout the interview not only helps people to retain what has been said, but also enables misunderstandings to be corrected, and demonstrates that the professional has been listening. The professional may then wish to introduce a new topic from the mutual agenda agreed at the beginning of the interview.

Ending the interview and goal-setting

The end of an interview is as important as its beginning. It is a time to summarize what has been discussed and agreed, with a view to developing or revising a 'road map' of future care. The professional should restate concerns that have been raised and how they will be addressed by themselves, the patient, or someone else. There should always be a final invitation to patients and any loved ones present to ask further questions or make comments.

Clear plans should be made and, as in breaking bad news, the summary should always emphasize what *can* be done rather than what cannot. No matter what the subject under discussion, no one should leave an interview feeling hopeless; being deprived of hope is a kind of mental pain. By working collaboratively with patients to achieve shared goals, the professional conveys hope.

Encourage the patient to prioritize the concerns that have been identified, and promote the use of simple problem-solving skills to find the optimal resolution to each concern. Some solutions may be provided by the professional themselves (e.g. changing medication). Some plans require the help of other people, such as other professionals or family members. Some may involve the patient taking action of their own (e.g. increasing daily exercise, obtaining or reading further information, etc.). There may also be occasions when it is productive to focus on the nature of the patient's own thoughts and feelings. By clarifying and challenging the assumptions that patients use to interpret their situation, the professional can help patients to view their options in a more productive and balanced light (*see* Clarifying and Challenging Assumptions).

Finally, encourage patients to anticipate setbacks and obstacles so that, if they do occur, the patient does not feel defeated by them.

End the interview with an agreement about the time, date, and place of your next meeting at which you will review the patient's concerns and their progress at resolving them.

Problem-solving

Problem-solving is little more than structured common sense, so can be used in a wide variety of contexts, including routine clinical interviews. Although simple in principle, problem-solving is often surprisingly effective in helping people to recognize and garner their options and resources. Healthcare staff can help patients and carers structure their thoughts along the following lines:

1. What is the nature of the problem or concern facing you?
2. Brainstorm a list of possible options without limiting yourself to 'sensible' or logical options.
3. Describe the pros and cons of each option by imagining its consequences.
4. Decide upon the best solution, all considered.
5. Describe the steps needed to implement this plan.
6. Implement the plan if possible within an agreed timeframe.
7. Evaluate how well the outcome solved the problem and return to the brainstormed list to consider further options if needed.

People are more likely to follow-through with a planned course of action if they feel they have the support and encouragement of a healthcare worker who is interested in the outcome. Having an action plan tends to be intrinsically motivating, particularly if the goal is realistic and attainable. If the problem is large, break it down into smaller, more manageable chunks. Help the patient anticipate obstacles so they are ready for them, and consider how they would handle setbacks so that they are not overly disappointed if they do occur. Finally, encourage them to regard setbacks as an opportunity to learn more about the problem (i.e. 'challenges' not 'failures').

Alongside this focus on solving problems, the patient should be encouraged to identify and acknowledge the resources they are already using. In a crisis people often assume that their distress is a function of their failure to cope with the crisis rather than a natural expression of it. By focusing on what the patient is already doing well, and the personal and social resources at their disposal, a more solution-focused perspective can emerge. How would the patient know if their problems and concerns were starting to be resolved? What is going already well? What would have to change for a particular concern to be resolved? What state of affairs is the patient wanting to achieve and what is the most direct way of getting there? From the perspective of some point in the future, what would be helpful to be doing now and in the immediate future?

Clarifying and challenging assumptions

As we explored in Chapter 1, people interpret their experiences on the basis of their assumptions about the world. Sometimes these biases lead to unrealistic optimism about the future, the self, and other people, but sometimes they lead to a negative distortion of events—drawing unhelpful conclusions that result in emotional distress. For example, people may underestimate their own resources and, as a result, feel helpless in response to the challenges they face.

Examples of negative bias include:

- **All or nothing thinking** *If I cannot be cured, it means I am going to die imminently.*

- **Selective filtering of information** Rather than consider the fact that chemotherapy may increase the chance of a cure, the patient dwells on the prospect of losing their hair.

- **Conceptual leaps (mind-reading)** *Because the doctor would not tell me I am cured it must mean that I am dying. If I ask too many questions, the staff will think I'm a nuisance.*

- **Over-generalizing** *My father died of cancer so I am bound to die.*

- **Catastrophizing** Focusing on what is possible rather than what is probable. *I just know I am going to be one of the 5% for whom this treatment does not work. If my chemotherapy is delayed another week, the cancer will take hold again.*

People's underlying assumptions may be as obvious and explicit as the examples above, but often they must be inferred from things the patient has said. By carefully listening to the subtext of what patients say, one can learn to detect implicit assumptions and make them explicit: *When you say that no one could ever love you now that you've had cancer, I was wondering what you were thinking about in particular.*

Having established the underlying assumption, or heartfelt belief, one can then move on to challenge it by looking at its evidence base and alternative possible conclusions: *You seem to be saying that there is no man on earth who would be interested in having a relationship with someone who has lost her fertility. Do you think that is one hundred per cent true, or perhaps just true of some men?* This leads to the exploration of less catastrophic and overgeneralized ways of anticipating the future, without trivializing the significant challenges to be faced.

Challenging someone's underlying assumption is best achieved using a Socratic method of questioning, allowing the patient to observe and discover their own way of thinking rather than confronting them with it. By helping people to see the link between the way they think and their subsequent distress, professionals can encourage patients to use more creative ways of construing their concerns. Furthermore, this approach can lead patients to become more aware of their own personal resources and sources of social support. Subsequent testing in the real world (a 'behavioural experiment') enables people to check whether their assumptions are true or false. For example, a woman who feels conspicuous and different may assume that people are some-how aware of her mastectomy. By going to the supermarket and deliberately observing whether people are in fact staring at her, she can test this probably mistaken assumption.

Specific communication issues

Giving bad news

> They sat down and then Mr. W. [surgeon] confirmed the unthinkable; that they suspected I had indeed some form of breast cancer. I must have glanced at Dr. M. [oncologist] and the other women to see if they could offer me a comforting smile, but I vaguely recall that they were looking at the floor with serious expressions, and couldn't look at me directly as I was given the news. I think I uttered 'right' and 'ok' and then A. was introduced to me as a breast-care specialist and Macmillan nurse, the latter giving me the shakes a bit. I immediately envisioned emaciated bodies being wheeled around in beds in hospices … And then I thought of G. [husband] and I. [daughter] – what on earth was going to happen to us? How was I going to tell G.?

Informing someone that they have a life-threatening illness or a recurrence of their cancer is probably the most unpleasant duty any doctor has to perform. Some level of distress to patients and their families is unavoidable but, as in any other area of medicine, clinical skill can do a lot to minimize the damage. Effectiveness in breaking bad news not only benefits the patient's long-term adjustment,[2, 41, 92] but enhances the patient–physician relationship. And it may even reduce the job-stress of physicians.[93]

In most settings it is the most senior doctor who delivers critical diagnostic and prognostic information, though other healthcare staff are often required to inform patients of disappointing setbacks to their treatment. The decision as to who delivers bad news of any sort must be documented and made explicit within the healthcare team so as to avoid any confusion. Similarly, every patient should be clear whom they can speak to if they later require clarification or further information.

A large proportion of hospital complaints about doctors are to do with communication problems, especially about the breaking of bad news.[7] Little more than 10 years ago, one American study found that 23% of cancer patients had been given their diagnosis over the telephone.[94] In a more recent UK study, the police were rated as more sympathetic than both doctors and nurses, when breaking bad news, probably because the police have had some training in this area.[95]

A great deal has been written about the bad news interview, though little of it has been based on empirical research or derived from theory.[42] Most writings on the subject have taken the professional's point of view. The few empirical studies which have ascertained what *patients* liked and disliked about their bad news interviews identified (1) a private interview, (2) in a quiet location, (3) free of jargon, (4) compassionately conveyed, with (5) some measure of hope, as being the most important factors.[42]

How does the way in which bad news is conveyed have long-term consequences for the patient's psychological adjustment? Some authors have argued that the terrible nature of the news that doctors must deliver dwarfs the issue of the way in which it is conveyed.[96] Others have argued that the way in which bad news is delivered can influence whether someone develops anxiety or depression, and there is growing evidence that some of the trauma of the diagnostic interview can be mitigated if the doctor practises some fairly simple procedures.[41]

In order to minimize the traumatic impact of the bad news, it may help to recall the following six principles:

1. Imparting bad news should be a gradual process.

2. The doctor should be caring and emotionally supportive.[2]

3. The patient should be warned that bad news is on the agenda.

4. The manner and language used to convey bad news should be sensitive to individual and cultural expectations (i.e. patient-centred).

5. The patient should exercise control over the rate at which they absorb the bad news.

6. The doctor should convey a sense of direction and safety without conveying false hope.

Dr Peter Kaye has advocated a 10-step approach to conducting a bad news interview.[97] We draw strongly upon this approach in the following.

1. Preparation

Ensure that you know the medical facts before the meeting and who, if any, the patient wants with them during the interview. Not everyone wants someone else present so this must be ascertained in advance, not assumed. A survey of 65 000 UK cancer patients conducted in 2000 found that 54% did not want anyone else present during the consultation.[17] Where cognitive function may already be compromised, the doctor needs to have a rough idea what the patient is capable of understanding. In any event talk to the patient, while including the person with them, rather than the other way round. The patient's condition should be as stable as possible (e.g. not still recovering from neurosurgery). Ensure that there is a quiet and private setting and that you have sufficient time set aside. Remember that patients will be hanging on to your every word. This is an interview they will probably remember for the rest of their lives. In the large national survey of UK cancer patients mentioned above, as many as 21% of patients had been given their diagnosis in less than 10 minutes, a wholly inadequate length of time given the importance of the interview.

> I really think that it is wrong to ask a woman to undress when she comes to the Breast Clinic to get the results of her tests. Unfortunately I already felt very vulnerable and this just added unnecessarily to my distress. If the purpose of this pantomime was to prepare me for bad news, it was a useless manoeuvre: the nurse with a set smile talking about the weather made it absolutely plain to me that the lump on my breast wasn't benign.

2. What does the patient know?

Ask the patient to tell you their narrative of events—'*How did you become aware that you* were *ill?*' Some patients claim to know very little, perhaps because they wish to corroborate what they do know. Gentle prompts such as '*What happened next?*' lead to further information about what the patient understands, and the words they use to express it. You are then in a better position to shape your explanations in order to dovetail with the patient's model. One can also pick up areas of frank misunderstanding and fear. '*Have you had any ideas about what your illness might be?*'

3. Is more information wanted?

> *Would you like me to tell you more about your illness (your recent tests)?*

There is a tension or conflict within the patient between wanting to reduce the uncertainty by learning more about their condition, and wanting to protect themselves from the bad news itself (denial and avoidance). Never impose information when it is clear that the patient would prefer not to know, but always offer further opportunities to discuss. Sadly, patients are often told they are going to die even after they have made it clear that they do not wish to be told.[98]

4. Give a warning shot

> *Well, I'm afraid that the results suggest that it's looking quite serious.*

The warning shot enables the patient to prepare their psychological resources. Like post-traumatic stress, the more unexpected an event is, the more its traumatic impact. The possibility that the diagnosis may be cancer may or may not already be in the patient's mind. For example, the patient may have been primed already by their GP for the possibility of bad news. However, no assumptions about the patient's expectations are entirely safe. The warning shot enables a further negotiation to occur and for the patient to let the doctor know what level of new understanding they can absorb at that particular moment.

5. Respect the defence of denial

Psychological defences are there for a reason. For most people denial is temporary, vacillating and inconsistent and, as indicated in Chapter 1, is a natural part of the early process of adjustment. It allows people to titrate or filter the amount of information they absorb.

Patients have a *right* to know, but they do not have a *duty* to know. For those who make it clear that they do not want further information, for example those who change the subject or say they have enough information, or ask you to do what you think is best, let them know that they can always obtain further information whenever they wish and how they can contact you.

6. Provide a clear, simple explanation if requested

Avoid *brutal* honesty but never mislead.

Brutal statistical 'reality' is not what people are always asking for. At the other extreme, the tractor beam of sincerely wanting to give patients only good and hopeful, if dishonest, news can feel irresistible. Getting the balance right is a reflection of how well the professional understands the patient and their context. (This is the function of the first three points.)

Try to remain sensitive to the patient's preferences regarding how much information is disclosed. Work towards narrowing the information gap between what you understand and what the patient understands, arriving at the patient's optimum level of understanding. Robert Buckman[99] has referred to this stage as like steering an oil tanker: you cannot expect the patient's understanding to keep up with you if you make sudden lurches. Constantly check the patient's understanding with what you have said, not *if* they understand but *what* they understand.

Try to retain a delicate mixture of hopeful encouragement and acknowledgement of the grim reality of the new situation. Make it clear you have a plan, but acknowledge first the patient's shock and fear. If you appear to be unwilling to discuss the seriousness of the illness or its prognosis, it may convey to the patient that the situation is too terrible to be discussed.[32]

Use plain English. Do not assume that everyone understands terms like 'prognosis' let alone 'metastasis'. This is even more important where the patient's comprehension may be already compromised because of the disease, surgery, a learning difficulty, or where English is not their native language. Although the use of euphemisms is widely condemned in the interests of clarity, terms like 'tumour' or 'growth' can provide a way of avoiding cultural taboos associated with the word 'cancer'.[13]

Above all show sensitivity to the impact that your words are having. The emotional supportiveness of doctors during bad news consultations is associated with less depression, post-traumatic symptoms, and general distress in their patients.

> The consultant succinctly and carefully tells me what they've found from the bits of my breast tissue they've examined. Malignant cells in various parts of my breast. He speaks softly and unequivocally: 'I'm afraid it's cancer.' He looks straight into my eyes and there is a connection. I am grateful for that, though I really want him to stuff those words back into his mouth and say something different. After a pause he sticks the mammogram X-ray up on the wall and we all swivel our heads to look at it illuminated. It's the minutest bit steadying to look at the areas of shade and light on the transparency – for a split second it's as if the problem is all out there, in front of us, and manageable.

7. Elicit concerns

What concerns you the most in what we've talked about?

Allow the patient time to explore their immediate concerns in order that they can prioritize them into more manageable elements. You may wish to ask the patient to tell you what they understand from what you have said. What have they immediately assumed when the word 'cancer' (or recurrence) was mentioned? Avoid lengthy explanations at this point, but clarify unhelpful misunderstandings.

For example, patients with a brain tumour are likely to be particularly concerned about physical disablement, loss of mobility, role changes (e.g. greater dependency), and loss of dignity as they lose their ability to care for themselves. Fear of personal disintegration associated with dementia is also common among patients and families dealing with a diagnosis of brain cancer.

8. Ventilation of feelings

Can you say what you are feeling at the moment?

Help the patient try to name their feelings. In Chapter 1 we considered why emotional expression is both powerful and important for most people. By expressing even quite powerful feelings and naming them, people begin to feel a sense of control over them. At the same time, one must respect the fact that some people may regard it as undignified or even shameful to express their feelings openly. By giving the patient sufficient time to talk, doctors convey that they are not overwhelmed but are nonetheless moved by their patient's emotions. Listening with empathy does not require an expert. If this were someone you loved, how would you wish for them to be cared for by their doctor? Remember that this is merely the beginning of a period of adjustment to the bad news you have just imparted; it may take the patient considerable time to absorb and integrate it into their mental maps of the world.

> I can't take in what he's saying. My head is swirling with waves of shock as I try to absorb a piece of fact for which there is no appropriate slot in my mind.

9. Summary and plan

The patient's immediate sense of safety can be enhanced by the doctor showing leadership and a belief that they have something useful to offer. The summary should encapsulate the patient's concerns, the individuality of the patient's situation, and the management options available to the doctor. The plan should include immediate treatment plans, a 'road map' for the medium-term future, further opportunities to discuss the situation, and encouragement of the patient to use whatever social support they have available.

The summary should emphasize what *can* be done rather than what cannot. Retain a clear sense of hope without giving false reassurances. Above all, never convey the impression that nothing more can be done. Helping people to problem-solve even one of their concerns (e.g. where to get help with financial matters) can be a symbolically important achievement, in that it can give the person a sense of agency and control.

Hope is a complex emotion and involves something more than a simple belief that one can be cured; it also involves a sense of momentum and striving towards something. Believing that one's situation retains some element of hope is essential for mental adjustment.[100, 101] In one Scandinavian study, the highest incidence of suicide was found among cancer patients who had been offered no further treatment, and no further contact with the health care system.

10. Offer availability

After hearing the word cancer, many patients are unable to take in any further information since they are in shock. Write down for the patient the time and date of the next meeting which will be used for further explanation, and an opportunity to meet with other relatives (since, clearly, bad news affects the whole family, some of whom will be required to care for the patient).

Discussing resuscitation

The main aim of palliative care is to promote quality of life and to support a peaceful death when the time comes.[103] The main aim of cardiopulmonary resuscitation (CPR) is to restore life when a patient's cardiorespiratory function has stopped. It is arguable how much these two aims are compatible in light of one review that found that from 1268 CPR attempts, no patient with metastatic cancer survived to discharge.[104] The use of CPR may reverse the process of death if a patient has a sudden cardiac or respiratory event but is not always in the patient's best interests when it prolongs suffering in a patient who is slowly deteriorating and dying. Indeed, unsuccessful CPR can lead to a distressingly technological end, which is in contrast to the peaceful and dignified death that most people wish for. And it can be distressing and demoralizing for the healthcare team involved.

Cardiopulmonary resuscitation is often used in hospitals, where the culture dictates that lives must be saved at all costs. By contrast, CPR is rarely used in hospices or in the patient's home. It is not that CPR is inappropriate in palliative care. It should be considered if its success is likely to result in an acceptable quality of life for the patient, especially among pre-terminal palliative care patients.[103] The ethical issues have less to do with whether CPR would be 'futile' if successful, and more to do with whether successful CPR is likely to benefit the patient by enabling them to achieve a level of recovery that would justify the potential liabilities of the treatment.[105]

Most well people, if given a choice, would unquestioningly choose to be resuscitated if their heart stopped. The portrayal of CPR in television dramas, heroically bringing people back to life promotes unrealistic over-optimistic expectations.[106] However, if they were suffering and knew they were dying and were sensitively told about the possible impact of CPR on the quality of life and the probability of its success, they might well choose differently. For example, one study of geriatric patients found that 94% did not want CPR once they were told about the probability of survival.[107]

Gone are the days when a decision not to resuscitate a patient was made by their doctor. The choice of whether to be resuscitated is ultimately the patient's (or family's where the patient is no longer competent), because the patient is the best judge of their own quality of life. So doctors need to discuss these issues with patients and families, preferably early enough for it to still be considered an appropriate option.[105] Yet the limited evidence that exists suggests that these discussions rarely take place,[108] probably because most professionals find it distressing and difficult to do.[109] Locally agreed policies are therefore essential and training should be available to support this delicate aspect of communication.

Discussions about the appropriateness of CPR should occur as part of an ongoing supportive relationship between the senior doctor and the patient. Like bad news, it is rarely completed within a single consultation but is part of a longer process of negotiation. Some authors have advocated that 'Do not attempt to resuscitate' (DNAR) discussions should occur within more general conversations about the aims of treatment.[105] They argue that it may be easier for doctors to discuss CPR when this is still an appropriate and realistic option. As the aims of treatment change from curative intent to those of palliating symptoms and maximizing quality of life, the doctor can reintroduce the topic as a natural element of continuing care. Just as surgery and chemotherapy may no longer be appropriate, so too CPR if explained sensitively can be seen as contrary to the patient's best interests or their wish for a dignified death.

It may help to explain that CPR as a technique was developed in response to sudden cardiac arrest rather than as a treatment to be used in advanced cancer. It is also important to stress that a decision by the patient not to be resuscitated will in no way compromise other aspects of their palliative care (i.e. other treatments will not be withheld).[105] As far as possible, relatives should be included in these discussions and provided with the same information as the patient so that any misgivings they have can be aired and discussed. Finally, like informed consent, the process of DNAR discussions and any resulting decision should be fully and clearly recorded in the patient's medical notes, and the decision should be shared among the nursing and medical teams.

Identifying vulnerability

No particular pattern of factors accurately predicts psychological or social distress within an individual, just as no particular pattern of factors determines protection against it.[110] Each person must be assessed with reference to their own norms and expectations, as well as those of their family and cultural background. People are individuals and may have all sorts of distinctive reasons why they become distressed. Nonetheless, a number of authors have attempted to ascertain general factors that tend to predict later psychological distress.

The level of anxiety, depression, and intrusive thoughts during the early phases of cancer has been found to predict anxiety and depression six months later, though the type of 'coping strategies' people used were poor predictors.[111, 112] Although some authors have dismissed the evidence for age, marital status, or social class as significant risk factors,[110] studies of long-term cancer survivors suggest that older people may be more likely to become depressed and that the most significant factor related to this was the presence of cancer-related symptoms.[113] Indeed, emotional distress tends to increase with advanced disease associated with physical symptoms like pain, physical disability, and fatigue. Uncontrolled pain and hopelessness in people with advanced cancer are particularly high-risk factors for suicide.[114]

Previous psychiatric history is widely thought to be an indication of someone's vulnerability in the face of current stress.[115] Social deprivation (poverty, poor housing, social exclusion, or dislocation) embodies a number of concurrent stresses and concerns that increase the likelihood of significant distress. Similarly, social isolation (a lack of social support) means that individuals have few confidants with whom to make sense of unfolding events, and few people to provide them with love and practical care. On the other hand, distress in one's partner can be a source of additional distress (see Chapter 3). Finally, a history of substance abuse (alcohol, drugs) often suggests a tendency to avoid confronting difficult challenges, thus making it more difficult to respond effectively to the implications of cancer and the requirements of its treatment.

In view of the unique nature of each person's concerns, personal history, and social context, it would be unwise to set too much store by risk factors alone. However, the number and severity of patient's concerns do seem to predict later distress[1] so it is helpful to elicit these concerns so as to assist the patient in resolving them as early as possible (see Eliciting Concerns). Understanding some of the core adjustment issues that patients and their loved ones are facing enables the healthcare professional to normalize and support people in resolving these concerns. As we argue throughout this book, inherent in these core processes of adjustment are the seeds of prolonged and more severe distress: the ability of people to maintain their motivation through having plans and goals; their concerns for and support from their loved ones; their sense of value and control in the world; their feelings about their body; and their existential/spiritual concerns (see Chapter 1—Core Assumptions).

The use of questionnaires as a method of screening for psychological distress holds an obvious appeal, though questionnaires are relatively crude and impersonal at best and their specificity is often unimpressive. Furthermore, questionnaires can only target a specific range of concerns and inevitably limit the patient's responses to these constructs (e.g. anxiety and depression). Even where questionnaires do identify high levels of distress, the specific nature of this distress and its source must always then be explored and assessed in a clinical interview. Sensitivity to the presence of emotional distress, moreover, should be inherent in all communication between healthcare professionals and patients, rather than such distress being merely identified using questionnaires. Nonetheless, although their primary value is in research, a brief outline of some common self-report questionnaires is presented in Appendix 1.

The presence of emotional distress per se obviously does not always indicate pathology, and nor should it be used as a pretext for clinical intervention unless this is carefully negotiated with the person concerned. Emotional distress can have many causes, is usually understandable, and is unique to given the individual's personal circumstances and social context. What healthcare staff can do is to help patients (and relatives) articulate their specific concerns, consider how they might be tackled, and weigh up what additional resources, if any, are required. Finally, professionals should be able to identify higher levels of distress so as to make appropriate referrals for more specialist and intensive psychosocial help.

It may be helpful to think of different levels of psychosocial assessment and support:

Level	Group	Assessments	Intervention
1	All health and social care professionals	Recognition of emotional distress	Information-giving, preparation and guidance; compassionate, respectful and responsive communication
2	Health and social care professionals with additional expertise. Trained volunteers	Eliciting physical, psychological, social and spiritual concerns	Helping patients to articulate their concerns and consider possible solutions. Simple interventions such as relaxation training. Volunteers can be trained to provide emotional support through listening to patients' experiences
3	Trained and accredited professionals with training in specific interventions	Eliciting physical, psychological, social and spiritual concerns, and teasing out more complicated concerns	Counselling and specific psychological: cognitive-behaviour therapy, solution-focused therapy, and other techniques delivered according to a particular theoretical framework
4	Psychosocial specialists (clinical psychologists, psychiatrists, social workers, chaplains)	Assessment of Multiple or more Complex problems. Couple and family assessment	Specialist psychological, psychiatric, spiritual, or social interventions (e.g. social work), involving work with individuals, couples, families.

Adapted from the UK's National Institute for Clinical Excellence (NICE) Improving Supportive and Palliative Care for Adults with Cancer, 2004, London: NICE

Working with people with special needs

(*see* also Chapter 5—Head and Neck Cancers—Communication in the Context of Speech Difficulties)

People with learning disabilities[116]

In general, people with learning disabilities tend to have considerably more health problems associated with respiratory and cardiovascular conditions than with cancer. However, they have higher levels of unrecognised illness and reduced access to preventative screening measures and health promotion programmes as compared with the general population.[117] And, as people with learning difficulties move from residential institutions into community-based care, they often have less consistent access to medical care and supervision. They also may be exposed to a more carcinogenic lifestyle: excessive eating, drinking, and use of tobacco.

Among long-term residents of institutions there is a higher incidence of gastrointestinal cancers, which is probably due to the high rates of infection by the very carcinogenic bacillus *Helicobacter pylori* found in such institutions. People with Down's syndrome are thought to have a twenty to thirty-fold greater risk of leukaemia compared with the general population[118] yet have a relatively low incidence of breast cancer. However, over the past fifty years the life expectancy of people with learning disabilities has increased and, overall, the incidence of death caused by cancer is considerably lower than in the general population.[119] On the other hand, because of communication difficulties, people with learning disabilities may not always be able to articulate changes within their bodies (e.g. pain) with the result that their symptoms are not identified until later in the disease trajectory.

People with learning disabilities are as diverse a group as any other section of the population, with widely varying levels of disability. Those with mild to moderate intellectual disabilities may live fairly independently and have good communication skills, while those with severe disabilities may have no verbal communication skills at all and therefore greater needs for support. People with learning disabilities, even more than the rest of the population, may have outdated views about cancer. Many people may believe that cancer is an inevitable death sentence while people with a more profound disability may have a limited understanding of death.[120]

Information must therefore be available in a number of formats, languages, and media that reflect the diversity of their needs. Pictorial representations[121] (diagrams, drawings, photographs, etc.) go a long way to reinforcing what may be said with words, although other media should also be considered (interactive CD-ROMs, video, etc.). Furthermore, an introductory visit to the hospital or department may help allay anxiety, as well as the assignment of a particular cancer professional to work as the patient's key worker. Those caring for people with learning disabilities (professional care workers, family members) may be well placed to help cancer professionals understand the optimal communication, information, and emotional needs of the individual. They should therefore be routinely consulted for their views and advice. However, too often there is a lack of mutual understanding of the respective roles of specialists in cancer and learning disability.

Patients should always be spoken to directly, even though the involvement of carers and families is often crucial in ensuring that any information conveyed can be reviewed later if necessary. Cancer professionals should be wary of making judgements about the patient's ability to understand or deal with a diagnosis of cancer. People with learning disabilities, by definition, have lower IQ scores but their feelings and emotions are not impaired. They have a right to be treated the same way as other people but given special consideration because of their special needs.[122]

The family member or care worker's prior knowledge of the patient is often valuable in articulating the symptomatic history of the individual with a learning disability, as well as their psychosocial concerns. Pain, for example, is sometimes expressed as hyperactive behaviour or even self-injury among people with learning disabilities so is more likely to be recognized by the individual's carer rather than a cancer professional.[120]

Nonetheless, the person with learning disabilities should be as fully involved as they wish to be in decisions regarding their treatment, and their consent to treatment or clinical trials should be sought whenever possible.

In some instances it is the professional carer who is given the full explanation of the diagnosis and expected to break the news to the patient. Yet, despite their closer relationship with the person with a learning disability, the care worker may lack the training or experience to undertake this role, let alone the emotional support in doing so. Care workers, like family members, may have a long relationship with the patient and the diagnosis may cause them considerable distress. Thus they should also have easy access to further information and support throughout the course of the patient's illness.

Visually impaired patients

Despite the fact that visually impaired or blind people lack the visual cues that sighted people take for granted (facial expression, body posture, etc.), they often compensate by using other highly developed strategies. The visually impaired person is more likely to rely on nuances of tone, hesitations, and the sound of body movements to interpret the mood, character, and attitudes of the person they are speaking to.

When working with someone who is visually impaired, tell them a little about the surroundings where you have taken them, be it an office or medical consulting room. If appropriate, explain where major items of furniture are and where the door is in relation to where the person is sitting. Introduce clearly other people who are present and encourage them to say a few words so that the visually impaired person can establish their voice pattern. It may be helpful to invite the patient to explain briefly the extent of their visual impairment so as to avoid any misunderstanding.

Blind people are often spoken to in a patronizing way, as if they are unable to understand normal adult language, and not surprisingly they find this offensive. So speak in a normal manner and do not raise your voice or change its normal pace.

Hearing-impaired patients

One in seven people have some form of hearing loss. It can be particularly daunting for people with a hearing impairment to attend a hospital appointment when not only is cancer on the agenda, but they may have to absorb complex information from professionals and are in danger of being misunderstood by them. It is therefore important that healthcare staff feel confident about communicating with people with a hearing loss.

It is often helpful to set aside more time for a consultation with a patient with a hearing impairment and establish as soon as possible the extent of the impairment. The majority of people with a hearing loss will be those with mild to severe impairments, who will depend largely on hearing aids and lip-reading. This group comprises predominantly older people, who are more likely to have visual impairments as well. The minority are those who and profoundly deaf and more likely to depend on sign language as their preferred method of communication. These patients should be provided with a qualified sign language interpreter. However, all deaf people who have sight are likely to use a number of further methods for communicating, including: lip-reading, writing (pen and paper), facial expression, gesture, and body language.

The following are practical guidelines for working with people with hearing impairments:[123]

- Prepare for your interview by establishing the patient's preferred methods of communication.
- Ensure you have the person's attention before speaking. Speak predominantly to the patient rather than the person they may have brought with them.
- Maintain your gaze and eye contact with the patient and ensure that you do not obstruct your face or turn away while speaking.
- Avoid your face being silhouetted by light from a window behind you.
- Minimize background noise and echoes.
- Ensure that those with hearing aids are using them.
- Speak clearly and slightly more slowly than usual, but not so slowly as to distort your speech patterns.
- Do not exaggerate lip movements or shout, but rather speak in a slightly louder voice than normal. Lip-reading is tiring so provide breaks if the conversation is long. Lip-reading is also more difficult if the patient and the professional are not facing one another at the same level (i.e. avoid the patient lying down when you speak).
- 'Signpost' your conversation by clearly introducing the new topic when you change the subject.
- Do not dominate the conversation but enable the patient, like any other, to voice their concerns.
- Rephrase rather than repeat if the patient does not understand, and always check that you have been understood. Write things down if you are unable to communicate in other ways.
- Provide a written back-up of important information you have conveyed.
- Avoid jargon.
- Ensure that all members of the team are aware of the patient's communication needs.

Psychiatrically ill patients

One in four people is considered to have a mental health problem at some point in their lives, and cancer is clearly an enormous strain on anyone's mental and emotional resources.[124] For some people cancer exacerbates or rekindles existing problems while for others it precipitates new ones. People with mental illnesses (schizophrenia, manic-depression, etc.) face high levels of discrimination, negative coverage in the media, and misunderstanding within the community. Only about half of one British community sample, surveyed in 1996, knew the difference between a psychiatric disorder and a learning disability,[125] and young people in particular are inclined to characterize people with a mental illness as being aggressive, violent, or old—prejudices for which there is no evidence.[126] Approximately 13% of people with mental health problems are employed compared with about a third of people with long-term physical health problems[126] and they frequently face more social hardship than the rest of the community.

Many people with psychiatric disorders are in remission or receiving long-term treatment that enables them to function productively in the community. Given the discrimination that people with psychiatric histories often face, they appreciate being treated the same as anyone else in the community. In order to avoid treatment conflicts (e.g. drug interactions) it is wise to contact the patient's treating doctor (having first obtained the patient's permission). The opinion of a psychiatrist should be sought if the patient is in distress and requesting psychiatric help, if their behaviour is causing distress to others, or if there is concern that either their psychiatric or cancer treatment may be compromised without such psychiatric advice.

Recommended strategies for improving mental health[124] interestingly, would also seem to hold promise in the face of cancer:

- learning to relax
- taking exercise
- learning to assert yourself
- setting goals
- expressing feelings
- facing up to problems
- finding someone to talk to
- keeping an open mind.

Working with someone clinically depressed or suicidal

Clinical depression is not the same as 'feeling depressed' or 'sad', and nor is it an inevitable consequence of having cancer. Unlike episodes of sadness, grief, or feeling low, clinical depression is more pervasive and unrelenting; it rarely offers any chinks of hope to enable people to transcend its gloom. Estimates of clinical depression among people with cancer vary widely, depending on the methods of assessment chosen. For example, among 505 randomly selected female cancer patients (mostly ambulatory outpatients) one American study found only 5.3% with major clinical depression.[127] However, other studies have reported higher rates[128] and the incidence seems to increase with advancing disease.[114] Yet much of it goes undetected.[128]

The assessment of clinical depression is rarely straightforward in people with cancer. For one thing cancer involves considerable loss and, in the context of loss, sadness is a normal and adaptive emotion. In Chapter 2 we describe some of these losses and the many possible reasons why people develop feelings of hopelessness and despair. For many people cancer resonates with previous losses and reawakens associated feelings and thoughts. Unresolved problems from the past frequently assume an urgency that compounds the stress of cancer. Past separations, deaths, and illnesses in the family become 'active' again and both patients and their relatives often feel the need to reconsider these past losses as well as the current crisis of cancer.

Such sadness, however, can develop into the more sustained state of clinical depression that can ultimately lead to the hopelessness associated with suicidal feelings. In assessing 'clinical' depression, one cannot rely on typical physical symptoms such as loss of appetite, weight loss, or sleep disturbance because these can be caused by the cancer or its treatment. Instead, one must rely more heavily on psychological features such as an inability to experience pleasure (anhedonia), feelings of guilt, and a sense of worthlessness. Patients who blame themselves for being a burden on others or those with a pervasive sense of hopelessness and despair are also more likely to be depressed. Rather than focus solely on whether or not the patient is clinically depressed, healthcare staff should spend time ascertaining what may have contributed to the depression and what may be maintaining it because some of these factors may be resolvable. For example, some forms of chemotherapy can lead to depression (for medical factors associated with depression *see* Chapter 5—Depression).

Key symptoms of depression among people with cancer

- dysphoric mood (sadness)
- loss of the ability to enjoy things (anhedonia)
- hopelessness which is pervasive, with a sense of despair or despondency
- helplessness and passivity
- loss of self-esteem, self-loathing, or self-disgust
- withdrawal; the person uncharacteristically prefers to spend more time alone
- feelings of worthlessness and/or guilt. People who are depressed feel they have always been worthless, not simply that they are being a burden on other family members.
- suicidal thoughts, or a wish for death.

In assessing someone who shows some of these features, it is important to note when these feelings began, how quickly they began, and what the patient believes to be their cause. How does the depression 'sit' within the context of what the patient has been through, both physically and emotionally? What meaning does this illness have for the patient in view of their life experiences and expectations (e.g. other deaths from cancer)? Are there particular themes (e.g. guilt) that emerge from what the patient says?

How much support has the patient had over the course of their illness? What concurrent stresses are they facing? Does this crisis resonate with previous events in the patient's life? Is there a previous history of depression either in the individual or the family? How long has the patient had these symptoms?

Treatment

The issue of how to treat clinical depression is more contentious. Although there is only a handful of relatively small controlled trials to indicate that antidepressant drugs are effective in treating depression in cancer,[129] there is considerable clinical support for such treatments[128] and there is little reason to think they would be any less effective in cancer care than elsewhere. Antidepressants should be offered when a clear diagnosis can be made, but they should always be prescribed within the context of a supportive thera-peutic relationship in which the doctor has elicited the psychosocial concerns of the patient. When antidepressants are merely used with the aim of a 'quick fix' for emotional distress they do little to help a person and their loved ones make the necessary adjust-ments to the crisis they are facing. Psychological, social, and emotional support should therefore always accompany the use of psychotropic medication.

Antidepressants usually take two to three weeks to work and, unlike minor tranquil-lizers (benzodiazepines) with which they are often confused by the public, they are not addictive. They all have side-effects of some kind but it is rare that people are unable to tolerate them. They sometimes fail to work because their dose has been set too low. If there is any doubt about their use, the advice of a psychiatrist should be sought.

Equally effective, psychological (talking) approaches to the treatment of depression have the advantage that patients are active contributors to a treatment that is tailor-made to their specific circumstances. And they appear to work. A meta-analysis of 20 studies of psychological interventions for depression in cancer found a moderate positive effect size.[130] Treatments such as cognitive-behaviour therapy focus on the concerns brought by the patient, couple, or family and encourage people to make full use of their existing resources. They try to disentangle the reasons a person may have developed depression and help the person resolve these concerns whenever possible (e.g. see Chapter 1 for a description of core assumptions that are often violated by cancer). Psychological therapists can help patients unearth and address unresolved problems and losses from the past, while providing support to the patient as they tackle the current challenges of cancer.

Suicidal thoughts

Although cancer patients carry twice the risk of committing suicide as the general pop-ulation, the risk is still very low and suicide is rare in clinical practice. Those who com-mit suicide usually do so by taking an overdose of analgesic or sedative drugs.[131] The extent to which the individual has already made clear plans of how they would commit suicide is a good indicator of the seriousness of their intentions. Many of the factors that have been associated with increased risk of suicide are preventable, or amenable to intervention, so it is important to explore fully the possible reasons for wanting to commit suicide.

To have suicidal thoughts at some point during a cancer illness is common, but they should always be explored because they can be an expression of a more enveloping depression. People sometimes imagine that it would be better to take control of their life by ending it, rather than endure the suffering that they envisage lies ahead; suicide may at least offer some measure of control. Patients also understandably wish to avoid having to face a wasting, unremittingly painful death, let alone expecting their families to have to witness it as well. Once again, it is the idiosyncratic images that cancer provokes in people that determine their responses to it. They may feel overwhelmed by the scale of the loss they face (e.g. facial disfigurement, amputation, loss of speech, or other profound disability, etc.) or feel guilty at the level of dependency that their illness has left them with.

Suicide risk factors among people with cancer[114,131]

- hopelessness
- helplessness, lack of control over events
- uncontrolled pain or other physical suffering
- depression
- advanced disease/poor prognosis
- prior suicidal attempts, either by the patient or a member of their family
- exhaustion and fatigue
- lack of social support/social isolation
- substance or alcohol abuse.

Not surprisingly, hopelessness about the future is a key risk factor; in one study hopelessness was a better predictor of suicidal thoughts than depression.[132] In this regard it is worth recalling a Scandinavian study that found that the highest incidence of cancer suicide was among patients who had not been offered further treatment or further contact with the health care system.[102] Healthcare professionals have a key role not only in eliciting such feelings of hopelessness about the future, but also in helping to shape achievable realistic targets for patients to aim for, and never allowing the patient to feel abandoned.

The main rule of thumb for assessing the likelihood that someone will attempt suicide is the degree to which they have begun to make viable or realistic plans for carrying it out. In assessing a person's risk of suicide, it helps to use a series of graded questions:[133]

- *Do you ever feel you don't want to wake up in the morning?*
- *Do you feel that life is not worth carrying on?*

- *Have you ever felt so low you have wanted to end your life?*
- *Have you thought about how you would go about it?*
- *How prepared are you?*

It is important to stress that encouraging people with suicidal impulses to talk about their thoughts and feelings in no way encourages them to act upon them. On the contrary, it can be a relief to talk to someone about these thoughts and impulses, particularly if they are taken seriously and given respect. Talking about their thoughts is likely to help the suicidal patient reconsider their views as they contemplate the very real anguish for their survivors if they were to act upon them. Moreover, by helping patients talk about their desperate feelings, professionals can begin to assess the history and reasons behind them. If poorly controlled symptoms are driving these feelings, the professional may be able to alleviate them with analgesia, or reassure the patient about the considerable resources of palliative care should they be needed in the future. If the patient feels unable to face the distress of all that they have lost, the professional may be in a position to kindle better care and support for the patient to help them overcome hurdles and adapt to unavoidable or irrevocable changes. If the patient feels they have lost control over their lives, the professional should help the patient identify areas where they can still exert their influence and power, or demonstrate their competence and effectiveness. If the patient is profoundly depressed, the use of an antidepressant in conjunction with psychological support should be considered.

Working with denial and avoidance

As we explored in Chapter 2, denial and avoidance are common strategies we all use to manage particularly difficult news such as the death of a loved one, the diagnosis of a life-threatening illness, or a poor prognosis. It is a way of maintaining one's existing model of the world while gradually absorbing the implications of what one has been told. It is typically a short-term defence mechanism, though people often alternate between denial and acceptance for a more prolonged period.

The choice not to receive a frank diagnosis may soften or change with time as treatment begins, the imminent threat recedes and the patient begins to feel safer. Many people therefore desire opportunities to explore, at their own pace, the meaning and implications of the difficult news.

Rather than being in denial, people who choose not to receive a full disclosure of their diagnosis may be reflecting cultural norms that regard such information as an unfair burden on patients (*see* Consent, Collaboration, and Choice). Even when denial is obviously present, it may pose no problem if patients accept whatever treatment is offered and are otherwise able to communicate openly with their loved ones. Moreover, those who accept their diagnosis but choose not to have further treatment are not necessarily in denial, though it is possible they may be hopeless and depressed and therefore require careful assessment.

There are times, however, when denial in patients may 'jeopardize aspects of their physical well-being, intimate social attachments, and ultimate prognosis'.[134] (Wool 1988, p. 38) People who delay reporting symptoms or deny the need for treatment because they say they are well or merely suffering some minor ailment, may well be jeopardizing their own prognosis. In such circumstances, denial is a problem that probably requires intervention.

People may seem to be in denial when they refuse to talk with their family about their illness, the future, or their feelings. However, patients may be expressing false hope in order to spare their families distress, and other family members may even share this strategy particularly when they are highly dependent upon one another (so-called 'enmeshed families'). These issues are discussed further in Chapter 3.

Patients who tenaciously hold on to denial may doubt their ability to cope with the information they are keeping at bay (though admittedly there is a circularity to this argument: to know that something is dangerous implies that one already knows what 'it' is). It is the horrific assumptions that people have acquired about cancer and its treatment that provoke denial in the first place. Thus, the way in which bad news is conveyed (e.g. offering the patient strength, hope, and support) may help mitigate the need for denial. For those unable to relinquish denial, the offer of ongoing support is essential.

To summarize, denial and avoidance are normal features of adjustment to difficult information. Although there may be fluctuations between denial and acceptance, 'solid denial' is usually short-lived. In most instances, denial should be respected as a normal defence mechanism and not challenged unless it is causing serious problems for the patient or their loved ones.[135] However, staff should ensure they do not collude with denial by providing false hope, but ensure that further information is always on hand whenever the patient is ready to absorb it.

Challenging denial

Where denial jeopardizes the patient's well-being or is creating serious problems for the patient or their relatives, it may be necessary to challenge it. Before doing so, however, one should establish that the individual has, indeed, been given the information in question, and that there is no one in the team in whom they may already be confiding a more realistic understanding. Then, carefully explore the meaning of the denial to the individual. Consider:

- 'What form does the denial take?
- To whom is the denial communicated?
- What are the circumstances in which denial is expressed?
- What is threatened?'[136] (Weisman 1972, p. 63)

1. Establish what the patient understands from what they have been told: '*Would you mind running through with me what you have been told about your illness? ... What do you understand by this?*'

2. Using what the patient has said, gently challenge them to expand on any areas which have been left vague, open or inconsistent: '*You used the phrase 'if all goes well'. I was wondering whether we could look at this for a moment. What do you think it would mean if things didn't go so well?*'

3. A useful technique is to express the ambivalence the patient may be feeling: the tension between acceptance (fearful reality) and denial (safe fantasy): '*It seems that part of you feels that your illness may be quite trivial, yet part of you seems to accept that you are in hospital and not at all well*'.

4. If the above strategies do not appear to work, more pointed questioning may reveal 'windows'[135] of acceptance: '*Do you ever worry that things might be worse than you have said they are?*'

5. Remember that the goal is not for the patient to be able to say 'I have cancer' or 'I do not have long to live' but rather for them to be able to communicate with others about issues of importance to the patient. Ultimately it remains an ethical question as to how far one should confront a patient with 'the truth' and, where there is any doubt, the family should always be consulted and the issues discussed within the entire healthcare team.

Anxiety, worry, and uncertainty

(*see* Chapter 5—Intense Fear)

Fear is an instinctive response to threat and uncertainty, while anxiety is a clinical term for fear in the absence of 'real' or objective danger. Here, however, we use fear and anxiety synonymously because the distinction between real and imagined threat is often hard to distinguish in the context of cancer. Not surprisingly, anxiety is common among people with cancer, especially at times of crisis like diagnosis, recurrence, in advanced disease [137] and at times of high uncertainty, for example when worrying about the results of medical tests and starting new treatments. However, anxiety can have a large number of causes that need to be carefully assessed. Some fears even pre-date the cancer and must therefore be understood within the personal context of the individual.[138] Perhaps the most common fear is that of the unknown. By its nature, the unknown contains more potential for threat than what is known. Living with uncertainty is therefore one of the hardest challenges facing people with cancer.

Fear is a normal emotion that is marked by changes in three related systems: physiology, thinking, and behaviour. Ideally, treatment involves tackling all the three systems simultaneously: helping people to keep their bodies calm (physiological), identifying and challenging their unhelpful thoughts and assumptions (cognitive), and confronting difficult or avoided situations (behavioural).

The physiological symptoms of arousal include muscle tension, palpitations, rapid breathing, perspiration, etc.; in other words, the body's automatic preparations for running away from a threat or having to defend itself from the threat (the 'fight or flight' response). Anxiety also makes people more vigilant for further threats and this can lead to a state of prolonged physiological arousal. This state of chronic vigilance (e.g. generalized anxiety disorder) can even seem normal for the individual suffering with it, who may have little idea that they are 'living on their nerves'. Learning to relax the muscles and breathe more calmly is the most effective way of reducing overall arousal in the body. Relaxation training is the most widely researched method but a number of other approaches draw on similar principles: massage, meditation, yoga, etc. Relaxation therapy involves selectively tensing, and then releasing, all the groups of muscles throughout the body. By learning to notice stored muscle tension and practising how to release it in the situation in which it occurs, patients can reduce their ambient levels of physiological arousal.

When people are anxious they naturally have thoughts associated with the threat, though not always accurate ones ('a cancer diagnosis means I am going to die'). Simply reassuring an anxious person is rarely a productive strategy,[139] and may even lead people to seek repeated reassurances to the point where this behaviour can be a problem in its own right. Worry causes distress because frightening thoughts and images of the future can induce all the physiological arousal as if the threat were already occurring in the present. As we saw in Chapter 1, worrying is unique to humans and is an adaptive mechanism for survival, closely related to anxiety. It enables people to imagine the future so they can prepare for it or avoid it completely. Often merely putting nebulous fears into words (either by speaking to someone or writing them down) has the effect of giving them 'shape' and thus making them seem more controllable,[32] turning the unknown into the predictable (see Worrying about Children, Chapter 3, for an example of decatastrophization).

Cognitive therapy techniques attempt to disentangle what is driving the anxiety by asking the patient to describe the thoughts that precede the episode of anxiety and that occur during it. By learning to identify the unhelpful thoughts that provoke anxiety, and by challenging their underlying assumptions, the individual can discover how to replace them with more realistic and helpful ways of thinking.[140]

However, some areas of uncertainty are even more avoidable. Because people with cancer do not always choose to obtain full information, they may retain beliefs about their disease or its treatment that are considerably worse than those of the medical team treating them. Carefully presented information whenever the individual is ready for it can therefore reduce anxiety.

Finally, people tend to avoid and, indeed, escape from threats if they are able to. Thus, people who find social situations anxiety-provoking will tend to avoid them, and people with agoraphobia prefer to avoid leaving the safety of their homes. This is the behavioural component of anxiety. Avoidance tends to maintain fears, while exposure to the potential threat (even in words) tends to lessen the fear, particularly if the individual approaches the threat in gradual steps of increasing difficulty, enabling them to learn to feel safe about each step before moving on to the next (see Chapter 5—Intense Fear).

Working with someone acutely confused or cognitively impaired

In cancer care, delirium, sometimes known as 'acute confusional state', is more common than dementia, which is a form of irreversible brain deterioration. It is frequently the result of a drug reaction or systemic poisoning associated with a tumour, and when this is resolved most people recover quickly. However, confusion may not be obvious and can therefore be easily missed (the distinctions between delirium, dementia, and depression are discussed in Chapter 5—Focus on CNS Tumours).

Acute confusion is characterized by:

(1) a relatively rapid onset;

(2) an altered level of consciousness that is often worse at night. The person may appear distracted, drowsy, or drifting in and out of sleep;

(3) poor concentration and memory, with evidence of slow, muddled thinking;

(4) disorientation of time and place;

(5) mistaking the surrounding environment, especially at night, leading to further confusion. Hallucinations and delusions are common;

(6) mood changes such as tearfulness and agitation;

(7) restlessness.

Common factors that can lead to delirium include:

- dehydration
- medication
- severe chest or urinary infection
- vitamin B12 deficiency, leading to anaemia
- hyperthermia or hypothermia
- constipation
- tumour toxins
- diabetes
- drug or alcohol withdrawal

For those with acute confusion, it is a matter of providing reassurance and safety while the underlying causes are being resolved. People who are acutely confused are likely to have similar needs to those who are cognitively impaired or suffer with dementia. They may have moments of clarity when they become aware of their failing ability or confusion, and become anxious and distressed in response to this alarming insight. Due to failing memory, they may also find themselves in situations that seem strange and unfamiliar. They therefore need the reassurance, guidance, and comfort of someone showing them concern.

In contrast to acute confusion, which is usually temporary, dementia is a chronic condition. People with dementia are often avoided by other people and over time their social lives can dwindle away, yet their need for social contact may be as strong as ever. Likewise their sense of 'agency', the ability to make things happen, is core to a person's sense of self-esteem and value yet, though this may be intact, it can be undermined when others assume the patient is incapable of any structured activity. The main task of caring for people with dementia is one of maintaining the dignity of their personhood by showing them respect, care, and knowledge of their past, even if the individual has difficulty retaining their own personal history.[141] A secure caring relationship goes a long way to replenishing the individual's sense of lost identity and reducing their fear and uncertainty.

Angry, difficult, or disliked patients

Any professional in the course of their work will meet people they find objectionable or awkward to deal with. They may have poor personal hygiene, or simply remind the professional of someone they do not like. Some people may appear unduly angry, hostile or uncooperative during every encounter. The behaviour of people from unfamiliar cultures may initially grate with a staff member's own personal assumptions about the world, leading them to feel uncomfortable or anxious. Some people may even seem beyond the pale (e.g. neo-Nazis). At the same time, all professionals share an ethical responsibility to do their best for every patient. How can one manage these conflicting feelings? There are a number of strategies that can help professionals work with angry, difficult, or disliked patients.

Acknowledgement

We usually label people as 'difficult' when their behaviour hinders our own goals. They are seen as obstructive, awkward, or non-compliant. From their point of view, however, the patient may be reacting in the most adaptive way they know. The fact is that 'difficult' patients are usually trying to communicate something. Thus, spending a few minutes attempting to understand the patient's perspective is time well spent. Familiarity with the concerns and issues in their life may lead to a clearer understanding of (and even empathy with) why they behave the way they do.

Behind anger and hostility there is often fear and insecurity. The individual may have had a long history of feeling their needs have been neglected, especially by healthcare professionals. They may believe that they will not be respected unless they exercise control through their 'difficult' behaviour. The patient may feel intimidated by the healthcare team and powerless in relation to them, and their disease may have left them feeling lost and confused about themselves and their future. 'Difficult' behaviour can therefore represent an attempt to exert control, attract attention, or gain respect; indeed, there may be many different sources of concern within the context of the patient's life.

Anxiety is often expressed as anger, and vice versa. Anger and anxiety are flip sides of the fight–flight response. Whether someone is angry or anxious, it helps to offer them a suitable time and place to express their feelings openly so as to understand the reasons driving these strong emotions. Rather than act defensively by arguing back, it is far more productive to start by acknowledging the feelings and the events that have led to their distress. Once the person's feelings and views have been fully acknowledged and understood, they will often dissipate. The professional may then be in a position to help the patient look at other feelings they may be having, including underlying feelings of fear and loss.

Of course, there can also be justifiable anger, as when a patient feels that healthcare professionals have neglected their needs. Patients sometimes have good reasons for complaining so it is therefore important that people's experiences are not merely rationalized away by professionals, providing yet more fuel for the patient's perception that they have not been listened to. Instead, staff members should listen carefully to the patient's story, convey that they have understood the feelings and concerns, and support the patient in deciding an appropriate course of action (e.g. lodging a formal complaint).

Boundaries

Every institution and relationship has rules and boundaries. Boundaries are simply written and unwritten social rules (e.g. it is offensive to swear in public). If a patient is drunk and disorderly, abusive or violent, the institution is entitled to enforce its rules regarding these behaviours. Curiously, this clarifying of boundaries can often be reassuring ('containing') to the patient, especially when the individual concerned is unconsciously testing the strength and cohesion of the team treating them. Just as healthcare professionals are not angels, patients carry responsibilities too. Institutions that are clear about their boundaries also communicate respect for the integrity of their patients.

Similarly, when a patient is abusive or hostile towards a member of staff, it is reasonable for the staff member to tell the patient how they are genuinely left feeling: '*I often feel you are quite angry with me. Is this something we could talk about?*' This may elicit a clearer picture of what the patient is feeling, and the assumptions they may be harbouring about the professional. If this fails to resolve the problem, an offer to transfer care to someone else should be made. At the very least it may be helpful for the professional to assert politely how he or she wishes to be treated: '*I would be grateful if you would not shout at anyone while you are with me or in this clinic*'.

Support

Sometimes, patients are difficult or disliked for reasons that are difficult to fathom. Paradoxically, they may even be 'difficult' because one feels especially attracted to them, or they share characteristics with a loved one. Some patients may seem irritating, exasperating, or upsetting to one member of staff even though everyone else in the healthcare team considers their behaviour benign. In such instances, it helps to obtain clinical supervision and support from a colleague. The process of describing and talking through one's feelings and reactions to the patient often helps to reveal one's underlying associations and assumptions concerning them (*see* Chapter 7—Reducing Stress—Clinical Supervision).

Finally, at times the healthcare team treating the patient can become split in their views towards the patient, causing unfamiliar conflict between team members, yet there may be nothing obvious in the patient's behaviour to cause this. If the healthcare team itself is in conflict over a particular patient, it may help to call upon a psychosocial specialist to assist the team in unravelling the source of the 'split' feelings.

Professional issues in communication

Communication between professionals

Poor communication between professionals leads to low morale and higher stress[142] but communication between professionals also has a direct and obvious impact on patient care. Professionals are required to communicate with one another throughout every stage of a patient's care. Where they do not communicate effectively with one another, the patient invariably suffers. Surgeons and oncologists who work to different treatment plans confuse patients and undermine their confidence in their safety. Nurses who have not been involved with the doctor's medical decisions regarding a particular patient may be more reluctant to comply with them. General practitioners who are not given information about the physical and psychosocial needs of their patients (or even that patients have been discharged from hospital) are clearly unable to provide adequate care in the community. All staff need to be able to ascertain how much the patient and family members understand about the diagnosis, prognosis, and future treatment. Effective systems of staff communication are therefore critical to patient care.

The head of the team is ultimately responsible for telling the patient important news such as diagnostic and prognostic information, but it helps every member of the team to know how much the patient has been told and how much they understand. The team must work to a consistent and co-ordinated plan that is agreed by everyone at regular team meetings (including the patient in as far they want to be involved). This plan must be openly available to the patient if they wish to have access to it. Patient-held records offer an innovative way forward in this regard.

Conventionally, information is exchanged between professionals through word of mouth, letters, and written patient records. The difficulty with written medical notes is that they quickly become huge and unwieldy, making it time-consuming to retrieve the information one needs. They frequently contain gaps, repetitions, and discrepancies, and rarely provide a concise summary of the patient's medical history, current stage of treatment, or current understanding of their condition and prognosis. Staff are seldom given guidance on where and how to write in medical notes. Some members of the medical team maintain their own separate records that may or may not be summarized in the medical notes. In short, medical record-keeping is a minefield of confusion.

This is still the case for the majority of hospitals, but computerized patient records offer promise for the future. The potential advantages of computerized patient records are clear: they can be constantly updated as the patient receives services and treatments at different sites within a healthcare network, and the stored information can be within easy reach of any member of the network—surgical units, radiology and lab facilities, oncology treatment centres, general practitioners, and potentially even the patient's own home. In these notes the head of the team can provide a terse summary of the patient's medical history and the treatment care plan that has been agreed with the patient, with sections devoted to communication with the patient and their psychosocial needs.

Every healthcare team, especially in cancer, should have a clear structure that defines how communication is transmitted throughout the team, and between the team and the patient and their family. A team leader, given their other responsibilities, is not always best placed to maintain an overview of all the patients under their care. A key worker system, in which different members of the team assume the role of care co-ordinator for specific patients, has the advantage of ensuring that someone maintains an up-to-date overview of the patient's situation and needs, and takes responsibility for collating and disseminating information concerning the patient's care.

Healthcare teams and patient confidentiality

Every patient has the right to privacy, yet there is also a need to share relevant clinical information between members of the healthcare team so that the best care can be given to the patient. But what is 'relevant' information?

Ultimately it is up to the patient to decide what, how much, and to whom they wish to disclose. Therefore, where there is any doubt as to whether the best interests of the patient are being served by sharing information between professionals, the views of the patient should always be sought. This is perhaps less of an issue with strictly medical information, but it becomes more important when intimate personal and social information comes to light. This information may have the potential to compromise the patient or prejudice other staff members' views of the patient. For example, is it in the best interests of the patient for every team member to know that a patient has a past psychiatric history? Is it relevant for all staff to know that a patient is a sex worker or from any other marginalized sector of the community? Where the patient poses a threat to themselves or others, a breach of confidentiality may be unavoidable, but some situations are less straightforward. Consider the following incident.

A student nurse was assigned to care for a 70-year-old man dying of lung cancer on an oncology ward. The man's daughter unexpectedly arrived on the ward one afternoon and was shown to his room. Ten minutes later she left, leaving the man in tears. Over the next two hours he explained to the student nurse that he had sexually abused his daughter when she was a child and that she had just come to the hospital to tell him she hated him. He then asked the student nurse not to tell anyone his shameful secret.

The student nurse was left in conflict, feeling repulsion towards her patient's past actions, yet moved by his distress. She also felt vaguely violated by his request that she not mention the incident to her colleagues. She knew that to tell even one colleague would probably turn them all against him, a helpless dying man, so she said nothing until he had died but was forced to contain her own conflicting feelings.

Healthcare poses many such ethical questions for professional staff, and cancer care is no exception. However, following a complicated clinical situation or difficult death, it helps the morale and cohesion of the entire team to reflect on the ethical and emotional issues raised. Such a meeting also helps to support the individual staff members involved. So rather than leaving professionals to face these questions alone, healthcare teams should find regular opportunities to review their practices and reconsider their policies.

Communication training

Learning to communicate effectively takes time and practice. It is not ideally learned from books like this but through receiving feedback about one's actual behaviour. Communication skills training is most effective when it is run in uni- or multiprofessional groups drawn from particular clinical teams, using a combination of didactic and experiential methods, such as teaching, role play, feedback, group work, and discussion. Workshops which use video feedback, role-plays, and actors to simulate patients in highly emotional clinical situations[143] can lead clinicians to adopt better communication skills.[144] They also enable professionals to consider their own concerns and anxieties, such as fear of causing distress to their patients, exposing themselves to the distress of their patients, lacking the support of others, etc.

Considerable evidence has accrued to show that such groups can be effective in altering staff–patient interactions[145] leading to better patient satisfaction with care,[146, 147] better symptomatic outcome (emotional health, symptom resolution, function, and pain control),[148] and more patient-centred care.[88] Good supportive care is only likely to be maintained, however, if professionals receive adequate support and clinical supervision (see Chapter 7).

References

1. Parle M, Jones B, and Maguire P. (1996). Maladaptive coping and affective disorders among cancer patients. *Psychological Medicine* **26**:735–44.
2. Mager WM and Andrykowski MA. (2002). Communication in the cancer 'bad news' consultation: patient perceptions and psychological adjustment. *Psycho-Oncology* **11**:35–46.
3. Radley A. (1994). *Making sense of illness: the social psychology of health and disease.* London: Sage.
4. ORI Research (1999). *Information and support – a survey of people with cancer 1999.* London: Macmillan Cancer Relief.
5. Cape J. (2002). Consultation length, patient-estimated consultation length, and satisfaction with the consultation. *British Journal of General Practice* **52**:1004–6.
6. Fallowfield L. (1993). Giving sad and bad news. *The Lancet* **341**:476.

7. Royal College of Physicians of London (1997). *Improving communication between doctors and patients: a report of a working party*. London: Royal College of Physicians of London.

8. Cassileth BR, Zupkis RV, Sutton-Smith K, and March V. (1980). Information and participation preferences among cancer patients. *Annals of Internal Medicine* **92**:832–6.

9. Kemp N, Skinner F, and Toms J. (1984). Randomized clinical trials of cancer treatment ... a public opinion survey. *Clinical Oncology* **10**:155–61.

10. Jenkins V, Fallowfield L, and Saul, J. (2001). Information needs of patients with cancer: results from a large study in UK cancer centres. *British Journal of Cancer* **84**:48–51.

11. Bonnet V, Couvreur C, Demachy P, Kimmel F, Milan H, Noel D, *et al.* (2000). Evaluating radiotherapy patients' need for information: a study using a patient information booklet. *Cancer Radiotherapy* **4**:294–307.

12. Detmar SB, Aaronson NK, Wever LDV, Muller M, and Schornagel JH. (2000). How are you feeling? Who wants to know? Patients' and oncologists' preferences for discussing health-related quality of life issues. *Journal of Clinical Oncology* **18**:3295–301.

13. Mitchell JL. (1998). Cross-cultural issues in the disclosure of cancer. *Cancer Practice* **6**:153.

14. Mizushima Y, Kashii T, Hoshino K, Morikage T, Takashima A, Hirata H, *et al.* (1990). A survey regarding the disclosure of the diagnosis of cancer in Toyama Prefecture, Japan. *Japanese Journal of Medicine* **29**:146–55. Cited in Mitchell JL. (1998). Cross-cultural issues in the disclosure of cancer. *Cancer Practice* **6**:153.

15. Richards MA, Ramirez AJ, Degner LF, Fallowfield LJ, Maher EJ, and Neuberger J. (1993). Offering choice of treatment to patients with cancers. A review based on a symposium held at the 10th annual conference of the British psychosocial oncology group, December. *European Journal of Cancer*, 1995 **31A**:112–6.

16. Brennan JH and Sheard TAB. (1994). Psychosocial support and therapy in cancer care. *European Journal of Palliative Care* **1**:136–9.

17. Airey C, Becher H, Erens B, and Fuller, E. (2002). Cancer national overview 1999/2000. London: UK Department of Health.

18. Higby DJ. (1985). The doctor and the cancer patient: Sources of physician stress. In: DJ Higby (ed.) *The cancer patient and supportive care,* Boston: Nijhoff Publishers.

19. Salmon P. (2000). *Psychology of medicine and surgery: a guide for psychologists, counsellors, nurses and doctors.* Chichester: Wiley.

20. Klein GA, Orasanu J, Calderwood R, and Zsambok CE. (1995). *Decision making in action: models and methods.* Ablex, NJ: Norwood; Cited in Michie S, Smith D, McClennan A, and Marteau TM. (1997). Patient decision making: an evaluation of two different methods of presenting information about a screening test. *British Journal of Health Psychology* **2**:317–26.

21. Ramirez AJ, Richards MA, Rees GJG, O'Neill WM, Wilkinson S, Young J, *et al.* (1994). Effective communication in oncology. *Journal of Cancer Care* **3**:84–93.

22. Fallowfield LJ, Hall A, Maguire P, Baum M, and A'Hern RP. (1994). Psychological effects of being offered choice of surgery for breast cancer. *British Medical Journal* **309**:448.

23. Pocock SJ. (1983). *Clinical trials: a practical approach.* Chichester: John Wiley & Sons.

24. Tobias JS and Souhami RL. (1993). Fully informed consent can be needlessly cruel. *British Medical Journal* **307**:1199–201.

25. Luker K, Leinster S, Owens G, Beaver K, and Degner L. (1993). *Preferences for information and decision making in women newly diagnosed with breast cancer.* Final report. Liverpool: Research and Development Unit, University of Liverpool Department of Nursing. Cited in Fallowfield LJ, Hall A, Maguire P, Baum M, and A'Hern RP. (1994). Psychological effects of being offered choice of surgery for breast cancer. *British Medical Journal* **309**:448.

26. Degner L and Sloan J. (1992). Decision making during serious illness: what role do patients really want to play? *Journal of Clinical Epidemiology* **45**:941–50.

27. Degner LF, Kristjanson LJ, Bowman LD, Sloan JA, Carriere KC, O'Neil J, *et al.* (1997). Information needs and decisional preferences in women with breast cancer. *Journal of the American Medical Association* **233**:1485–92. Cited in Maguire P. (1999). Improving communication with cancer patients. *European Journal of Cancer* **35**:1415–22.

28. Cumming SR and Harris LM. (2001). The impact of anxiety on the accuracy of diagnostic decision-making. *Stress and Health* **17**:281–6.

29. Maguire P. (1999). Improving communication with cancer patients. *European Journal of Cancer* **35**:1415–22.

30. Blumberg B, Kerns P, and Lewis M. (1983). Adult cancer patient education: an overview. *Journal of Psychosocial Oncology* **1**:19–39.

31. Michie S, Smith D, McClennan A, and Marteau TM. (1997). Patient decision making: an evaluation of two different methods of presenting information about a screening test. *British Journal of Health Psychology* **2**:317–26.

32. Spiegel D. (1990). Facilitating emotional coping during treatment. *Cancer* **66**:1422–6.

33. Akkerman D. (2002). Director of Information, Cancer Council Victoria. Personal communication.

34. Henman MJ, Butow PN, Brown RF, Boyle F, and Tattersall MH. (2002). Lay constructions of decision-making in cancer. *Psycho-Oncology* **11**:295–306.

35. Ley P. (1997). Compliance among patients. In: A Baum, D Newman, J Weinman, R West, and C McManus (ed.),*Cambridge handbook of psychology, health and medicine*, Cambridge: Cambridge University Press.

36. Fredette S. (1990). A model for improving cancer patient education. *Cancer, Nursing* **13**:207–15.

37. Carlsson ME and Strang PM. (1997). Facts, misconceptions, and myths about cancer: What do patients with gynecological cancer and the female public at large know? *Gynecological Oncology* **65**:46–53.

38. Mills ME and Davidson R. (2002). Cancer patients' sources of information: use and quality issues. *Psycho-Oncology* **11**:371–8.

39. Leydon G, Boulton M, Moynihan C, Jones A, Mossman J, Boudioni M, *et al.* (2000). Cancer patients' information needs and information seeking behaviour: in depth interview study. *British Medical Journal* **320**:909–13.

40. Maguire P. (1992). Improving the recognition and treatment of affective disorders in cancer patients. *Recent Advances in Clinical Psychiatry* **7**:15–30.

41. Maguire P. (1998). Breaking bad news. *European Journal of Surgical Oncology* **24**:188–99.

42. Ptacek JT and Eberhardt TL. (1996). Breaking bad news: a review of the literature. *Journal of the American Medical Association* **276**:496–502.

43. Coulter A, Entwistle V and Gilbert D. (1999). Sharing decisions with patients: is the information good enough? *British Medical Journal* **318**:318–22.

44. Meredith C, Symonds P, Webster L, Lamont D, Ryper L, Gillis CR, *et al.* (1996). Informational needs of cancer patients in West Scotland: cross sectional survey of patients' views. *British Medical Journal* **313**:724–6.

45. Fallowfield LJ, Baum M and Maguire GP. (1986). Effects of breast conservation on psychological morbidity associated with diagnosis and treatment of early breast cancer. *British Medical Journal* **293**:1331–4.

46. Mills ME and Sullivan K. (1999). The importance of information giving for patients newly diagnosed with cancer: a review of the literature. *Journal of Clinical Nursing* **8**:631–42.

47. Eardley A. (1988). Patients' worries about radiotherapy: evaluation of a preparatory booklet. *Psychology and Health* **2**:79–89.

48. Hyatt J. (1994). *In it together: promoting information for shared decision making.* A report for the London: King's Fund Centre, King's Fund.

49. Finlay IG and Wyatt P. (1999). Randomised cross-over study of patient-held records in oncology and palliative care. *Lancet* **353**:558–9.

50. Cornbleet MA, Campbell P, Murray S, Stevenson M, and Bond S. (2002). Patient-held records in cancer and palliative care: a randomized, prospective trial. *Palliative Medicine* **16**:205–12.

51. National Cancer Alliance. (2003). *The teamwork file.* Oxford: NCA (www.teamworkfile.org.uk).

52. Shelby RA, Taylor KL, Kerner JF, Coleman E, and Blum D. (2002). The role of community-based and philanthropic organizations in meeting cancer patient and caregiver needs. *CA: A Cancer Journal for Clinicians* **52**:229–46.

53. Ley P and Florio T. (1996). The use of readability formulas in healthcare. *Psychology, Health and Medicine* **1**:7–28. Cited in Ley P. (1997). Written communication. In: A Baum, D Newman, J Weinman, R West, and C McManus (ed.), *Cambridge handbook of psychology, health and medicine.* Cambridge: Cambridge University Press.

54. Ley P. (1997). Written communication. In: A Baum, D Newman, J Weinman, R West, and C McManus (ed.), *Cambridge handbook of psychology, health and medicine.* Cambridge: Cambridge University Press.

55. Office for National Statistics. (2002). *Living in Britain – Results from the 2000/01 General household survey.* London: The Stationery Office.

56. Eiser JR and Eiser C. (1996). *Effectiveness of video for health education: a review.* London: Health Education Authority.

57. Thomas R, Daly M, Perryman B, and Stockton B. (2000). Forewarned is forearmed – benefits of preparatory information on video cassette for patients receiving chemotherapy or radiotherapy – a randomised controlled trial. *European Journal of Cancer* **36**:1536–43.

58. Ford S, Fallowfield L, Hall A, and Lewis S. (1995). The influence of audiotapes on patient participation in the cancer consultation. *European Journal of Cancer* **31**:2264–9.

59. McHugh P, Lewis S, Ford S, Newlands E, Rustin G, Coombes C, *et al.* (1995). The efficacy of audiotapes in promoting psychological well-being in cancer patients: a randomised, controlled trial. *British Journal of Cancer* **71**:388–92.

60. Ong LML, Visser MRM, Lammes FB, van der Velden J, Kuenen BC, and de Haes JCJ. (2000). Effect of providing cancer patients with the audiotaped initial consultation on satisfaction, recall, and quality of life: a randomised, double-blind study. *Journal of Clinical Oncology* **18**:3052–60.

61. Knox R, Butow PN, Devine R, and Tattersall MH. (2002). Audiotapes of oncology consultations: only for the first consultation? *Annals of Oncology* **13**:622–7.

62. Williams ER, Potts HW, Young T, Davidson R, Boudioni M., Brennan J, *et al.* (2002). *Are men missing from cancer information and support services?* Unpublished study – Cancer Research UK London Psychosocial Group; Guy's, King's & St Thomas' Medical School.

63. Brennan JH and Bullock A. (2001). A problem shared… *Newsletter of the British psychosocial oncology society*, September issue, 1–4.

64. Smith SD, Nicol KM, Devereux J, and Cornbleet MA. (1999). Encounters with doctors: quantity and quality. *Palliative Medicine* **13**:217–23.

65. Doyle D and Jeffrey D. (2000). *Palliative care in the home.* Oxford: Oxford University Press.

66. Middleton JF. (1995). Asking patients to write lists: feasibility study. *British Medical Journal* **311**:34.

67. Stein HF. (1985). Whatever happened to countertransference? The subjective in medicine. In: HF Stein and M Apprey (ed.), *Context and dynamics in clinical knowledge*, Charlottesville: University of Virginia Press.

68. Frank. (1973). *Persuasion and healing.* Baltimore: Johns Hopkins University Press. Cited in Stein HF. (1985). Whatever happened to countertransference? The subjective in medicine.

In: HF Stein and M Apprey (ed.), *Context and dynamics in clinical knowledge*, Charlottesville: University of Virginia Press.

69. Figley CR. (1985). (ed.) *Compassion fatigue: coping with secondary traumatic stress disorder in those who treat the traumatized.* New York: Bruner/Mazel.

70. Maguire, P. (1985). Barriers to psychological care of the dying. *British Medical Journal* **291**: 1711–13.

71. Heaven C and Maguire P. (2003). Communication issues. In: M Lloyd-Williams (ed.), *Psychosocial issues in palliative care*, Oxford: Oxford University Press.

72. British Medical Association. (2003). *Communication skills education for doctors: a discussion paper.* London: BMA.

73. Rolland JS. (1994). Working with illness: clinicians' personal and interface issues. *Family Systems Medicine* **12**:149–69.

74. Butow PN, Dunn SM and Tattersall MH. (1995). Communication with cancer patients: Does it matter? *Journal of Palliative Care* **11**:34–8.

75. Jones GY and Payne S. (2000). Searching for safety signals: the experience of medical surveillance amonst men with testicular cancer. *Psycho-Oncology* **9**:385–94.

76. Dakof GA and Taylor SE. (1990). Victims' perceptions of social support: what is helpful from whom? *Journal of Personality and Social Psychology* **58**:80–9.

77. Leventhal H, Meyer D, and Nerenz D. (1980). The common-sense representation of illness danger. In: S Rachman (ed.), *Contributions to medical psychology*, Vol. 2, New York: Pergamon Press, pp. 7–30.

78. Galanti G. (1991). *Caring for patients from different cultures: case studies from American hospitals.* Philadelphia: University of Pennsylvania Press.

79. Enelow AJ, Forde DL, and Brummel-Smith K. (1996). *Interviewing and patient care*, 4th edn, Oxford: Oxford University Press.

80. Henley A. (1987). *Caring in a multiracial society.* London: Bloomsbury Health Authority.

81. Chapman K, Abraham C, Jenkins V, and Fallowfield L. (2003). Lay understanding of terms used in cancer consultations. *Psycho-Oncology* **12**:557–66.

82. Ley P. (1988). *Communicating with patients: improving communication, satisfaction and compliance.* London: Chapman and Hall.

83. Cull A, Stewart M, and Altman DG. (1995). Assessment of and intervention for psychosocial problems in routine oncology practice. *British Journal of Cancer* **72**:229–35.

84. Ward SE, Goldberg N, Miller-McCauley V, Mueller C, Nolan A, Pawlik-Plank D, *et al.* (1993). Patient-related barriers to management of cancer pain. *Pain* **52**:319–24.

85. Heaven CM and Maguire P. (1997). Disclosure of concerns by hospice patients and their identification by nurses. *Palliative Medicine* **11**:283–90.

86. Söllner W, DeVries A, Steixner E, Lukas P, Sprinzi G, Rumpold G, *et al.* (2001). How successful are oncologists in identifying patient distress, perceived social support, and need for psychosocial counselling? *British Journal of Cancer* **84**:179–85.

87. Passik S, Dugan W, McDonald MV, Rosenfeld B, Theobald DE, and Edgerton S. (1998). Oncologists' recognition of depression in their patients with cancer. *Journal of Clinical Oncology* **16**:1594–600.

88. Fallowfield L, Lipkin M, and Hall A. (1998). Teaching senior oncologists communication skills: Results from Phase I of a comprehensive longitudinal program in the United Kingdom. *Journal of Clinical Oncology* **16**:1961–8.

89. Dr Jill White former Director of the National Youth Orchestra of Great Britain – personal communication.

90. Dowsett SM, Saul JL, Butow PN, Dunn SM, Boyer MJ, Findlow R, *et al.* (2000). Communication styles in the cancer consultation: preferences for a patient-centred approach. *Psycho-Oncology* **9**:147–56.

91. Balint M. (1957). *The doctor, his patient and the illness.* London: Pitman.

92. Roberts CS, Cox CE, Reintgen DS, Baile WF, and Gibertini M. (1994). Influence of physician communication on newly diagnosed breast patients' psychological adjustment and decision-making. *Cancer* **74**:336–41.

93. Ramirez AJ, Graham J, Richards MA, Cull A, and Gregony WM. (1996). Mental health of hospital consultants: the effect of stress and satisfaction at work. *Lancet* **347**:724–8.

94. Lind SE, Del Vecchio Good M, Seidel S, Csordas T, and Good BJ. (1989). Telling the diagnosis of cancer. *Journal of Clinical Oncology* **7**:583–9.

95. Finlay I and Dallimore D. (1991). Your child is dead. *British Medical Journal* **302**:1524–5.

96. Persaud R. (1993). Breaking bad news. *Lancet* **341**:832–3.

97. Kaye P. (1996). *Breaking bad news – a ten step approach.* Northampton: EPL Publications.

98. Rogers A, Karlsen S, and Addington-Hall J. (2000). 'All the services were excellent. It is when the human element comes in that things go wrong': dissatisfaction with hospital care in the last year of life. *Journal of Advanced Nursing* **31**:768–74.

99. Buckman R. (1998). Communication in palliative care: a practical guide. In: D Doyle, GWC Hanks, and N MacDonald (ed.), *Oxford textbook of palliative medicine*, Oxford: Oxford University Press.

100. Weisman AD and Worden JW. (1976). The existential plight in cancer: significance of the first 100 days. *International Journal of Psychiatry in Medicine* **7**:1–5.

101. Carver CS, Pozo C, Harris SD, Noriega V, Scheier MF, Robinson DS, *et al.*(1993) How coping mediates the effects of optimism on distress: a study of women with early stage breast cancer. *Journal of Personality and Social Psychology* **65**:375–90.

102. Boland C. (1985). Suicide and cancer: II medical and care factors in suicide by cancer patients in Sweden 1973–1976. *Journal of Psychosocial Oncology*, **3**:17–30 Cited in Breitbart W, Chochinov HM, and Passik S. (1998). Psychiatric aspects of palliative care. In: D Doyle, GWC Hanks, N MacDonald (ed.), *Oxford textbook of palliative medicine*, Oxford: Oxford University Press.

103. Willard C. (2000). Cardiopulmonary resuscitation for palliative care patients: a discussion of ethical issues. *Palliative Medicine* **14**:308–12.

104. Faber-Langendoen K. (1991). Resuscitation of patients with metastatic cancer. Is transient benefit still futile? *Archives of Internal Medicine* **151**:235–9.

105. Reid C and Jeffrey D. (2002). Do not attempt resuscitation decisions in a cancer centre: Addressing difficult ethical and communication issues. *British Journal of Cancer* **86**:1057–60.

106. McDermott A. (2002). Involving patients in discussions of do-not-resuscitate orders. *Professional Nurse* **17**:465–8.

107. Murphy DJ, Burrows D, Santilli S, Kemp AW, Tenner S, Kreling, B, *et al.* (1994). The influence of the probability of survival on patients' preferences regarding CPR. *New England Journal of Medicine* **330**:545–9.

108. Thorns AR and Ellershaw JE. (1999). A survey of nursing and medical staff views on the use of cardiopulmonary resuscitation in the hospice. *Palliative Medicine* **13**:225–32.

109. Morgan R and Westmoreland C. (2002). Survey of junior doctors' attitudes to cardiopulmonary resuscitation. *Postgraduate Medical Journal* **78**:413–5.

110. Ronson A and Body J-J. (2002). Psychosocial rehabilitation of cancer patients after curative therapy. *Supportive Care in Cancer* **10**:281–91.

111. Nordin K and Glimelius B. (1999). Predicting delayed anxiety and depression in patients with gastrointestinal cancer. *British Journal of Cancer* **79**:525–9.

112. Nordin K, Berglund G, Glimelius B, and Sjoden PO. (2001). Predicting anxiety and depression among cancer patients: a clinical model. *European Journal of Cancer* **37**:376–84.

113. Deimling GT, Kahana B, Bowman KF, and Schaeffer ML. (2002). Cancer survivorship and psychological distress in later life. *Psycho-Oncology* **11**:479–94.

114. Breitbart W, Chochinov HM, and Passik S. (1998). Psychiatric aspects of palliative care. In: D Doyle, GWC Hanks, and N MacDonald (ed.), *Oxford textbook of palliative medicine*, Oxford: Oxford University Press.

115. Harrison J and Maguire P. (1994). Predictors of psychiatric morbidity in cancer patients. *British Journal of Psychiatry* **165**:593–8.

116. Hogg J, Northfield J, and Turnbull J. (2001). *Cancer and people with learning disabilities.* Kidderminster, UK: BILD Publications.

117. Howells G. (1986). Are the medical needs of mentally handicapped adults being met? *Journal of the Royal College of General Practitioners* **36**:449–53.

118. Powers LW and Register MK. (1991). Down syndrome and acute leukemia: epidemiological and genetic relationships. *Laboratory Medicine* **22**:630–6. Cited in Hogg J, Northfield J, and Turnbull J. (2001). Cancer and people with learning disabilities. Kidderminster, UK: BILD Publications.

119. Cooke LB. (1997). Cancer and learning disability. *Journal of Intellectual Disability Research* **41**:312–16.

120. Tuffrey-Wijne I. (2003). The palliative care needs of people with intellectual disabilities: a literature review. *Palliative Medicine* **17**:55–62.

121. Donaghey V, Bernal J, Tuffrey-Wijne I, and Hollins, S. (2002). *Getting on with cancer.* London: Gaskell and St George's Hospital Medical School, .

122. Read S. (1998). The palliative care needs of people with learning disabilities. *International Journal of Palliative Nursing* **4**:246–51.

123. Hearing Concern (2002). *Communication with deaf and hard of hearing patients – A guide for professionals.* London: Hearing Concern.

124. Mind (2001). *Understanding mental health.* London: Mind (The National Association for Mental Health).

125. Wolff G, Pathare S, Craig T, and Leff J. (1996). Community knowledge of mental illness and reaction to mentally ill people. *British Journal of Psychiatry* **168**:191–8.

126. Mind (2001). Public attitudes to mental distress: a mind fact sheet. London: Mind (The National Association for Mental Health).

127. Lansky SB, List MA, Hermann CA, Ets-Hokin EG, DasGupta TK, Wilbanks GD, *et al.* (1985). Absence of major depressive disorder in female cancer patients. *Journal of Clinical Oncology* **3**:1553–60.

128. Maguire P. (2000). The use of antidepressants in patients with advanced cancer. *Supportive Care in Cancer* **8**:265–7.

129. Berney A, Stiefel F, Mazzocato C, and Buclin T. (2000). Psychopharmacology in supportive care of cancer: a review for the clinician. III Antidepressants. *Supportive Care in Cancer* **8**:278–86.

130. Sheard T and Maguire P. (1999). The effect of psychological interventions on anxiety and depression in cancer patients: results of two meta-analyses. *British Journal of Cancer* **80**:1770–80.

131. Massie MJ and Popkin MK. (1998). Depressive disorders. In: JC Holland (ed.). *Psychooncology*, Oxford: Oxford University Press.

132. Chochinov H, Wilson K, Enns M, and Lander S. (1998). Depression, hopelessness and suicidal ideation in the terminal ill. *Psychosomatics* **39**:366–70.

133. Dr Jonathan Evans – personal communication.

134. Wool MS. (1988). Understanding denial in cancer patients. *Advances in Psychosomatic Medicine* **18**:37–53.

135. Maguire P and Faulkner A. (1988). Communicate with cancer patients: 2 Handling uncertainty, collusion and denial. *British Medical Journal* **297**:972–3.

136. Weisman A. (1972). On dying and denying: a study of psychiatric terminality. New York: Behavioral Publications. Cited in Wool MS. (1988). Understanding denial in cancer patients. *Advances in Psychosomatic Medicine* **18**:37–53.

137. Noyes R, Holt CS, and Massie MJ. (1998). Anxiety disorders. In: JC Holland (ed.), *Psychooncology*, Oxford: Oxford University Press.

138. Brennan JH. (2000). Changing tack: the importance of the therapeutic relationship. *Primary Care and Cancer* **20**:31–4.

139. Stark DPH and House A. (2000). Anxiety in cancer patients. *British Journal of Cancer* **83**:1261–7.

140. White CA. (2001). Cognitive behaviour therapy for chronic medical problems. *A guide to assessment and treatment in practice*, Chichester: Wiley.

141. Kitwood T. (1997). Dementia reconsidered. *The person comes first*. Buckingham: Open University Press.

142. Firth-Cozens J. (2001). Interventions to improve physicians' well-being and patient care. *Social Science and Medicine* **52**:215–22.

143. Razavi D, Delvaux N, Marchal S, DeCock M, Farvacques C, and Slachmuylder J-L. (2000). Testing healthcare professionals' communication skills: the usefulness of highly emotional standardized role-playing sessions with simulators. *Psycho-Oncology* **9**:293–302.

144. Fallowfield L, Jenkins V, Farewell V, Saul J, Duffy A, and Eves R. (2002). Efficacy of a cancer research UK communication skills training model for oncologists: a randomised controlled trial. *Lancet* **359**:650–6.

145. Jenkins V and Fallowfield L. (2002). Can communication skills training alter physicians' beliefs and behaviour in clinics? *Journal of Clinical Oncology* **20**(3):765–9.

146. Klein S. (1999). The effects of the participation of patients with cancer in teaching communication skills to medical undergraduates; a randomised study with follow-up after 2 years. *European Journal of Cancer* **35**(10):1448–56.

147. Tierney WM, Dexter PR, Gramelspacher GP, Perkins AJ, Zhou XH, and Wolinsky FD. (2001). The effect of discussions about advance directives on patients' satisfaction with primary care. [see comments]. *Journal of General Internal Medicine* **16**(1):32–40.

148. Stewart MA. (1996). Effective physician-patient communication and health outcomes: a review. *Canadian Medical Association Journal*, **152**:1423–33.

Chapter 7

Professional context

Part 1 365
  Stress and burnout in healthcare professionals. 365
    Sources of stress 365
    Effects of stress 366
    Burnout. 367
  Cancer professionals. 368
    Doctors 369
    Nurses. 375
    Radiographers 377
    Other healthcare professionals 379
    Medical secretaries, receptionists, and porters. 379
  Preventing burnout and reducing stress 380
    Management strategies to prevent burnout. 380
    Strategies to reduce stress in healthcare 381
    Team functioning 384
Part 2 386
  User-involvement 386
  Voluntary support 387
  Complementary therapy and alternative medicine 389
    Informed consent. 391
    Guilt and responsibility 392
    Spiritual abuse 392
    Colluding with denial 393
  References 393

Are professionals who work in cancer care any different from other people?

Almost any member of the community will tell you that cancer is a tough area of healthcare in which to work. They immediately recognize that working with people who face the certainty, or even the possibility, of their death must take its toll on the staff. They assume that because cancer professionals are dealing every day with profound anguish and distress, they must be personally affected themselves. And they are right. People who work in cancer care show high levels of stress and emotional burnout. But paradoxically, the emotional distress of working in cancer care is rarely acknowledged by the very professionals themselves or by the healthcare institutions in which they work.

In recent years there has been growing evidence that there may be a personal cost of working in cancer care, and that changes to the way that healthcare is practised is not only needed for the benefit of the patients but for the staff too. One of the main reasons professionals become burned out is that they are indeed emotionally affected by the work they do. Cancer units are resonant with emotion. As professionals, and as people, healthcare staff are there to assist other people through particularly terrible times in their lives. And healthcare is mostly delivered by people who want to care—who want to provide medical *care*, nursing *care*, and palliative *care*. They want to have enough time to know their patients a little, to ease their distress and suffering, as well as cure their cancer. For many professionals this desire to care was their 'calling', the very reason they were drawn to their profession.

But unfortunately there are other sources of stress in modern healthcare that professionals must also deal with. It may be both emotionally draining and rewarding work but cancer care is becoming crowded out by other time-consuming pressures, and by increasingly tight financial margins. So perhaps it is not surprisingly that those who work in the field experience high levels of stress and burnout.

In Part 1 of this chapter we examine some of the evidence concerning stress among cancer professionals. We consider how these staff can sustain the supportive care of their patients without themselves becoming unduly stressed and burned out. The culture of medicine rarely recognizes vulnerability among its practitioners, nor encourages time for reflection and repair. Yet if healthcare professionals of any discipline are to provide supportive care to their patients *and sustain it*, they also need time to consider the impact of their clinical work on themselves as people, lest they become poor clinicians.

In Part 2 we acknowledge that patients and professionals encounter other players in the world of cancer care, notably those working in the voluntary sector and those who offer complementary therapies and alternative medicine. We speculate whether people with cancer are increasingly turning to these 'folk' practitioners because scientific healthcare no longer has the time to offer the supportive care they need, or has simply lost touch with these needs. Healthcare institutions have developed over decades, or even centuries, and their institutional practices are often out of touch not only with the current needs of their service users, their patients, but also with the professional staff working within them.

If people with cancer are 'voting with their feet' by searching for supportive care elsewhere, how can healthcare institutions learn to be more responsive to their patients' needs? One way to be more responsive, and to cut through the sluggish torpor of institutionalization, is to involve the people who use the service to reflect on their experiences and to advise on how systems and practices might be changed. The perspective of healthcare service users, which can also include that of healthcare staff, has only recently been finding its voice. Yet it is the collaboration of patients and professionals that offers one of the most promising ways of improving supportive care in cancer.

Part 1

Stress and burnout in healthcare professionals

Stress among healthcare providers can have a decisive impact on the supportive care of people with cancer because, as we shall see, when professionals are chronically stressed (burned out) they often protect themselves by emotionally withdrawing from their patients and colleagues.

What is stress? Most people have an understanding of the term 'stress' but ask them to define it and they may find it hard to articulate. The lack of an adequate common definition is a fundamental problem in stress research. What is stressful for one person may not be stressful to another, and what is stressful to a person one day may not seem so stressful the next. One working definition is to say that *stress occurs when there is an excess of demands over the individual's resources to meet them*. Both the demands and the resources can be *internal* (from within the individual) or *external* to them (other people, equipment, etc.). However, it is important to state from the outset that suffering from stress is not a sign of 'weakness', just as managing to cope with a high level of stress is no measure of one's personal strength.

Besides the difficulty in defining stress, there is the obvious problem of measuring it. As Firth-Cozens has noted, if you ask doctors to complete a stress questionnaire, they will say that work overload is the main source of stress; if you ask them to write about recent stresses they have faced they will typically write about difficult clinical incidents involving death and dying, relationships with senior colleagues, or making a mistake.[1]

Sources of stress

Despite these difficulties with the concept of stress, a consensus is emerging that the amount of stress people experience in relation to their work is related to three primary factors:

- the demands of the work
- the degree of control they have over it
- the amount of support they feel they receive in their personal and professional lives.

For example, these three factors have been shown to predict the amount of distress reported by 5704 American physicians.[2] It is also interesting to note that these factors parallel the main issues affecting distress among people with cancer: multiple concerns, control over events, and social support. A number of related factors have also been associated with work stress. These are useful to review when considering one's own work environment. They include:[3]

- **factors intrinsic to the job**
  - long hours
  - work overload

- poor working conditions
- responsibility for people's lives
- time pressures
- emotional strain of the work
- **role in the organization**
  - role ambiguity or conflict
  - responsibility for people as opposed to things
- **relationships at work**
  - lack of trust or support
  - criticism
  - lack of delegation
  - excessive competition
  - poor leadership
  - crowded workspace
  - abrasive personalities, etc.
- **career development**
  - job security
  - career ceiling, etc.
- **organization structure and climate**
  - lack of autonomy
  - lack of organizational participation or involvement in decision making
- **home–work 'spillage'**
  - events at work or home spill over into one another

Effects of stress

The negative effects of stress are well-documented although, interestingly, again fairly non-specific.[4] Some of the many effects of stress are listed here to illustrate its widespread damaging nature.

Behavioural-social
- increased consumption of tobacco, coffee, alcohol, drugs
- impulsive, emotional behaviour
- difficulty making decisions
- poor relationships at home and work
- emotional withdrawal leading to social isolation

Physical
- poor general health
- insomnia
- tiredness
- fast shallow breathing
- palpitations
- muscle tension
- irritable bowel syndrome
- headaches

- family and relationship problems
- increased incidence of suicide

- skin disorders
- restlessness
- nausea
- hypertension
- ulcers

Cognitive

- anxiety
- boredom
- irritability and aggression
- depression
- inability to concentrate; distractible
- poor memory
- apathy
- loss of confidence

Organizational

- higher absenteeism
- more sick leave
- poor time-keeping
- poor productivity and decision making
- low morale
- poor co-operation and more industrial disputes
- higher rate of accidents

Burnout

Sustained or chronic stress leads to a phenomenon called 'burnout', a term first applied to the work setting by Freudenberger[5] in 1974. Since then, burnout has been widely investigated, particularly among human service occupations such as healthcare, in which sustained stress is thought to be largely due to the emotional nature of the relationship between staff and patients.[6] Burnout refers to the end result of chronic stress though it is often used as if it were a direct measure of stress, perhaps because there is a widely used psychometric tool for measuring it among groups of people.[7] Yet despite its usefulness in describing particular work environments or staff groups, one should be wary about applying the term to an individual because no reliable method exists for 'diagnosing' burnout in individuals.[6]

Burnout has three primary features:

(i) **Emotional exhaustion** A depletion of emotional resources whereby people feel they have little more to give. Patient contact may be experienced as oppressive and burdensome. There is a loss of energy for the work and a general sense of fatigue.

(ii) **Depersonalization** A negative, callous or excessively detached attitude towards patients or colleagues. Individuals with burnout may appear irritable or distant, and there is often cynicism or lack of idealism.

(iii) **Loss of personal accomplishment and job satisfaction** A loss of confidence in one's competence, and achievements, involving a loss of productivity, creativity, and motivation. Burnout leads to low morale, withdrawal, and an inability to cope.

Burnout is ultimately a way of coping with sustained stress, rather than a 'failure to be professional'.[6] Cancer care is intrinsically an emotive area of work, assuming professionals allow themselves to be touched by their patients' experience. There are many moving and rewarding moments in working with people facing adversity, but the highs are more than balanced by the lows.

Most healthcare professionals have not had training or preparation for the emotional impact of their clinical role and there is little formal recognition of the emotional strain of the work. There are many clinical situations, however, when the most appropriate course of action for the professional is to do little other than 'stay with' the patient's distress and offer their emotional support. Without training and support, this important act is seen as 'doing nothing', perhaps leaving professionals feeling helpless and a failure. However professionals can reduce the emotional distress such situations bring about by learning how to manage their feelings of helplessness and appreciate the therapeutic value of support and clinical supervision.

Being 'professional', especially in medicine, is sometimes equated with not being personally affected by the work, yet to achieve this requires the very detachment found in professionals who are emotionally burned out. This is not what patients need and it is not the kind of care that most healthcare professionals aspire to give. If 'familiarity breeds contempt' then professionals must work actively to avoid patients' suffering becoming so familiar as to engender little reaction, or for them to use distancing tactics to maintain excessive professional distance (*see* Chapter 6—What is Appropriate Professional Distance?).

Cancer professionals

Professionals are people first, professionals second. Like anyone else, healthcare staff must balance the aspirations and responsibilities of their professional lives with those of their personal lives. Cancer care is inherently stressful and makes significant demands on the professional staff who work in it. Oncology and palliative medicine have become highly complex and technical at a medical level, but no less distressing at a personal level. Being faced daily with the mortality of others affords little refuge from looking at one's own.

Being compassionate and caring ultimately comes at a price. Too often the price is overtaxed healthcare staff who are emotionally drained and fearful for their own health. For example, in one sample of French nurses, nearly two-thirds admitted having persistent fears of developing cancer themselves.[8] Healthcare staff work with people at an extraordinarily vulnerable time in their lives and consequently are expected to be proficient at using a number of sophisticated interpersonal skills, whilst showing sensitivity to the emotional pain of their patients. But stress can also arise from a mismatch between what is expected of one's working life and what it turns out to be like.

Increasingly there is evidence that nurses, doctors, and radiation therapists (radiographers) suffer high levels of stress and burnout and an imbalance between their professional and personal lives. When people are stressed, their decision making is impaired, they more easily feel overwhelmed and become uncreative in their thinking and behaviour. When healthcare staff are burnt out, they are likely to respond to their distress by becoming emotionally distant from their patients, with obvious consequences for patient care. And people who are burnt out also frequently end up feeling dissatisfied with their performance which, in turn, increases their feelings of stress. When workplace stress goes unrecognized and unexpressed, people put up defences against it; they idealize their own roles, become manically driven by the demands of throughput, emotionally withdraw, or project their difficult feelings onto others (patients, colleagues, institutions, etc.).

In Chapter 1 we argued that change is stressful because it involves people having to alter their mental maps of the world. Change can be rejuvenating and refreshing when the results are seen to be positive and helpful, but when change is continuous, unrelenting, and ambiguous, fatigue and burnout are natural results. For decades professional staff working in the UK's National Health Service (NHS) have experienced the upheaval of repeated organizational restructuring with little time to consolidate changes before more have been introduced. In the United States, compared with non-health-related employees, healthcare workers also report less job satisfaction, support, autonomy, and role clarity.[9] Managed healthcare has meant less time for patients, while fewer and fewer healthcare staff are fired by enjoyment or satisfaction derived from their job. Efficiency and speed have edged out time for human contact and compassion; it is hard to establish a caring relationship with someone based on little more than a few minutes chat every few weeks. And factory work is ultimately monotonous.

Change within organizations and individuals is an inevitable fact of life, and often a positive one, but large changes which occur too rapidly for people to alter their internal maps are likely to meet with resistance. Just as the patient with cancer may use avoidance and denial to slow down the absorption of change, healthcare workers, like any others, will do what they can to retain continuity and coherence in their working lives. For change to be integrated with the least amount of stress, the same principles apply: adequate information, preparation, participation, achievable goals, and support.

Doctors

Society has high expectations of physicians and surgeons. As a society, we expect doctors to give their patients potentially life-saving treatments, and to intervene in people's bodies with scalpels, X-rays, hormones, and poisons. The achievement of scientific medicine in the face of such a wily and resistant disease as cancer is a testimony to man's creative intellect. But as Gjerløw has asked, 'will the brain continue to grow, and the heart shrink?'[10] The clinical application of all these impressive advances remains a stressful business, and stressed physicians are more likely to treat patients poorly, both medically and psychologically.[11, 12] Stress has a very negative effect on the accuracy of diagnostic decision making, quite apart from its impact on the quality of life and job satisfaction of doctors.[13]

Doctors generally suffer from higher levels of psychological distress, alcoholism, and depression than other segments of the working population.[12] In one small study of 76 hospital doctors a 'direct link' was found between the number of hours worked by doctors and their stress levels.[14] However, there was a difference in the profile of senior and junior doctors. Junior doctors felt a huge pressure to succeed in their careers and to be well regarded by their seniors in order to secure promotion. Senior doctors, who have higher status and more autonomy and control over work demands, reported less stress than their juniors but also felt less supported by colleagues.

One senior oncologist has described the anguish of having to break devastating news to their patients:

> I personally experience almost a physical pain at seeing a patient collapse with grief at the sudden understanding that soon they are going to die, and that any attempts are doomed to fail. But it's a responsibility that we as oncologists can't shirk.

Doctors face a number of increasing demands:[14]

- time constraints
- co-ordinating increasingly complex packages of care
- responding to the diverse and changing needs and concerns of their patients
- increasing administrative demands
- mounting clinical pressures to see more patients in less time
- needing to stay abreast of scientific and clinical developments
- having to tell people that they may be fatally ill
- having to administer treatments which not only make people more ill for a time but sometimes kill them
- conducting clinical research and inviting people to join clinical trials
- teaching junior medical staff
- clinically managing a team of staff.

Cancer medicine can be emotionally draining work and there is clearly a limit to the range of skills and roles we can expect doctors and surgeons to perform. Understandably, doctors often lack the 'management skills' to deal with such an unreasonably wide range of demands.[15] In fact, society probably expects too much of clinical cancer medicine in view of the limited time and resources it is given. Clinical oncologists in the UK annually see two and a half times more patients than their European or American counterparts,[16] leading to a particularly oppressive level of work overload. High demand, low control, and lack of social support at work are thought to be additive in their stressful effects,[17] similar to the way that multiple stresses in people with cancer increase their likelihood of psychosocial distress.

A high level of stress seems to be common among cancer doctors. Among a survey of 393 UK cancer doctors, 31% reported high levels of emotional exhaustion with 28% having distress scores indicative of a psychiatric disorder.[18] Factor analysis revealed four main issues:

- feeling overloaded and its effect on home life
- having organizational responsibilities/conflicts

- dealing with patients' suffering
- being involved with treatment toxicity and errors.

Interestingly, palliative care doctors reported the lowest levels of stress and burnout, perhaps because they tend to work in more close-knit multiprofessional teams, and have more time to care for their patients. This same survey also revealed that although dealing with patients' suffering is an important source of stress for cancer doctors, contact with patients and relatives, when done well, was also the most important source of job satisfaction. The authors noted that their study 'exemplifies the 'double-edged' nature of stress, according to which a task can be stressful if done badly, but rewarding if done well'[18] (Ramirez *et al.* 1995, p. 1268). It also highlights the importance of training in communication skills both to reduce the stress and to enhance the satisfaction of working with patients.[15] Ultimately, however, doctors need time to provide adequate supportive care.

There is little evidence about whether male and female doctors face different types of stress though, anecdotally, there seems to be an expectation from patients that female doctors will provide more time to attend to their emotional needs. It is also likely that female doctors often have to work harder than male doctors to engender the cooperation of their nursing colleagues.

Burnout among doctors

An American study of burnout among cancer doctors found that of the 598 respondents, 56% reported a degree of burnout in their professional lives.[19] Burnout appeared to be stronger among those with more patient care. The most widely cited reason for burnout was lack of sufficient personal and vacation time—once again, an imbalance between the professional and personal life. Furthermore, 53% said they felt that continuous exposure to fatal illness was a factor, describing their burnout as 'frustration or sense of failure'. A more recent American study found that house staff suffered the highest levels of burnout, more emotional exhaustion, and more emotional distance from their patients.[20] A French study of general practitioners found that over 80% felt a sense of failure, and one in two were reminded of their own mortality.[21]

What is the source of this high level of burnout? Consider some of the less visible stresses that cancer doctors chronically have to deal with:

- reconciling the first rule of medicine 'Do no harm' with the fact that so many cancer treatments cause unmitigated physical discomfort and distress;
- managing a personal sense of disappointment and failure in the face of a patient whose cancer has recurred, and loss when they have died;
- responding to an increasingly educated public (often thanks to the Internet), encouraged by news reports of cancer breakthroughs, when, realistically, what can be offered falls short of expectations;

• How should the doctor reconcile their wish to do their best for their patients with what they are told to do? Doctors are increasingly restrained by protocols from using their clinical judgement when faced with the evident uniqueness of each individual patient. As James McCormick has written,

> Guidelines derive from population studies and are not always applicable to the unique person who decides to consult. All might be well if guidelines were securely based and if they were perceived as giving advice rather than mandatory instruction. Unfortunately, many guidelines are insecurely based, and doctors, sometimes fearing medico-legal consequences, are motivated towards slavish adherence to them.[22]

Along with the loss of their individual clinical judgement comes the progressive lack of opportunity to establish any meaningful level of contact with patients. Hospital doctors in the UK are increasingly engaged in factory levels of throughput. Conveyor-belt medicine is not what most doctors expected from their careers. Like poor quality of life, stress in healthcare staff can be the result of a mismatch between what the professional wants to achieve and what they are able to do, given their existing time and resources: a mismatch of expectation and experience (*see* Chapter 1).

Unfortunately, the way doctors deal with the stress of cancer medicine is commonly counter-productive (e.g. drugs and alcohol).[12] Rather than standing together (e.g. to protect their own quality of life, or to argue alongside patients for better resources), doctors sometimes withdraw from one another and rely on their own strategies for coping. One such strategy is an addiction to work, 'workaholism', a manic defence in which the doctor achieves short-term rewards (the admiration of less active colleagues, self-worth obtained from high productivity, etc.) at the expense of personal stress and ultimate burnout.[15] Another strategy is emotional distance from patients and/or colleagues that may reduce emotional strain in the short-term but ultimately lead to poorer care, less job satisfaction, and less support from colleagues.

Managing stress

In managing stress, it is important to tackle both its causes and its effects. The causes of stress among cancer doctors are largely to do with the excessive and multiple demands on their time and resources and, not surprisingly, a lack of balance between their professional and personal lives. It seems that junior doctors are subject to more clinical pressures, a lack of clarity as to what is expected of them and a lack of recognition of their achievements. Senior doctors, by contrast, are more likely to find themselves with little or no access to support, and few opportunities to reflect on their clinical practice. These causes are not merely structural but embedded in the history and culture of medicine. Like patient-centred care, creating a 'person-centred work environment' is a significant unmet goal of modern medicine,[2] but tackling the effects of stress may require challenging something of the historical culture of medicine.

Balancing personal and professional life   As one might expect, one study has found that maintaining a 'balanced and healthy lifestyle' is associated with lower scores on a measure of 'psychiatric disturbance'.[23] In this survey of 882 UK hospital consultants vigorous exercise and involvement in hobby and leisure activities were two of the several 'coping strategies'. *Not* working long hours, and talking to family, friends, and colleagues were also found to help. Twenty-six per cent coped by drinking alcohol 'quite a lot'—a low figure in our anecdotal view though, alas, this group was associated with higher levels of mental health disturbance too.

Examining belief systems   The core beliefs and assumptions that doctors bring to their encounters with patients affect how they listen, interpret, and judge patients' stories and how they empathize with patients and support them.[24] In Chapter 1 we considered how every person's 'mental maps' of the world shape how they perceive and respond to events and other people. This is as true for doctors as it is for anyone else.

Doctors also commonly believe that:[25]

- lack of knowledge is a personal failing;
- doctors must bear responsibility on their own;
- one should be altruistically devoted to work and be prepared to deny one's own needs;
- to be 'professional' one must keep one's uncertainties and emotions to oneself.

A central question for doctors is therefore to do with how they see their role. If the personal vocation of medicine is primarily to cure disease then oncology may invoke feelings of frustration and failure when this aspiration is not achieved. Training in the palliative care of advanced illness is likely to help redress some of these concerns if the result is that doctors can sustain the sense that they have something valuable to offer.[19]

Assumptions, beliefs, and expectations are picked up throughout a person's life but they are rarely examined. For example, how does a doctor's role in their family of origin affect their role in relation to the patients and families they treat? How often do doctors have the opportunity to explore their cultural belief systems and how much do these beliefs affect their attitudes to a patient's ethnicity, race, gender, age, social class, and sexuality? Only regular periods of reflection are likely to elucidate these influences. However, by sharing these sort of beliefs and assumptions within routine case discussions, mutual trust is more likely to develop between members of the clinical team with the result that there is more support and understanding on hand for *any* member.

Support, recognition, and reflective practice   Social support at work is more effective at alleviating *work*-related stress than support derived from home.[14] Junior doctors are particularly prone to emotional strain, poor sleep, poor diet, and feelings of depression, and often they feel that their senior colleagues do not appreciate their good work.[26] General practitioners often face the death of patients they have known for years with little support from colleagues yet nearly 90% in one survey acknowledged that it is a source of personal suffering for them.[21] In fact, it seems that the culture of clinical medicine rarely acknowledges, praises, or supports colleagues but, on the contrary, is more preoccupied with issues of blame and litigation. Yet, on the whole, doctors are more than happy to give their support if a colleague approaches them for it.

Junior doctors with higher levels of distress also show higher levels of empathy, perhaps typifying the double-edged meaning of the word sensitivity. Those who protect themselves through maintaining a distance from their patients may derive less job satisfaction as a result of having patients who are less satisfied with their care. Those doctors who are more empathic, however, are also more affected by their work unless sufficient support and supervision are available. As others have argued, it is surely better to safeguard the latter type of doctor rather than promote the former.[26]

At least junior doctors seem to provide more support to one another, and may derive support from non-medical colleagues. Senior doctors are more at risk of stress because they lack the opportunity to talk through their decisions or the emotional impact of their work; their position of authority precludes any expression of doubt or vulnerability regarding the burdens they carry. It is natural for either senior or junior doctors to feel grief at the death of a patient for whom they have cared for many years, yet rarely is there a professional context in which this can be expressed or even acknowledged.

It is not easy for doctors to recognize when a patient triggers a personal issue in them, and even more difficult to learn how to let their own emotional reactions towards patients inform their judgements in a helpful way.[27] Systems of clinical supervision and case discussions, however, ensure that medical staff of all grades have confidential opportunities to explore their achievements, lack of knowledge, clinical difficulties, or emotional distress without fearing they will be judged or their professional image tarnished.

Perhaps it is a tall order in the pressured competitive climate of clinical medicine, but unless medical practitioners develop the trust to reflect openly about their work with one another, their feelings and fears are likely to go underground. The results are predictably defensive: psychologically tough doctors who are distant, intimidating, workaholic, alcoholic, or insensitive, with little support to and from their colleagues.[28] Until doctors learn to care for one another better, they will be forced to rely on their own ways of coping and the sad old adage 'Physician, heal thyself'.

Managing mistakes Only gods are infallible; human beings make mistakes. Yet with ever-increasing medical litigation, a medical culture of blame has developed. As the most senior member of the healthcare team, the onus is on the senior doctors and hospital managers to encourage a more supportive culture concerning mistakes. Where there is a culture of blame, people are more likely to conceal their ignorance or doubt, let alone mistakes they may have made. The manager may be angry at the subordinate who has made a mistake but no good is served by the subordinate being humiliated. While mistakes obviously need investigating to reveal their cause, those responsible for them may need considerable support as they prepare for the consequences. Regular team reviews of difficult clinical situations can create a safer, more supportive environment if the most senior members of the team are prepared to take the lead in sharing their doubts and errors with their colleagues. Similarly, patients are less likely to litigate if they learn about mistakes from their doctors openly and promptly, rather than discovering them through other sources at a later date.[29]

Nurses

Nurses represent the largest single professional group in oncology and are central to the care of people with cancer. Although the time patients spend in hospital has been reduced in recent years, they are often more ill and require more intensive specialized nursing.[30] Cancer nursing has also developed rapidly from being largely ward-based to embracing a plethora of roles (e.g. clinical nurse specialists working in palliative care or particular disease sites, or those specially trained to administer chemotherapy), while the support of district nurses in the community fulfils a vitally important role in cancer care.

By virtue of the high level of contact and the physically intimate nature of their care, many nurses form emotionally close relationships with their patients.[20] Therefore, not surprisingly, nurses are especially vulnerable to the emotional strain of caring, and can be particularly distressed when a person they have cared for dies. It is perhaps all the more distressing if the patient is young or the death sudden.[30] Fears of developing cancer themselves are also common among nursing staff,[8] and it is perhaps little wonder that newly qualified nurses working in cancer are an especially stressed group.[31]

Among all professional groups, nurses have one of the highest rates of suicide and psychiatric outpatient referrals.[1] The fact that most nurses are women is significant in light of the fact that employment tends to benefit the health of unmarried women more than married women.[32] Like doctors, general nurses seem to struggle with the balance between home and working life, with older nurses reporting more stress than younger ones, perhaps because of multiple additional commitments such as family and domestic responsibilities.[8, 33]

UK nurses, like their medical colleagues, have felt more stressed in recent years as a result of increased workload, staff shortages, and structural changes in the NHS.[30] Shorter hospital admissions, more patient throughput, and greater use of outpatient treatments have taken nurses away from bedside care. Instead, they are often required to administer painful, debilitating treatments in which small errors of judgement can have catastrophic consequences.[34] They have less time to provide emotional care which, for many, was their main calling or motivation for going into nursing.[8]

An American survey of 7301 self-selected nurses found that 65% believed there was less time for direct patient care, while less than 10% reported there was more time.[35] Seventy-five per cent of nurses believed that the quality of nursing care had declined over the previous two years. Importantly, half of those surveyed reported feeling 'exhausted and discouraged' on leaving work, and almost as many felt 'discouraged and saddened' by what they could not provide for their patients. In the context of such disillusionment and stress, it is perhaps not surprising that nurses have been found in some studies to show low levels of empathy.[36] While the nurse–patient relationship is held to be a cornerstone of healthcare, these trends have disturbing implications for patient care.

Managing stress

Alleviating the effects of stress is not as helpful in the long run as tackling its causes, but in the case of cancer nursing this is no simple matter. Cancer nursing is an inherently stressful job because it is about intensively caring for people who may be critically ill or dying. However, recruiting and retaining trained nurses in such a stressful area of medicine will always be challenging unless the stress of cancer nursing is first acknowledged.

Nursing often involves physical care that also requires sensitive communication skills so as to preserve the dignity of patients and to prevent unnecessary psychosocial distress. This emotionally draining aspect of nursing care needs to be acknowledged through the provision of adequate systems of support and clinical supervision.

The need of professionals to reflect on their belief systems and the assumptions they hold is as important for nursing staff as it is for doctors. In view of their central role in cancer patient care nurses need to be especially reflective about the cultural assumptions that they bring to their contact with patients. This is especially true regarding the intimate physical care that nurses provide which must always strive to be sensitive to the diverse cultural expectations of patients.

Management

Stress could be reduced, of course, if throughput were balanced by adequate resources (staffing levels, facilities, time, etc.), taking us back to the definition of stress (see page 365). Increasing nurses' sense of control over their work (autonomy and participation in decisions, etc.) can often help to reduce stress levels, although one must ensure that greater autonomy does not compromise the ability to obtain support. The way nurses work affects their levels of stress and job satisfaction. In primary nursing care, for example, nurses are usually assigned the care of specific patients. When working in this way, nurses report feeling more autonomy, less management control, and more involvement, cohesion, and support than do nurses organized in teams in which each member of staff has particular tasks to perform but no key worker role.[9]

Contact with employers also seems to affect job satisfaction. Among 106 ward-based UK nurses (of 340 who were approached), those with low job satisfaction tended to feel more anxious and depressed and often felt undervalued by their organization.[37] They reported low levels of contact with managers, a sense that their opinions were not sought on clinically relevant issues, as well as poor communication with other professionals. The combination of high effort and low rewards in terms of status and pay is a recipe for feeling undervalued. Flexible working schedules which accommodate childcare responsibilities are an obvious first step in creating a person-centred work environment for nurses.

Managements solutions must be tailored to the particular context, but a participative management style promotes a clearer, more innovative, and task-focused climate in which nurses feel their views are being heard and respected. Managers who are supportive, flexible, and responsive are exemplifying the style of communication that they wish to foster in their subordinates. The ideal is for information to flow smoothly up and down the nursing hierarchy.

Support

Historically, nurses have worked in teams which offer the potential for peer support. Most nurses do seem to use their colleagues for support provided ward managers create an atmosphere that encourages such emotional disclosure.[30] A lot of the time people informally find their own trusted 'soul-mates' within the organization, someone in whom to confide. However, while this is obviously to be encouraged it cannot be assumed that every member of the team has the support they need. A more structured approach in which there are regular opportunities to review clinical situations that have been confronted (perhaps including a consideration of the wider ethical issues) ensures that particularly distressing incidents are acknowledged, and those involved are offered support. This is also likely to reinforce a sense of team cohesion (*see* Teams).

Increasingly, nurses are being deployed in more peripatetic specialist roles such as clinical nurse specialists and nurse consultants, providing specialist skills, information, and support. Similarly, community nursing staff are often faced with making decisions of enormous responsibility with limited emotional or medical support. All these staff play a crucially important role in the psychosocial support of people with cancer. But while an increase in autonomy may have increased their job satisfaction, a reduction in peer support may have raised their stress levels. This needs research. In any event, it would seem prudent to ensure that specialist nurses, like any other isolated healthcare professionals, have regular opportunities to review their clinical work and caseload, and receive support for the more distressing aspects of their work (*see* Clinical Supervision).

Nurses sometimes feel that their medical colleagues leave them to manage some of the hardest tasks in cancer care: dealing with the aftermath of bad news, or caring for a dying patient. This lack of support raises the stress level of nursing staff by leaving them feeling unvalued and exploited.[8] Opportunities to review clinically complex or distressing events should include all relevant members of the healthcare team. A death on the ward should be acknowledged in the context of a staff meeting, preferably one that allows key healthcare workers to reflect on what occurred and air any residual feelings and ethical questions they may be left with. This encourages any misgivings about the patient's care to be voiced and addressed, rather than buried as a lingering resentment. While conflict with doctors may have diminished over the past few years, at least in Britain,[30] the nurse–doctor relationship remains an evolving one.

Radiographers

Therapy radiographers, or radiation therapists as they are known in the United States, form the third key professional group in cancer care. Given their importance, it is a mystery that so little has been written about them as a professional group.

Radiographers perform a technically skilled job that requires high level of accuracy. They work with dangerous ionizing radiation and must attend to stringent safety measures. Their working conditions are rarely pleasant in that radiotherapy departments are usually underground and devoid of natural light, a small but important added stress that most people would prefer to avoid. Historically, radiographers have had relatively little autonomy over the treatments they administer which are largely prescribed by doctors, and they have little control over the rate of patient throughput. However, they usually work in teams where there is the opportunity for good mutual support.

Radiographers frequently have daily contact with patients over many weeks, affording them a rare opportunity to develop excellent relationships with their patients and to monitor their psychosocial and physical concerns over time. For other patients, radiographers provide shorter but no less valuable palliative treatments. Radiographers derive a lot of their job satisfaction from caring for patients. However, increasing demands for ever greater throughput challenge the radiographer's ability to perform their highly technical role without compromising their caring relationship to patients. Many radiographers are under pressure to spend less time per patient and, as the quality of the overall care they give deteriorates, they consequently feel decreasing job satisfaction and more symptoms of burnout.

Like nurses, the majority of radiographers are female. Although little evidence is available, it is likely that the positive association between age and stress level found among nurses holds true for radiographers. That is, as women get older they are required to juggle the multiple and increasing pressures of their home and working lives.

The limited evidence that exists suggests that, as a professional group, radiographers experience high levels of stress and burnout, even higher than those of nursing staff.[38] In an American study of 603 radiation therapists (only 50% of those who were sent questionnaires), over half reported high levels of emotional exhaustion: feeling depleted or drained of emotional resources, overextended and exhausted by their work. About 45% were characterized as having developed negative, callous, or cynical attitudes towards their patients, even though over 40% continued to maintain high professional self-esteem. Once again, workload was a major source of stress.

Managing stress

Radiotherapy departments probably vary as much as the individuals who work within them, and each should be assessed as to its own sources of stress and burnout. However, certain issues should be routinely considered. Working patterns should be flexible enough to enable people to balance work commitments with family responsibilities. A balance must be struck between the need for efficiency of throughput, with the need to maintain a caring clinical environment in which radiographers can also obtain personal job satisfaction. Task variety and change helps to ensure that radiotherapy staff do not become bored or stagnant. Like nurses, radiographers need to feel that their clinical opinions are acknowledged and taken seriously and that their role within the organization is valued. Mutual support between radiographers should be encouraged and time made available for this.

Other healthcare professionals

Physiotherapists, speech and language therapists, occupational therapists, social workers, psychologists, psychiatrists and counsellors, and other professionals are important, if less numerous, players in cancer care. Although there is a dearth of research on the stress faced by these allied healthcare professionals, their peripatetic and often professionally isolated roles within cancer care can lead them to *feel* more peripheral or less valued than their medical, nursing, and radiotherapy colleagues.

Due to their small number, these professionals sometimes find it difficult to feel part of any one team if their work is divided among several teams. Consequently they may find it harder to influence organizational decisions and must often obtain support from colleagues within their own profession who may have limited knowledge of the clinical and organizational pressures they face. Allied healthcare professionals also work in response to the unpredictable demands of their cancer colleagues and therefore have little control over work demands, though this may be balanced by greater autonomy over the work they do.

Most of these professionals have intense personal contact with their patients, often involving matters of deep emotional concern. The one-to-one nature of much of their work provides safe conditions for intimate topics to be discussed and, as a result, they are frequently exposed to the myriad powerful feelings experienced by patients and their families. Lacking the support of a wider team, these staff are likely to be particularly vulnerable to emotional fatigue.

Medical secretaries, receptionists, and porters

It would be unwise to overlook the importance of the many ancillary staff who also have frequent contact with patients: secretaries, receptionists, porters, and catering and cleaning staff. These staff members often represent a valuable source of information and support for patients and their families, and all are subject to the same emotional reactions as their professional colleagues when a patient they have known dies, or the person they are speaking to is in distress. Rarely are these staff groups given training and support for this aspect of their roles, yet they too may be facing highly stressful jobs. Frequently they have a heavy workload with little control over its flow, low status, poor pay, and little recognition.

Managers and staff teams can help by acknowledging the contribution of these staff to the overall service and include them as much as possible in staff training and social events. The 'trojan horse' of an occasional training session in communication skills can be an opportunity to engage ancillary staff in conversations about difficult experiences they have had and the different stresses they face.

Preventing burnout and reducing stress

Face-to-face contact with distressed patients is an inevitable source of emotional strain for oncology healthcare staff, but its stressful effects should at least be minimized and addressed. Healthcare managers need to encourage their staff to develop ways of sustaining their ability to care, rather than becoming emotionally detached and distant as a way of coping. They should also ensure that professionals have sufficient opportunities to 'off-load' their stress while in the workplace rather than allow it to accumulate or be taken home.

Management strategies to prevent burnout

- Provide new staff working in cancer care settings with an induction training that emphasizes self-care and the responsibility of individual staff member to raise concerns about their own levels of stress.
- Provide training for all staff in the psychosocial aspects of cancer care. By developing expertise in communication skills, professionals feel more confident and competent at handling difficult emotional situations.[39]
- Clarify the parameters of what is expected in each person's role so as to reduce stressful ambiguity within jobs (where does the job end?) and between professionals (respect for different professional roles).
- Encourage staff to balance the demands of their work and personal lives so as to reduce feelings of guilt in the context of heavy work demands. Among other things, caseload management, for example, can ensure that professionals take proper lunch breaks and go home on time, etc.
- Allow people areas of autonomy and responsibility within their work so as to promote creativity, innovation, and personal commitment. Having a diversity of roles also helps to sustain interest (e.g. opportunities for research).
- Provide opportunities for further training and personal development.
- Encourage participation in organizational decision making to ensure that staff feel a sense of control and that their voice will be heard.
- Create a mutually supportive workplace in which staff are encouraged and given the time to talk about and reflect on their work. Enable emotional concerns to be aired and worked through rather than suppressed. This can occur in a number of forums: informal contacts, case discussions, team meetings, clinical supervision, etc.

A work environment that does not acknowledge the implicit stress of cancer care is more likely to promote a culture of emotional detachment, distance, and lack of support between staff. If emotional distress is not expressed it is likely to go underground. By contrast, a workplace culture that encourages staff to talk through difficult clinical experiences and mutually support one another is one which enables professionals to remain emotionally involved in their work, while continuing with other fulfilling areas of their lives.[40]

Strategies to reduce stress in healthcare

Like burnout, it is far better to reduce stress in the workplace by anticipating and preventing it, than by having to react to a crisis.

(i) **Be aware of your own feelings** It is hard to predict when patients or family members will trigger powerful emotional reactions. You may find yourself identifying with a particular patient because they remind you of an important figure from your past, someone currently important to you, or even an aspect of yourself. Such feelings can be difficult to understand because they are implicitly or unconsciously held. You may feel angry towards a patient for no apparent reason, upset by them, or want to rescue them, or find yourself feeling over-involved, bored, or coldly detached. The point to note is whether you can explain these feelings in view of what has occurred between you or whether they have arrived 'out of the blue', or are out of proportion to the situation. Clinical supervision is an ideal forum in which to unearth and understand these feelings (see below), often to the benefit of patient care.

(ii) **Be aware of your stress level** Keep a mental tally of how your work pressures rise and fall. Consider the list of stress symptoms at the beginning of this chapter with a view to becoming aware of when you are becoming generally over-stressed. Some sources of stress are obvious and inevitable, such as when a ward team has to manage a number of deaths over a short period, but others may be more obscure, such as when a patient is angry and hostile, or when on top of work pressures your own children are unwell. How do you feel at the end of the day? How much time do you think about your work when you are not there? How much time do you think about particular patients when you are not at work? If demands are becoming intolerable, speak to supervisors and colleagues. Maintaining a macho image of unyielding vigour and determination is ultimately self-defeating and potentially damaging to patients.

At an organizational level, it may be helpful to conduct a stress audit of a particular staff group to determine the levels and sources of stress. A number of paper and pencil tests are available to measure both stress[41,42] and burnout.[7] Engaging all parties to discuss the findings and to suggest solutions can promote a sense of team cohesion and participation.

(iii) **Be aware of stress in other members of the team** Support among professional colleagues needs to be reciprocal. When healthcare staff show concern for their colleagues and the stresses they have been dealing with in their professional and personal lives, everyone benefits. Furthermore, while no one is exempt from stress, some people are more isolated from support than others. Senior members of the medical team, hospital managers, secretaries, and porters may all experience stress in their workplace yet may feel inhibited about asking for support. A little extra concern for your colleagues reaps long-term rewards in the form of a more supportive workplace.

(iv) **Maintain the boundary between work and home life**   To be involved with cancer care involves a level of personal commitment to the intrinsic value of the work. Patients' needs *are* important and, while professionals are at work, they become their pre-eminent concern. However, the pressures of work can easily assume an almost moral imperative that edges out the 'selfish' needs of the individual professional. But to care for others effectively, healthcare professionals need to be sufficiently cared for themselves; maintaining a loving, happy, and stimulating home life is therefore as important as having a fulfilling and successful career. Try to prevent 'spillage' between personal and professional life by sticking to clear boundaries between the two (taking a proper lunch break, going home on time as much as possible, not taking work home, and so on).

(v) **Be aware of your sources of support**   Ideally, access to support should be a continuous feature of everyone's working life but, at stressful times, it is particularly helpful to be aware of your main sources of support. Talking about your experiences is a powerful way of integrating them with your own mental maps of the world (*see* Chapter 1), while at the same time dissipating their emotional impact. However, be aware of the difference between talk that relieves stress and complaining that reinforces it.

Be clear who you feel comfortable talking with on an informal basis and seek them out at moments of high stress, while not forgetting to reciprocate at other times. If possible, formalize this contact into regular meetings to discuss issues arising from your caseload and other work pressures.

Staff support groups are an option for teams who have the time, but they need to meet sufficiently frequently to feel relevant, and generally work best when led by someone external to the team who can provide the safety of structure and boundaries. However, a team leader can show concern for staff by arranging an impromptu meeting in response to an especially distressing incident or series of incidents.

An accessible option is to incorporate a supportive element into frequent team meetings. In the context of discussing clinical material, the team leader can introduce more general topics of relevance to everyone: how was the incident handled, how could care have been improved, how did it leave people feeling (especially those most involved), and are there ethical questions to be considered? By encouraging people to support one another in this way, the team leader promotes a non-blaming team culture in which mistakes can be openly discussed and rectified.

(vi) **Clinical supervision**   Clinical supervision is a particular form of staff support that also fulfils another important aim of professional healthcare: ensuring that the individual is practising at an appropriate level of expertise. It is therefore best done by someone within your own profession, though other professionals can sometimes be excellent substitutes. Staff of the same or a different grade can give supervision, provided the supervisor is clear as to the purpose of their role, and provided the person being supervised (and their patients) remains the central focus of attention.[43]

Clinical supervision is not management supervision but an opportunity for any professional to reflect on their primary skills as well as the broader pressures they are facing. It focuses on helping the receiver reflect on their clinical practice and explore alternative decision options, while receiving acknowledgement for tasks well done. It can involve learning to recognize blind spots and areas of difficulty, identifying unexamined assumptions brought to the work, discussing ethical doubts, or strong feelings about particular patients. At a more sophisticated level, clinical supervision can help healthcare staff use their emotional reactions to patients as a valuable additional source of information. Not surprisingly, this opportunity to talk through and integrate recent experiences is not only validating and supportive, but time well spent. Such reflective practice promotes self-regulation or corrective feedback. Yet although clinical supervision offers advantages in both quality control and staff support, it is still quite rare in many areas of healthcare.

(vii) **Staff appraisals and professional development** Formal appraisals by managers are valuable opportunities to identify sources of stress, provide feedback, and consider remedial action. They also enable staff to clarify ambiguous elements of their role and to set achievable targets to aim for. Managers can use this opportunity to acknowledge and praise the individual's work while helping to develop their range of skills through suggesting new initiatives: training courses, taking on different clinical roles, teaching, research, management, etc. Continuing professional development not only enables professional staff to stay up-to-date with clinical and academic knowledge, it also breathes the energy of fresh ideas into clinical practice that may have become tired and stale.

(viii) **Learn to dissipate the effects of stress** The option of relaxation may sound absurd as an antidote to stress when it merely constitutes the polar opposite. It is like saying that the best cure for being ill is to get well. In fact, there is more to it than this. Learning to relax may be a largely symptomatic response to stress but few people are aware of the ambient physical tension they carry with them from one situation to the next. It is the chronic nature of stored physical tension that seems to lead to many illnesses, so mastering the skills of releasing stored muscle tension can bring wide-ranging health benefits. People spontaneously release their bottled-up stress through talking, laughter, crying, and anger, while sport and physical exercise also carry additional health benefits.[44]

Forms of relaxation (meditation, yoga, etc.) have been used within a number of cultures for thousands of years, yet only relatively recently (Jacobson in 1929[45]) has Western medicine made scientific use of relaxation exercises as a natural antidote to stress. A number of different relaxation techniques exist (progressive muscle relaxation, autogenic training, biofeedback, meditational techniques such as mindfulness),[46] but their essence involves the subject learning how to release muscle tension and breathe more calmly so as to reduce autonomic arousal, while finding some 'psychological peace' through focusing on particular words or scenes. Cognitive techniques provide a more complete picture by focusing on the many ways people mentally amplify the pressures they face (*see* Chapter 6—Clarifying and Challenging Assumptions) and their behavioural responses to them.

For a simple example, think about how you are holding your body as you read these words. Which muscles are tensed and, importantly, which do not need to be tense (perhaps your shoulders or your arms)? Try to let these muscles relax. This simple measure, if repeatedly practised at different times throughout the day, can lead people to become more aware of the ambient stress they carry around with them and to release it as they feel it. After several weeks training, the body and brain learn to stay more generally relaxed.

Team functioning

Groups of people are powerful at influencing the individuals within them, so another approach to staff stress is to consider how the healthcare team functions as a whole. All healthcare teams are bound by the tasks and rules of the institution, and structured around hierarchies created by those in authority.[47] Leadership ensures that institutional systems enable members of the healthcare team to deliver their work effectively, efficiently, and to a high standard. But 'authority' in healthcare settings can sometimes be ambiguous, leading to potential conflict. Is it with the clinical team leader (frequently a senior doctor), one's professional head, or the institution's management team?

Cancer care is undoubtedly a mixture of triumphs and losses. The 'contagion' of distress from patient to professional is probably intrinsic to the work. Cancer care touches the professional's underlying fears, beliefs and behaviour, and probably their relationships with *their* loved ones. These powerful feelings (anxiety, loss, conflict) can be 'acted out' in the dynamics of working relationships.[48] For example, an observational study of a hospice[49] noted how dying patients were essentially isolated in single rooms behind closed doors while the communal areas of the hospice were empty. The emotional distress of dying was 'shuttered off' by the staff who, feeling helpless to prevent the inevitable, maintained a 'stoical brightness'. In other words, the distress of healthcare staff can be unconsciously expressed through 'blocking' practices that soon become institutionalized. It is beyond the scope of this book to explore these issues further, other than to note their importance.

Team working is based on the idea that by collaborating, team members with different professional skills are able to provide comprehensive and seamless care. The reality invariably drifts from this simple ideal. A diversity of perspectives within the team inevitably leads to some degree of conflict; team members not only have allegiances to the team but to their professional standpoint too.[50] For example, in the past nurses have complained that doctors leave them to care for patients in pain without adequate analgesia.[30] Their more continuous contact with patients meant that this was a significant source of stress for nurses. In fact, these previous conflicts between nurses and doctors seem to have decreased, perhaps as a result of doctors' improved knowledge and prescribing of palliative interventions for pain and symptom control.[30]

Of course, different perspectives also offer the potential for more creative discussions and decision making. Team collaboration implies a common understanding of healthcare goals, a common language, and a mutual understanding and respect between professionals with regard to each other's roles and areas of expertise. In other words, a well-functioning team develops a 'shared model' of its resources and purpose. Of course, every team in reality is active, fluid, and constantly changing so if it is to maintain a shared model, it must be able to reflect upon and review the assumptions on which the shared model is based. Teams, therefore, need to be self-reflective and adaptive about the ways they are functioning—constantly exploring different approaches to patient care.[50]

A successful and well-functioning team demonstrates:

A clear sense of leadership The aim of team leadership is to help the team to function effectively and supportively. It is not primarily one of control; authoritarian leaders only betray their anxiety. The style of the clinical or management team leader sets the tone for the rest of the team so all leaders should try to model what they expect from the rest of the team.

Contact and communication If there is limited contact between team members they will feel less comfortable communicating with one another. Frequent formal and informal contact helps to break down barriers and enables team members to support one another.

Opportunities to review its objectives, aims, and means of functioning Does the team have opportunities to consider its core goals and principles and the ethical principles guiding them? How does the team handle complicated issues of confidentiality? Is the team organized appropriately? Are members clear about one another's roles? Without clear role boundaries, there is scope for confusion, duplication, and omission. For example, one study revealed that the specialist breast care nurse was playing an 'unseen' role of having significant discussions of diagnosis and treatments with patients, while others in the team assumed her contact was more focused on psychosocial concerns.[51]

Respect for different perspectives Do team members really work together as a multidisciplinary team in which all perspectives are valued and respected, or is only lip-service paid to this ideal, with one or two people's views dominating and intimidating others? Does conflict between people within the team feel dangerous or is there a willingness to entertain a diversity of opinions?

Part 2

User-involvement

There has been a cultural shift in UK healthcare in recent decades. Healthcare is no longer simply seen as a service provided by professionals to patients, but one in which consumers increasingly commission and define the services they expect to get. In the United States, where market forces have long dominated healthcare, people who can afford healthcare are free in principle to shop around. By contrast, European healthcare has tended to be more co-ordinated within state welfare programmes, in which there is frequently less scope for choice and less consumer power. The cultural shift towards greater user-involvement in healthcare largely began in mental health services and took root when in the late 1980s and 1990s AIDS activists questioned the priorities of clinical research and practice.

The problem for any institution and individual is that particular ways of doing things quickly become habitual, 'the way things are done', the norm. The well-worn grooves of thinking and behaviour become ruts that are hard to transcend. The systems and relationships within a service or institution powerfully affect the atmosphere of the institution and the quality of care given, but rarely are there opportunities to reflect on these issues or the stresses faced by healthcare staff. To reflect on these issues is implicitly to invite change, and as described in Chapter 1, change is seen as stressful and threatening because it involves revising one's core assumptions and mental maps of the world. Consequently, institutionalized practices often go unchallenged, and the stresses faced by cancer patients (and, indeed, the staff caring for them) often go unrecognized.

User-involvement is the process of involving service users to help shape the way healthcare is delivered. Ultimately, user-involvement represents a continuum from the individual level of patient-centred care in which each patient's needs define the care and treatment they receive, to a more organizational or systemic level in which healthcare users (e.g. current or ex-patients, family members, general public, etc., depending on the context) advise on how services should be delivered. Whether at the individual patient care level or at the level of service development, the issue essentially becomes one of communication.

It is worth listing a few of the benefits of user-involvement:

- Feedback from patients and relatives about how they experience cancer services can reveal whether these services are organized for the convenience of professionals or service users. What are service users most happy and unhappy about regarding the services they have received? Are professionals perhaps adhering to institutionalized ways of doing things, or should other methods or systems be considered? User-involvement can lead to more sensitive and supportive healthcare, and can therefore be a lever for change.

- By involving not just patients but representatives of the wider community, gaps in services can be identified. For example, do healthcare practices and services reflect the diverse needs and wishes of patients and families in the served community: minority ethnic communities, the disabled, young and elderly people, those with drug and alcohol addictions, etc.?

- Enabling health service managers to make purchasing and allocation decisions on the basis of the perceptions and priorities of consumers in the community, not merely those of professionals, gives their decisions more democratic legitimacy. The same argument can be applied to lay involvement in setting healthcare research agendas.[52]

- Ensuring that services meet the real needs of people with cancer, rather than what professionals perceive these needs to be. Professionals work in their own particular area and therefore often have their own limited snapshot view of the patient's experience, with little knowledge of processes that extend over time (e.g. rehabilitation needs after treatment has ended). Issues like continuity of care, while important to users, may be invisible to professionals. In other words, what may seem like progress to the professional may seem like a backward step to the patient or their family.

The rationale and aims of a user-involvement project must be clearly defined and followed through. Frequently, the involvement of healthcare consumers is a single one-off activity that fails to engage participants throughout the entire cycle of identifying an issue, exploring options for resolving it, piloting a solution, and auditing the results. User-involvement may help to keep institutions healthy and honest but the involvement of users can be seen as unhelpful criticism if staff are also not involved, or not given the resources to carry out the changes that are needed. Unless professionals are engaged on equal terms in the process from the outset, they risk feeling undermined by the resulting decisions rather than party to them. Similarly users often find it intimidating to discuss healthcare services with professionals unless they are given training and support throughout the process (and have their time and travel costs paid for).

The tools of user-involvement should be appropriate to the questions they seek to address.[53] They range from focus groups, public meetings, in-depth qualitative interviews, running a workshop, a Delphi survey,[54] questionnaire sampling studies, and so on. Multiple approaches are often desirable. Likewise the participants of a user-involvement project should be as diverse as possible and include both users (current, past, and potential), healthcare providers, and institutional managers as well as sometimes family members, carers, support groups, lobby groups, voluntary and charitable organizations, community organizations (e.g. religious and ethnic), and hard-to-reach or marginalized groups such as the homeless.

Voluntary support

A growing number of voluntary self-help organizations offer support to people with cancer in the community. Between 1988 and 1992 the number of cancer support groups in the UK increased by nearly 30%.[55] Sixty per cent of all groups were started by someone with cancer in order to offer mutual support to other people coping with the disease. Voluntary support groups generally offer emotional support in the form of group meetings or one-to-one listening and befriending, telephone support, some form of information library, home and hospital visiting, and social activities.

In view of the growing number of long-term cancer survivors, voluntary self-help groups offer a potentially powerful form of community support. Yet, for all their potential, voluntary groups remain relatively little used by people with cancer, at least in the UK, and are sometimes derided as amateur or regarded with suspicion by healthcare staff.

Many volunteers are ex-patients who, having survived cancer, are motivated to 'give something back'. Some people may even be driven by their memory of the poor care and support they received at the time of their illness, but in our experience there is rarely any wish to criticize or undermine the healthcare that new members of the voluntary group may be receiving. Indeed, the survey mentioned above found that the majority of groups were keen to obtain the support and involvement of professionals. In particular, they were anxious for their group to be known more widely so that they could support and inform new patients. Healthcare professionals can therefore help community support groups by distributing their information in healthcare settings. Conversely, by liaising with voluntary support groups, professionals not only discover what local support groups are doing, they can also positively influence their practices by encouraging a few principles of care (e.g. confidentiality, never undermining a patient's medical care, not becoming emotionally over-involved, etc.) and providing some rudimentary training (e.g. listening skills, problem-solving, etc.). Excellent 'good practice' guides, aimed at both people affected by cancer and health professionals, now exist on the setting up and running of a group.[56] Increasingly, voluntary organizations in the UK are involved in commenting on local cancer services. In a CancerLink national survey published in 2000, half the groups had already been involved and over 80% of groups were keen to contribute to 'user-involvement' initiatives[57].

Volunteers are also commonly deployed in healthcare settings, though rarely are they cancer survivors. However, in one UK regional cancer hospital the information and support centre is staffed exclusively by ex-patient volunteers and carers.[58] This sends an important message to newly diagnosed patients, providing a source of hope and inspiration. It also provides them with support from people who know from first-hand experience something of what the patient or carer is going through. In this centre, volunteers must be at least a year beyond the end of their treatment, must be carefully vetted, and must undergo a six-day training programme which also serves to screen out people who are either unsuitable or not ready to provide support to others. Their travel expenses are paid in full. At the end of each session worked, volunteers are expected to receive clinical supervision from the paid co-ordinator, herself an ex-cancer patient. By blurring the distinction between volunteers, patients, and professionals, and trying to overcome an 'us-and-them' mentality, a more relaxed form of communication is possible. This can also lead to an informal type of user-involvement in which professional staff are able to discuss 'off-the-record' service development ideas with volunteers, and volunteers can offer their valuable perspective and feedback about services.

Complementary therapy and alternative medicine

A review of the evidence for complementary therapy and alternative medicine is considerably beyond the scope of this book, but we wish to acknowledge this increasingly important factor in cancer care. The use of complementary therapies by members of the public, including people with cancer, has grown consistently over the past quarter century in both Europe and North America.[59, 60] In 1998 a survey of 1023 women with breast cancer in south London found that a third of them had visited a complementary therapist since their diagnosis.[61] Over 70% of breast cancer patients in one small American study published in 2002 reported using at least one form of unorthodox treatment in the two to three years following their surgery, while two people in the study had used at least 10 forms of treatment.[62] Furthermore, a 1992 survey of hospices in central England revealed that 70% offered massage and aromatherapy services.[63] A national survey of 65 000 cancer patients in the UK, conducted in 2000, found that 12% of women and 4% of men had used a complementary or alternative treatment for their condition.[64]

Any discussion of complementary therapy and alternative medicine is unfortunately dogged by confusing terminology and lack of clarity. Modern biomedical healthcare, for example, is described as 'orthodox' or 'conventional', while a number of complementary and alternative approaches refer to themselves as 'traditional medicines'. Should acupuncture be considered an unorthodox treatment when, for example, 1300 medically qualified doctors are members of the British Medical Acupuncture Society,[59] and it is based on practices that stretch back 3500 years? Should relaxation therapy be considered a complementary therapy when its therapeutic value has been scientifically established by psychologists in numerous studies since the 1930s?

More importantly, it can be difficult for people with cancer to choose an appropriate treatment from the plethora of unconventional treatments available: reflexology, aromatherapy, Reiki, homeopathy, Yoga, visualization, acupressure, massage, herbalism, naturopathy, dietary supplements, healing, crystal therapy, iridology, etc. How can one be sure that the treatment is safe, and that the practitioner is properly qualified, in view of the paucity of regulatory bodies and the absence of disinterested third party advice?[60] Healthcare staff are usually no better informed than their patients, so often they find it uncomfortable when asked for their advice on such matters.[65] Fortunately sound information is gradually becoming available.[66]

There are several probable reasons why complementary therapies and alternative medicines are so popular, quite apart from the particular treatment method used.

To describe these as non-specific is in no way to detract from their importance. In fact, they highlight many of the shortcomings of modern healthcare practice.

- Most complementary therapies are delivered in a client-centred way, with sufficient time to draw the individual's wider needs and concerns into the discussion. The presenting problem is not considered in isolation but in the context of the person's unique life history and social context.

- Treatments are perceived as gentle and frequently tailored to the individual.

- The client is fully informed about what the treatment involves (though not always what it aims to achieve), and is encouraged to retain control and be a full and active participant in their own care.

- Health is considered more than the absence of disease. *Holistic* care includes consideration of a person's mind, body, and spirit, often using their own resources to regain a healthy balance in their lives.

- By focusing on spiritual concerns too, the complementary therapist, like any good therapist, enables people to explore the meaning of events as they gradually rethread them into their life narratives. The relatively long consultations that clients are usually given enable them to feel their concerns have been heard and acknowledged.

- Complementary therapies often provide clients with a model or rationale by which to understand their condition and the intervention being proposed.

- Finally, the practice of complementary therapies also frequently involves a strong element of physical contact between practitioners and patients, thus tapping into a potentially powerful, though much underused resource: human touch.

In fact, the central philosophical tenets of many complementary approaches are very similar to those of psychosocial oncology and palliative care. They share a belief that each person is unique, that people have creative and spiritual needs as well as physical and psychological ones, that people need a sense of meaning and purpose in their lives, and that illness also represents an opportunity for positive change.[67] Little wonder that complementary therapies are often very successful in restoring a sense of hope, control, and purpose to people's lives, the very things this book is advocating and which are currently too often absent in conventional medicine.

However, despite the recent adoption of the acronym CAM to denote both complementary and alternative medical approaches, there may be some benefit in retaining the former distinction whereby complementary therapies are defined as *additional* but *in harmony* with orthodox medical treatments, and alternative medicines are defined as *substitutes* for them. This distinction is particularly important in the context of life-threatening illness. Unless their quite different aims are distinguished from one another there is a danger that they will become confused by patients and professionals alike.

There is an ethical difference between those who purport to save or prolong life with merely 'anecdotal evidence' to support their claim, and those who offer a complementary therapy with the aim of improving quality of life or alleviating particular symptoms. People who offer any form of treatment are ethically obliged to be able to demonstrate its effectiveness using methods that are falsifiable by others. But this obligation is surely more pressing for those who recommend an alternative to orthodox medical treatments, which have accrued rigorous scientific evidence as to their efficacy.[65]

Complementary therapies often share a similarly limited evidence base to that of alternative medicine, but when their explicit and unambiguous aims are to control unpleasant symptoms and enhance quality of life, they are at worst ineffective and in most cases benign. In fact, there appears to be growing evidence that some forms of complementary therapy do indeed improve quality of life and reduce symptoms such as pain and nausea (acupuncture), anxiety (massage), and mild depression (St John's wort).[67] Despite claims to the contrary, however, there is little evidence that conventional research methods are inappropriate for the evaluation of complementary therapies and alternative medicine[68] though, equally, potential researchers in these areas may well find it more difficult to attract adequate research funding.

The final choice of treatment of course belongs to the patient, but if patients feel that their doctor is indifferent or hostile to their interest in complementary and alternative approaches, they are less likely to disclose them.[69] This may have damaging long-term effects on their communication and relationship. Healthcare professionals should therefore start the discussion from the patient's frame of reference, helping them to reflect on their beliefs and values regarding the source and nature of the treatment they desire.[65] An insistence on a scientific, evidence-based paradigm may be counterproductive and inhibit discussion.[69] Starting with such a polarized view is no more helpful than 'holistic fundamentalism'.[70] Rather, it is preferable to help the patient clarify the aims of treatment (e.g. cure vs. care) before moving on to a discussion of particular interventions that may help (whether orthodox or unconventional).

However, the ethical principles that apply in conventional medicine are equally applicable in unconventional settings, and healthcare professionals should not feel the need to abandon these in discussing any proposed treatment.[65]

Informed consent

A lack of clarity about treatment aims (to cure cancer or prolong life vs. improving quality of life) continues to afflict some areas of complementary therapy, sustaining the suspicion among healthcare staff in orthodox settings that practitioners of such therapies are misleading patients and their families by offering false hope. Clarity of purpose is core to the ethic of informed consent and this same ethic must apply to complementary therapies and alternative medicine.

In the face of the knowledge that one's cancer is incurable it is understandable that many people look beyond established scientific medicine. In such desperate circumstances, alternative practitioners are seen as confidently offering a way to keep one alive. Some may even rekindle the hope of an ultimate cure. The problem can be reduced to one of communication. Conventional medicine has been criticized for a lack of honesty towards cancer patients in the face of direct questions about the curability and prognosis of the disease. Providing false hope without evidence is unethical, and so is the insinuation of cure or increased survival. If this same test were applied to alternative therapies, should they not have the same ethical duty as orthodox medicine, to offer falsifiable evidence for their claims?

Unless communication is crystal clear, even complementary therapists may sound as if they have magical cures. Terms like 'remedy' and 'healing' can be particularly confusing and misleading in this regard. Too often the message is simply ambiguous: 'Regaining balance leads to healing'; 'We will help you learn that you can strengthen your immune system and enhance your potential for recovery.'[59]

Guilt and responsibility

A number of complementary therapies and alternative practitioners stress the fact that the way people look after their bodies and the way they behave influences their health and survival. This emphasis on self-healing has been described as a 'two-edged sword.'[67] It can enable patients to feel a sense of control, independence, and self-esteem by giving them an active role in 'fighting' their disease. But it can also leave people with an unfair burden of individual responsibility for their health,[71] and a deep sense of guilt and self-contempt when their illness does not improve or they sustain a recurrence of their disease. Are they not trying hard enough? Have they failed to eat the right things? Or have they simply not been good enough people? This insidious and dishonest message is a terrible legacy for people to die with.

Spiritual abuse

Tim Sheard has noted that spiritual deprivation is often to be found in orthodox biomedical cancer care with its apparently exclusive preoccupation with the body.[72] However, he also coined the term 'spiritual abuse' to refer to the practice of leading people in a vulnerable state of need to become spiritual devotees. Faced with bewildering uncertainty people with cancer, especially those whose disease is incurable, can be easily mesmerized into believing that a particular, often 'ancient' wisdom is within reach and that only their blind faith is required for their salvation. '*People desperate for a cure and in existential turmoil are very vulnerable to taking on new belief systems if that is the price of hope. In extreme forms this can be an abuse through the prescriptive adoption of a new world view which takes people away from their authentic selves, autonomy and wholeness*' (Sheard 1994, p. 2).[72]

Colluding with denial

Complementary therapists can often help people restore their sense of control, self-esteem, meaning, and hope. However, like orthodox healthcare staff, they must be careful to avoid clouding the purpose of their interventions, especially as the disease progresses. The unwavering pursuit of balance and harmony within the mind, body, and spirit can overshadow some of the more difficult emotions that people may also be experiencing as they face the possibility, and especially the prospect, of their death. Anger, regret, fear, and sadness. Colluding with the denial of these 'negative' but nonetheless important feelings, in deference to 'positive thinking' for example, can delay or thwart the individual's adjustment.[67]

There is no reason that complementary therapies should not conform to the same ethical standards of care expected of orthodox healthcare, and in many instances they do. Complementary therapies are gradually establishing more regulatory bodies to oversee and monitor their practitioners. No doubt these bodies will also look to the supervision and emotional support of their practitioners. Such moves are to be welcomed because with regulation comes the development of standards of care and the prospect of evaluation. Until more evidence has accrued, scientists need to keep an open mind about complementary therapies but, conversely, complementary therapists need to expose their practices to the scrutiny of others.

The fact that increasing numbers of patients are turning to complementary therapies suggests a dissatisfaction with the care they obtain in conventional healthcare settings. By integrating complementary therapies into routine cancer care, professionals may be in a better position to help complementary practitioners establish the value of their interventions, while ensuring that they conform to common ethical standards. Finally, rather than patients having to go elsewhere for their needs to be met, there may be much that professionals can learn by integrating complementary therapies within healthcare services.[73]

References

1. Firth-Cozens J. (1997). Stress in healthcare professionals. In: A Baum, D Newman, J Weinman, R West, and C McManus (ed.), *Cambridge handbook of psychology, health and medicine*, Cambridge: Cambridge University Press.
2. Linzer M, Gerrity M, Douglas JA, McMurray JE, Williams ES, and Konrad TR. (2002). Physician stress: results from the physician worklife study. *Stress and Health* **18**:37–42.
3. Cooper CL, Cooper RD, and Eaker L. (1988). *Living with stress*. London: Penguin.
4. NASS (1992). *The costs of stress and the costs and benefits of stress management*. UK: National Association for Staff Support.
5. Freudenberger H. (1974). Staff burnout. *Journal of Social Issues* **30**:159–65.
6. Maslach C. (1997). Burnout in health professionals. In: A Baum, D Newman, J Weinman, R West, and C McManus (ed.), *Cambridge handbook of psychology, health and medicine*, Cambridge: Cambridge University Press.
7. Maslach C and Jackson S. (1986). *Maslach burnout inventory*. Palo Alto, CA: Consulting Psychologist's Press.
8. Escot C, Artero S, Boulenger JP, and Ritchie K. (2001). Stress levels in nursing staff working in oncology. *Stress and Health* **17**:273–9.
9. Moos RH and Shaeffer JA. (1997). Health-care work environments. In: A Baum, D Newman, J Weinman, R West, and C McManus (ed.), *Cambridge handbook of psychology, health and medicine*, Cambridge: Cambridge University Press.

10. Gjerløw O. (2001). The physician role in transition: is Hippocrates sick? *Social Science and Medicine* **52**:171–3.

11. Arnetz BB. (2001). Psychosocial challenges facing physicians of today. *Social Science and Medicine* **52**:203–13.

12. Firth-Cozens J. (2001). Interventions to improve physicians' well-being and patient care. *Social Science and Medicine* **52**:215–22.

13. Cumming SR and Harris LM. (2001). The impact of anxiety on the accuracy of diagnostic decision-making. *Stress and Health* **17**:281–6.

14. Fielden SL and Peckar CJ. (1999). Work stress and hospital doctors: a comparative study. *Stress Medicine* **15**:137–41.

15. Fallowfield LJ. (1995). Can we improve the professional and personal fulfilment of doctors in cancer medicine? *British Journal of Cancer* **71**:1132–3.

16. Board of the Faculty of Clinical Oncology (1991). *Medical manpower and workload in clinical oncology in the United Kingdom*. London: Royal College of Radiologists. Cited in Ramirez A, Graham J, Richards MA, Cull A, Gregory WM, Leaning MS, *et al.* (1995). Burnout and psychiatric disorder among cancer clinicians. *British Journal of Cancer* **71**:1263–9.

17. Pelfrene E, Vlerick P, Kittel F, Mak RP, Kornitzer M, and De Backer G. (2002). Psychosocial work environment and psychological well-being: assessment of the buffering effects in the job demand-control (-support) model in BELSTRESS. *Stress and Health* **18**:43–56.

18. Ramirez A, Graham J, Richards MA, Cull A, Gregory WM, Leaning MS, *et al.* (1995). Burnout and psychiatric disorder among cancer clinicians. *British Journal of Cancer* **71**:1263–9.

19. Whippen DA and Canellos GP. (1991). Burnout syndrome in the practice of oncology: results of a random survey of 1,000 oncologists. *Journal of Clinical Oncology* **9**:1916–20.

20. Kash KM, Holland JC, Breitbart W, Berenson S, Dougherty J, Ouellette-Kobasa S, *et al.* (2000). Stress and burnout in oncology. *Oncology* (*Huntington*) **14**:1621–33.

21. Schaerer R. (1993). Suffering of the doctor linked with the death of patients. *Palliative Medicine* **7**:27–37.

22. McCormick J. (1996). Death of the personal doctor. *Lancet* **348**:667–8.

23. Graham J, Albery IP, Ramirez AJ, and Richards MA. (2001). How hospital consultants cope with stress at work: implications for their mental health. *Stress and Health* **17**:85–9.

24. Novack DH, Suchman AL, Clark W, Epstein RM, Najberg E, and Kaplan C. (1997). Calibrating the physician: personal awareness and effective patient care. *Journal of the American Medical Association* **278**:502–9.

25. Martin AR. (1986). Stress in residency: a challenge to personal growth. *Journal of General Internal Medicine* **1**:252–7. Cited in Novack DH, Suchman AL, Clark W, Epstein RM, Najberg E, and Kaplan C. (1997). Calibrating the physician: personal awareness and effective patient care. *Journal of the American Medical Association* **278**:502–9.

26. Firth-Cozens J. (1987). Emotional distress in junior house officers. *British Medical Journal* **295**:533–5.

27. McDaniel SH, Campbell TL, and Seaburn DB. (1989). Managing personal and professional boundaries: how to make the physician's own issues a resource in patient care. *Family Systems Medicine* **7**:385–96.

28. Rolland JS. (1994). Working with illness: clinicians' personal and interface issues. *Family Systems Medicine* **12**:149–69.

29. Witman AB, Park DM, and Hardin SB. (1996). How do patients want physicians to handle mistakes: a survey of internal medicine patients in an academic setting. *Archives of Internal Medicine* **156**:2565–9. Cited in Novack DH, Suchman AL, Clark W, Epstein RM, Najberg E,

and Kaplan C. (1997). Calibrating the physician: personal awareness and effective patient care. *Journal of the American Medical Association* **278**:502–9.

30. Wilkinson SM. (1995). The changing pressure for cancer nurses 1986–1993. *European Journal of Cancer Care* **4**:69–74.

31. Wilkinson SM. (1994). Stress in cancer nursing – Does it really exist? *Journal of Advanced Nursing* **20**:1079–84.

32. Waldron I and Jacobs JA. (1989). Effects of multiple roles on women's health – evidence from a national longitudinal study. *Women's Health* **15**:3–19. Cited in Bennett P, Lowe R, Matthews V, Dourali M, and Tattersall A. (2001). Stress in nurses: coping, managerial support and work demand. *Stress and Health* **17**:55–63.

33. Kirkaldy BD and Martin T. (2000). Job stress and satisfaction among nurses: individual differences. *Stress Medicine* **16**:77–89.

34. Papadatou D, Anagnostopoulos F, and Monos D. (1994). Factors contributing to the development of burnout in oncology nursing. *British Journal of Medical Psychology* **67**:187–9.

35. American Nurses Association (2001). *Analysis of American nurses association staffing survey.* Warwick, RI: Cornerstone Communication Group.

36. Reynolds WJ and Scott B. (2000). Do nurses and other professional helpers normally display much empathy? *Journal of Advanced Nursing* **31**:226–34.

37. Bennett P, Lowe R, Matthews V, Dourali M, and Tattersall A. (2001). Stress in nurses: coping, managerial support and work demand. *Stress and Health* **17**:55–63.

38. Akroyd D, Caison A, and Adams RD. (2002). Burnout in radiation therapists: the predictive value of selected stressors. *International Journal of Radiation Oncology * Biology * Physics* **52**:816–21.

39. Maguire P. (1985). Barriers to psychological care of the dying. *British Medical Journal* **291**: 1711–13.

40. Figley CR. (1998). Burnout as systemic traumatic stress: a model for helping traumatized family members. In: CR Figley (ed.), *Burnout in families: the systemic costs of caring*, Boca Raton, Florida: CRC Press.

41. Cooper CL, Sloan SJ, and Williams S. (1988). *Occupational stress indicator management guide.* Windsor: NFER-Nelson.

42. Tattersall A, Bennett P, and Pugh S. (1999). Stress and coping in hospital doctors. *Stress Medicine* **14**:1–4.

43. Hawkins P and Shohet R. (1989). *Supervision in the helping professions.* Milton Keynes: Open University Press.

44. Blair SN, Kohl HW, Gordon NF, and Paffenbarger RS. (1992). How much physical activity is good for health? *Annual Review of Public Health* **12**:99–126.

45. Jacobson E. (1929). *Progressive relaxation.* Chicago: University of Chicago Press.

46. Bruch MH. (1997). Relaxation training. In: A Baum, D Newman, J Weinman, R West, and C McManus, (ed.), *Cambridge handbook of psychology, health and medicine*, Cambridge: Cambridge University Press.

47. Obholzer A and Roberts VG. (ed.) (1994). *The unconscious at work: individual and organisational stress in the human services.* London: Routledge.

48. Hinshelwood RD and Skogstad W. (ed.) (2000). *Observing organisations.* London: Routledge.

49. Ramsay N. (2000). Sitting close to death – a palliative care unit. In RD Hinshelwood, and W Skogstad, (ed.) *Observing organisations.* London: Routledge.

50. Firth-Cozens J. (2001). Multidisciplinary teamwork: the good, bad, and everything in between. *Quality in Health Care* **10**:65–6.

51. Jenkins VA, Fallowfield LJ, and Poole K. (2001). Are members of multidisciplinary teams in breast cancer aware of each other's informational roles? *Quality in Health Care* **10**:70–5.

52. Entwistle VA, Renfrew MJ, Yearley S, Forrester J, and Lamont T. (1998). Lay perspectives: advantages for health research. *British Medical Journal* **316**:463–6.

53. Tritter J, Daykin N, Evans S, Sanidas M, Barley V, McNeill J, *et al.* (2002). *Improving cancer services by involving service users. Part two: user involvement tools*. Bristol: Avon, Somerset and Wiltshire Cancer Services.

54. Delbecq AL and van de Ven AH. (1975). *Group techniques for program planning. a guide to nominal group and delphi processes*. California: Sage.

55. CancerLink (Undated) *National survey of cancer support and self-help groups 1992*. London: CancerLink.

56. *Good practice resource pack for cancer self-help and support groups*. Cancerlink (now The Community Networks Team, Macmillan Cancer Relief).

57. Batten L. (2000). *Cancerlink report on results of research among support groups*. Crossbow Research: Unpublished manuscript.

58. Brennan JH and Bullock A. (2001). A problem shared. *Newsletter of the British psychosocial oncology society*, September issue 1–4.

59. Kohn M. (1999). *Complementary therapies in cancer care*. London: Macmillan Cancer Relief.

60. Walker LA and Budd S. (2002). UK: the current state of regulation of complementary and alternative medicine. *Complementary Therapies in Medicine* **10**:8–13.

61. Rees R. (1999). The use of complementary therapies by women with breast cancer in the South Thames region. Survey commissioned by the South Thames region. Cited in Kohn M. (1999). *Complementary therapies in cancer care*. London: Macmillan Cancer Relief.

62. Ashikaga T, Bosompra K, O'Brien P, and Nelson L. (2002). Use of complementary and alternative medicine by breast cancer patients: prevalence, patterns and communication with physicians. *Supportive Care in Cancer* **10**:542–8.

63. Wilkes E. (1992). *Complementary Therapy in hospice and palliative Care*. Sheffield: Trent Palliative Care Centre. Cited in Zollman C, and Thomson E. (1998). Complementary approaches to palliative care. In C Faull, Y Carter, and R Woof (ed.) *Handbook of palliative care*, Oxford: Blackwell Science.

64. Airey C, Becher H, Erens B, and Fuller E. (2002). *Cancer national overview 1999/2000*. London: UK Department of Health.

65. Adams KE, Cohen MH, Eisenberg D, and Jonsen AR. (2002). Ethical considerations of complementary and alternative medical therapies in conventional medical settings. *Annals of Internal Medicine* **137**:660–4.

66. Barraclough J. (ed.) *Integrated cancer care: holistic, complementary and creative approaches*. Oxford: Oxford University Press.

67. Zollman C and Thomson E. (1998).Complementary approaches to palliative care. In: C Faull, Y Carter, and R Woof (ed.), *Handbook of palliative care*, Oxford: Blackwell Science.

68. Rees R. (2001). Researching complementary therapies in cancer care. In: J Barraclough (ed.), *Integrated cancer care: holistic, complementary and creative approaches*, Oxford: Oxford University Press.

69. Tasaki K, Maskarinec G, Shumay DM, Tatsumura Y, and Kakai H. (2002). Communication between physicians and cancer patients about complementary and alternative medicine: exploring patients' perspectives. *Psycho-Oncology* **11**:212–20.

70. Sheard TAB. (1994). Unconventional therapies in cancer care. In CE Lewis, C O'Sullivan, and J Barraclough, (ed.) *The psychoimmunology of cancer*, Oxford: Oxford University Press.

71. Coward R. (1989). *The whole truth: The myth of alternative health.* London: Faber.

72. Sheard T. (1994). Complementary therapies, existential turmoil, spiritual abuse ... and spiritual deprivation. *Newsletter of the British psychosocial oncology group.* September issue.

73. Brennan J and Sheard T. (1994). Psychosocial support and therapy in cancer care. *European Journal of Palliative Care* 1:136–9.

Appendix 1

Common self-report questionnaires

Psychological and social distress 400
   Hospital Anxiety and Depression Scale. 400
   General Health Questionnaire 400
   Brief Symptom Inventory 400
   Beck Depression Inventory. 400
   State-Trait Anxiety Inventory 401
   Profile of Mood States 401
   Social Problems Inventory 401
Quality of life 401
   Functional Assessment of Chronic Illness Therapy. 401
   European Organisation for Research on Treatment for Cancer 401
World Health Organization Quality of Life assessment instrument 402
   Schedule for the Evaluation of Individual Quality of Life 402
   Short Form 36 402
   Life Evaluation Questionnaire 402
Symptoms 402
   Memorial Symptom Assessment Scale 402
   Edmonton Symptom Assessment Scale. 403
   Cancer Rehabilitation Evaluation System. 403
   Functional Assessment of Cancer Therapy—Fatigue. 403
   Brief Fatigue Inventory. 403
   Brief Pain Inventory 403
   McGill Pain Questionnaire 403
   Maslach Burnout Inventory 404
References 404

The following self-report measures are primarily useful in research studies that are trying to identify general trends among large numbers of people. Faced with an individual patient, they are of limited *clinical* value because they constitute little more than a snapshot assessment of a restricted number of variables. Determining a particular test's reliability (whether it consistently obtains the same result) and validity (whether it measures what it purports to measure) involves not just scientific but semantic and epistemological questions that are well beyond the scope and purpose of this section.

Some of these tests are nonetheless occasionally used as screening measures to detect psychological distress, though they should always be supported by a thorough clinical assessment, since on their own they are generally crude. Less formal, but perhaps more useful screening methods have been developed to detect high levels of distress. For example, in New York a self-report 'distress thermometer' has been used to assess concerns in terms of practical, family, emotional, spiritual, and physical problems.[1] Resulting scores can be used to trigger the appropriate referral to a social worker, mental health specialist, or pastoral counsellor who can then provide a more rigorous assessment.

Psychological and social distress

Hospital Anxiety and Depression Scale—HADS [2]

This is a 14-item (7 depression, 7 anxiety) scale that was developed for use with medical patients. Because physical symptoms of emotional distress can be caused by the illness or treatment, these clinical features (e.g. loss of appetite, sleep disturbance) are largely excluded in the HADS. Recent research with a large sample of cancer patients has confirmed that the HADS comprises two factors: anhedonia and autonomic arousal which are both related to a primary factor of psychological distress.[3] Scores on the depression and anxiety subscales can be summed to produce a more clinically useful measure of general psychological distress.[4] It has been widely used in psycho-oncology research.

General Health Questionnaire—GHQ[5]

There are several versions of this questionnaire ranging from the original 60-item form through 30, 28, 20, and 12-item versions, as well as different methods of scoring. It was designed to be a screening measure for the recent onset of psychiatric disturbance rather than the detection of long-standing problems. Physically ill patients tend to score higher on the GHQ so the authors recommend that thresholds be raised for these groups.[6]

Brief Symptom Inventory—BSI[7]

Although written for a sixth Grade reading level, the BSI comprises 53 items and as such may be too long for routine clinical use. The items allude to how the patient has been feeling over the past two weeks and are rated according to a five-point scale ranging from 'not at all' to 'always'. The scale produces a global severity index as well as nine psychiatric subscales such as 'paranoid ideation' and 'obsessive compulsive'. It also includes a 'somatization' scale that can be compromised by the patient's disease or treatment.

Beck Depression Inventory—BDI[8]

This 21-item scale has been used for many years as a measure of the severity of depression, though its use with medically ill patients is limited because it includes items that can be compromised by the effects of illness and treatment. It is particularly sensitive to low self-esteem and has good psychometric properties.

State-Trait Anxiety Inventory—STAI[9]

The two 20-item scales that make up this inventory differentiate between two aspects of anxiety: long-standing tendencies within individuals to be anxious (trait) and more transitory feelings of anxiety associated with the current situation (state). Again, this test has well-regarded psychometric properties with good reliability and validity.

Profile of Mood States—POMS[10]

The POMS is a 65-item list of adjectives describing various emotions, which the respondent rates according to a five-point scale depending on how much they have experienced the emotion over the past week. This generates scores that can be depicted along six mood states such as tension–anxiety, depression–dejection, anger–hostility etc. This may be useful for measuring various aspects of emotional distress over time in large research studies but its clinical utility is limited.

Social Problems Inventory—SPI[11]

Although still in development, this 21-item questionnaire addresses the relative paucity of tools for measuring social distress among people with cancer. It attempts to cover eight areas of social functioning including managing the home, health and welfare services, finances, employment, legal matters, relationships, sexuality and body image concerns, and recreational activities. Items are rated according to a four-point scale ranging from 'no difficulty' to 'very much'.

Quality of life

Functional Assessment of Chronic Illness Therapy—FACIT or FACT-G[12]

The FACIT scales are a collection of quality of life scales that target particular chronic illnesses. They build on the original Functional Assessment of Cancer Therapy—General (FACT-G) which comprises 27 items divided into four primary quality of life domains: Physical Well-Being, Social/Family Well-Being, Emotional Well-Being, and Functional Well-Being. There are separate questionnaires for many types of cancer including head and neck, lung and ovarian, as well as symptom-specific subscales such as anaemia and fatigue. These questionnaires have been translated into nearly 40 languages and have been extensively cross-validated. They generally have good reliability, validity, and can be understood by people with a Grade-6 education.

European Organisation for Research on Treatment for Cancer—EORTC[13]

Like the FACIT scales, there are a number of disease-specific EORTC modules which build on the original 30-item scale (known as the Quality of Life Questionnaire—QLQ-C30). It attempts to cover a wide area though a number of components of quality of life (e.g. trouble sleeping) are measured with only one item. It has been translated and validated in over 40 languages and has been widely used in research.

World Health Organization Quality of Life assessment Instrument—WHOQOL[14]

This international scale continues to develop and seeks to provide a cross-culturally valid measure of quality of life. It aims to determine the impact of disease and impairment on a person's life, and assesses both positive and negative aspects of quality of life. The full scale comprises 100 items though a 26-item version has been widely validated (WHOQOL-BREF). The WHOQOL attempts to measure six domains: physical, psychological, level of independence, social relationships, environment (safety, security, work and home environments, social resources), and spiritual.

Schedule for the Evaluation of Individual Quality of Life—SEIQoL[15]

The SEIQoL differs from other quality of life instruments by allowing the individual to specify what qualities of their life they value, rather than this being determined by other people. Patients are encouraged to identify five aspects of their lives that are most important to them, to rank their relative importance to one another and then to rate their current experience of each. In this way, the scale produces data that may be idiosyncratic to the individual but which can reflect meaningful changes to their quality of life over time.

Short Form 36—SF-36[16]

This scale is a short form of a longer questionnaire used by the Medical Outcomes Study to assess the outcome of medical care in the USA. The SF-36 measures health status along eight dimensions including physical limitations, pain, mental health, and energy level. As its name suggests this is a 36-item measure, each item being rated on a 5-point scale. It has even been translated from American into English.

Life Evaluation Questionnaire—LEQ[17]

This questionnaire, which is still in development, is an attempt to go beyond symptoms and level of daily functioning to reflect questions of meaning and positive growth among people confronting their possible death. Five principal components are measured: (a) freedom from restrictions imposed by the illness, (b) appreciation of life, (c) contentment, (d) resentment, and (e) social integration.

Symptoms

Memorial Symptom Assessment Scale—MSAS[18]

This scale is designed to provide a comprehensive symptom assessment. It requires patients to rate the frequency, severity, and distress associated with 32 common symptoms experienced by the patient over the previous seven days. Twenty-four items are rated according to their frequency, severity and distress while the remaining eight items are rated according to their severity, and distress. The scale yields a number of validated sub-scale scores covering global distress, physical symptoms, psychological symptoms, and a total MSAS score.

Edmonton Symptom Assessment Scale—ESAS[19]

This test is used for assessing the symptoms of patients receiving palliative care. The scale comprises nine items each of which is rated by the patient on a visual analogue scale. The nine items cover pain, activity, nausea, depression, anxiety, drowsiness, lack of appetite, well-being, and shortness of breath. An optional tenth item can be added by the patient.

Cancer Rehabilitation Evaluation System—CARES[20]

The CARES is designed to measure the quality of life of cancer patients with a view to identifying symptoms requiring rehabilitative care. The instrument comprises five scales for assessing rehabilitation problems and needs: physical, medical, sexual, marital, and psychosocial. These are rated according to a five-point scale ranging from Not at all (0) to Very much (4). The full CARES scale comprises 139 items while the short form contains 59.

Functional Assessment of Cancer Therapy—Fatigue—FACT-F[21]

This scale comprises the FACT-G with the addition of 13 fatigue items, totalling 41 items. In fact, the authors note that the 13-item fatigue subscale can be used alone as a brief measure of fatigue since it has shown to have adequate reliability and validity.

Brief Fatigue Inventory—BFI[22]

The Brief Fatigue Inventory models itself on the Brief Pain Inventory and was developed for the rapid assessment of fatigue in cancer patients. It reliably measures this one construct and contains nine items which are rated on a 1–10 numeric scale. Three items are concerned with the severity of fatigue and the other six assess how much fatigue has interfered with the patient's life over the past 24 hours.

Brief Pain Inventory[23]

This very widely used scale has been translated into many languages. Its short form comprises 15 items while the longer version has 56. The inventory measures the intensity of pain when it is at its worst, least, and at the current time. It reports the extent to which patients are experiencing pain relief from interventions, and how much pain is interfering with the patient's mood, functioning, and enjoyment of life.

McGill Pain Questionnaire[24]

The much lengthier McGill comprises 78 questions though shorter versions of the scale exist. This scale assesses the sensory and evaluative aspects of pain, as well as the individual's emotional response to it, though it does not measure the impact of pain on functioning. It is more widely used in the assessment of non-malignant pain than cancer.

Maslach Burnout Inventory[(25)]

The MBI-Human Services Survey attempts to measure burnout as it manifests itself in the staff members in human services institutions and healthcare occupations such as nursing, social work, psychology, and religion. Its 22 items consider emotional exhaustion, depersonalization and sense of personal accomplishment. The respondent answers each item in terms of the frequency (on a seven-point scale) with which they experience these signs of burnout. This self-report survey takes 15 minutes to complete.

References

1. Holland JC. (2000). An algorithm for rapid assessment and referral of distressed patients, In: MC Perry (ed.), *American society of clinical oncology education book.* (36th Annual Meeting). Alexandria, VA, ASCO.

2. Zigmond AS and Snaith RP. (1983). The hospital anxiety and depression scale. *Acta Psychiatrica Scandinavica* **67**:361–70.

3. Smith AB, Selby PJ, Velikova G, Stark D, Wright EP, Gould A, *et al.* (2002). Factor analysis of the hospital anxiety and depression scale from a large cancer population. *Psychology and Psychotherapy: Theory, Research and Practice* **75**:165–76.

4. Razavi D, Delvaux N, Farvacques C, and Robaye E. (1990). Screening for adjustment disorders and major depressive disorders in cancer in-patients. *British Journal of Psychiatry* **156**:79–83.

5. Goldberg D and Williams P. (1998). *A user's guide to the general health questionnaire.* Windsor: NFER-Nelson.

6. Bennett P. (2000). *Introduction to clinical health psychology.* Buckingham: Open University Press.

7. Zabora JR, Smith-Wilson R, Fetting JH, and Enterline JP. (1990). An efficient method for the psychosocial screening of cancer patients. *Psychosomatics* **31**:192–6.

8. Beck A, Ward C, Mendelson M, Mock J, and Erbaugh J. (1961). An inventory for measuring depression. *Archives of General Psychiatry* **4**:562–71.

9. Spielberger CD. (1983). *Manual for the state-trait anxiety inventory.* Palo Alto, CA: Consulting Psychologists Press Inc.

10. McNair DM, Lorr M, and Droppleman LF. (1971). *Profile of mood states.* San Diego: Educational and Industrial Testing Service.

11. Wright EP, Kiely MA, Lynch P, Cull A, and Selby PJ. (2002). Social problems in oncology. *British Journal of Cancer* **87**:1099–104.

12. Cella DF, Tulsky DS, Gray G, Sarafian B, Lloyd S, Linn E, *et al.* (1993). The functional assessment of cancer therapy (FACT) scale: development and validation of the general measure. *Journal of Clinical Oncology* **11**:570–9.

13. Aaronson NK, Ahmedzai S, Bergman B, Bullinger M, Cull A, Duez NJ, *et al.* (1993). QLQ-C30: a quality-of-life instrument for use in international clinical trials in oncology. *Journal of the National Cancer Institute* **85**:365–76.

14. Szabo S. (1996). The World Health Organization Quality of Life (WHOQOL) assessment instrument. In: B Spilker (ed.), *Quality of life and pharmacoeconomics in clinical trials.* Philadelphia: Lippincott-Raven.

15. Hickey AM, Bury G, O'Boyle CA, Bradley F, O'Kelly FD, and Shannon W. (1996). A new short form individual quality of life measure (SEIQoL-DW): application in a cohort of individuals with HIV/AIDS. *British Medical Journal* **313**: 29–33.

16. Ware JE, Snow KK, Kosinski M, and Gandek B. (1993). *SF-36 Health survey: manual and interpretation guide.* The Health Institute, Boston: New England Medical Centre.

17. Salmon P, Manzi F, and Valori RM. (1996). Measuring the meaning of life for patients with incurable cancer: the life evaluation questionnaire (LEQ). *European Journal of Cancer* **32**:755–60.

18. Portenoy RK, Thaler HT, Kornblith AB, Lepore JM, Friedlander-Klar H, Kiyasu E, *et al.* (1996). The memorial symptom assessment scale: an instrument for the evaluation of symptom prevalence, characteristics and distress. *European Journal of Cancer* **30A**:1226–36.

19. Bruera E, Kuehn N, Miller MJ, Selmser P, and Macmillan K. (1991) The Edmonton Sympton Assessment System (ESAS): a simple method for the assessment of palliative care patients. *Journal of Palliative Care* **7**:6–9.

20. Ganz PA, Schag CA, Lee JJ, and Sim MS. (1992). The CARES: a generic measure of health-related quality of life for patients with cancer. *Quality of Life Research* **1**:19–29.

21. Yellen SB, Cella DF, Webster K, Blendowski C, and Kaplan E. (1997). Measuring fatigue and other anaemia-related symptoms with the Functional Assessment of Cancer Therapy (FACT) measurement system. *Journal of Pain and Symptom Management* **13**:63–74.

22. Mendoza TR, Wang XS, Cleeland CS, Morrissey M, Johnson BA, Wendt JK, *et al.* (1999). The rapid assessment of fatigue severity in cancer patients: use of the brief fatigue inventory. *Cancer*, **85**:1186–96.

23. Daut RL, Cleeland CS, and Flanery RC. (1983). Development of the Wisconsin brief pain questionnaire. *Pain* **17**:197–210.

24. Melzack R. (1975). The McGill pain questionnaire: major properties and scoring methods. *Pain* **8**:277–99.

25. Maslach C and Jackson S. (1986). *Maslach burnout inventory.* Palo Alto, CA: Consulting Psychologist's Press.

Appendix 2

Managing the stress of cancer: a psychosocial guide for people with cancer

The following pages may be copied or adapted without copyright restriction.

The following booklet was written by the author in 2001. It was designed to normalize people's emotional experiences and reactions to having cancer, and to help patients and their partners consider how best to manage various common concerns. Indeed, it translates some of the key ideas of this book into a more patient-friendly format.

Information 408
Shock 408
    What can you do? 409
Out of control 409
    What can you do? 410
Who am I now? 410
    What can you do? 411
Feeling overwhelmed 412
Making sense 412
Taking control 413
Worrying 413
    Useless (unproductive) worrying 414
    Productive worrying 414
Getting on with living 415
Other people 415
    Changing relationships 415
Advice for couples facing cancer 416

For many people, having cancer is one of the toughest experiences they will ever have to face. There is probably no getting around this. The months following a cancer diagnosis can be a very stressful time, not just for the person with cancer, but also for anyone who cares about them. It can be a time of many changes from the way people normally live their lives, even though some of these changes may eventually turn out to be positive in the long run.

This short booklet will try to help you make sense of some of the changes and feelings you have had, and may persuade you that you are not alone—other people may have experienced similar changes and feelings. Cancer treatments may seem complicated at first but, in fact, people's lives are often a lot more complicated. Each of us has our own unique life story and our own unique combination of family and friends and each of *them* has *their* own complicated life story to tell. So is it not surprising that people have very varied reactions and feelings in response to cancer, whether they are a relative, friend, or the patient themselves. This booklet is about some of the main feelings and thoughts that people often have during the ordeal of cancer.

Information

The doctors have told you about your particular illness and how they are planning to help you. If you want to know more, or have not understood what you have been told, then you should certainly contact the medical team who are treating you. You should always have exactly as much information as you feel you want and the doctors should always be happy to provide it. Of course, it is important to remember that only *you* know *when* and *how much* new information you are ready to learn. Cancer and its treatment are often very complicated and it can take a long time to understand everything about the disease. General information about cancer and its treatment can always be obtained from …

Shock

Finding out that you have cancer is a series of events that you will probably remember forever. You found something, or felt it. It seemed curious. Some time later a doctor looked at it. The doctor asked you to have some tests. Later they said that you had cancer.

But, of course, it is never that simple.

It is often a time which leaves people with many questions both about the way in which the diagnosis came about as well as the speed with which this happened. Although many doctors do it well, almost all would agree that informing someone they have cancer is one of the most difficult jobs doctors have to do.

The reason it is so difficult is because the first thing most people think when they hear the word 'cancer' is that they are about to die. Unfortunately, this still seems to be the public's view of cancer, in spite of all the extraordinary medical advances in the treatment of cancer in the past few years. So it is not really surprising that people often remember the 'day of the diagnosis' as the most frightening day of their lives.

Some people describe the day of their diagnosis as like being plunged into a completely different world—a world in which all the rules seem to have changed. It is the start of 'the cancer journey' which can take months to complete. But then, after a while, the world begins to fall back into place, and things seem more familiar again …

Starting cancer treatment is therefore a time of huge changes with much to learn: meeting new doctors and other staff, undergoing strange tests and scary-sounding treatments, and *so many* hospital appointments. Your working life may have had to change, your lifestyle may have changed, and even your relationships may seem to have changed. This booklet is about some of those changes.

Change is *always* stressful, and stress can show up in a number of different ways. Look at this list:

- feeling fearful and tense
- insomnia (not being able to sleep)
- loss of appetite
- constant worrying
- feeling sad and hopeless
- getting cross with others

Do you recognize any of these? If you do, it is probably because you have been through a lot of stress recently.

What can you do?

- Do not bottle things up! Talking to someone you trust is one way of releasing your feelings. Find a good listener—this may not always be the first person you think of. Putting feelings into words almost always makes stressful situations seem easier to cope with.
- Find a time every day when you can relax. Relaxing does not necessarily mean doing nothing (although this is often the best kind of relaxation) but it does mean doing something pleasant and enjoyable, and giving your mind and body a time in which to calm down.
- As you read this, think about where in your body your muscles seem to be tense. Now try to release this tension and get in the habit of relaxing these muscles. This is much more important than it may sound. Ask your friends and family to help by reminding you, every now and again, to relax the muscles you do not need to be using.
- If you feel that anxiety is a particular problem for you, speak to a member of the healthcare team, who will arrange for a specialist to help you.

Out of control

Once treatment starts, events all seem to happen very quickly and it is easy to feel that your life has been completely taken over and that you are no longer in the driving seat.

Since my diagnosis, everything has changed. Everything feels upside down – I'm no longer the same person, I seem to have no control over my life, and I just don't know what to expect any-more. I want to go back to the person I used to be but I can't.

Some people say that the weeks following their diagnosis are a bit like being in a dream; the life they have known has been replaced by one that is new and strange. The months of treatment ahead can seem endless and there is a longing to feel in control of your life again.

What can you do?

When you are ready, it will be important to take back some control over your life again. One simple way of doing this, *if you feel ready for it*, is to obtain more information about your illness and its treatment. Another way is to learn what you can do to help yourself and the treatment. For example, think about one thing you could change to make your life healthier. Stopping smoking, if you still smoke, would be a good start, but a healthier diet or starting a gentle programme of increasing exercise can also help maximize your health. Never do more than is sensible (do not become a fanatic!) and, if you are not sure, always seek the advice of an expert, like the hospital dietician, a specialist nurse, your hospital doctor, or your GP.

Try to stay involved with things that you know you are good at. As we will see in the next section of this booklet, it is all too easy to let these things disappear when there are so many other things to think about. However, it is often the activities we are good at (like helping other people, achieving things in our work or hobbies, and doing our normal jobs at home) that tell us that we still have control over our lives.

If you are worried about your finances or housing, speak to a Social Worker or a Welfare Benefits Officer as soon as you can. It is reassuring to know you are getting whatever financial support you are entitled to.

Who am I now?

Another unfortunate consequence of long cancer treatments is that many people stop doing the things that they used to enjoy or do well. You may have stopped work, or cut down activities that involved contact with other people. These are activities that tell you every day that you are skilled, or needed, or talented, or funny, and so on. They remind you that other people value your personal qualities, your knowledge, and humour; in other words, these activities give you a sense of self-worth. As soon as you cut down on these sorts of activities, you are likely to feel less good about yourself and, surprisingly quickly, you may begin to lose confidence in yourself.

Another change that many people find difficult is seeing themselves as 'a patient', or 'a cancer patient'. It is as if being in the role of a patient sometimes makes people feel as if they are 'second-class citizens' and no longer as valuable as anyone else. They worry that *needing* other people means they have become dependent and that this means they are somehow being weak. In reality, of course, we all depend upon one another, however much we might like to think of ourselves as independent. Everyone is a patient at some stage in their life and there is certainly no shame in that; it is just a temporary role in one part of your life.

Adjusting to the loss of a part of the body (for example, a breast or testicle) or having to deal with other changes in the body can leave people feeling bereaved. In many ways, grief is an entirely appropriate reaction. Like bereavement, it can take considerable time to adjust to a change in your body and all the implications this has for how you see yourself and your life ahead. Gradually confronting these changes and talking them through with someone can help the process of adjustment. But, like bereavement, time is also a great healer.

Who am I for other people? Who are other people for me? The relationships we have with other people are extraordinarily important to how we feel about ourselves. Because these relationships change when someone becomes ill, it can cause difficulties and misunderstandings (*see* Other People). So this can also have an impact on how we feel about ourselves.

Finally, some people find that when they think about the future all they can see is months of treatment ahead and little else. Tests, treatments, and hospital appointments seem to dominate their lives, making it difficult to plan pleasant things to look forward to, or things to achieve. In fact, some people feel it is unsafe to make *any* plans for themselves because they fear being disappointed or because they worry that, by making plans, they would be tempting fate. It is an understandable reaction but a dangerous one! Without things to look forward to and things to achieve, life can feel pointless, and this can lead people to feel apathetic and depressed.

What can you do?

- A good place to start is to recognize how much your life has changed over the past few days or months and, considering all this, how well you have coped. You have had to deal with so many new experiences that it is little wonder that you may feel stressed, unhappy, or even lost at times. You have never had to cope with anything quite like this before. So, all in all, perhaps you should even feel proud of how well you have coped!

- Remember that, in spite of all the losses and changes that you may have had to cope with, *you are still the same person inside*. Your skills and qualities are still very much there, even if you have not had a chance to use them as much recently. For many people, the cancer journey can be a time of learning something useful, rather than losing anything within themselves.

- Try to *retain as much contact with your normal life* as possible. Maintain contact with work colleagues even if you have had to stop work. Try to fulfil your normal roles in life as much as you wish to (though prevent others from making unreasonable demands of you).

- *Do things you are good at and enjoy from time to time*; this will remind you that you are still the same person and it will preserve and restore your confidence in your skills and qualities.

- Try to *maintain activities that give you a sense of pleasure or fun*; this will give you something to look forward to (something we all need), as well as providing a short 'mental holiday' from the stress of thinking about cancer (e.g. reading a book, seeing a film).

- Above all, *try to prevent your illness and its treatment from becoming the central focus of your life.* Instead, see it as something you manage to fit into your otherwise busy life! Of course, there may be times when you do not feel up to being as active as usual and at those times it is important that you listen to your own body and do what you feel you need to do even if this means disappointing others. Only you know what you are capable of doing.

Feeling overwhelmed

One of the unfortunate consequences of cancer treatments is that they often take a long time. In fact, cancer treatments can sometimes seem *so* long and *so* exhausting that people end up feeling lost, frightened, and overwhelmed. It is at such times that people feel they want to withdraw into themselves, and become afraid of doing virtually anything.

If you feel you have hit this point, it may be helpful to remind yourself that it is not your fault. Feeling very low or afraid does *not* mean you are 'not coping', or that you are weak, or that you are letting anyone down. The treatment of cancer is very stressful, involving many changes, and there is a good chance that you are physically and emotionally exhausted.

If you are concerned about how withdrawn you have become, or how hopeless you feel at times, or if you feel constantly tense and anxious, you should tell a member of the healthcare staff treating you. Some people find it difficult turning to others for support, but if you are feeling overwhelmed in any of these ways, then it is best to talk about the difficulties you are having with someone neutral and independent who may be able to help.

It may be useful to have an understanding of how your mind is coping with all the changes brought about by your diagnosis. The following section provides some information about the mind which you might find helpful to think about.

Making sense

From the moment we are born, we try to make sense of the world around us. As babies, our ideas of the world are very simple but throughout our childhood we learn more and more complicated things about the world and how it works. We develop a sort of mental map of the world and this, of course, includes ideas about how *we* and other people fit into the world. These mental maps of the world are always changing because everyday something new happens which slightly changes how we see the world and ourselves within it. Some things in life, of course, are more dramatic and important and may force us to change the whole way we look at the world. This kind of change is always stressful. For example, leaving home for the first time, losing someone we love, becoming a parent, and retirement are all life-changing experiences, and there are lots of others. In all these experiences, we require time to adjust to the many ways in which the world appears to have changed.

Cancer is another experience that involves a lot of change. Cancer forces us to look again at the many things we may have taken for granted in our lives: our health, our goals in life, our relationships with other people, and even our sense of who we are, ourselves. We consider where we are in our lives. Reflecting on these things can be rewarding but stressful, and it may take time to draw the right conclusions. Changing the way you look at your life, yourself, and other people is almost always difficult and this is why getting cancer can be so stressful. Cancer involves so many changes to what is *normal* in someone's life that most people find it hard to keep up. This is why talking about your feelings and thoughts is always so important at times of change. It helps us to make sense of what is happening and find a way forward. This period of transition in your life will take time, it may have its highs and it is lows, but it can *also* be an opportunity for something positive to occur.

Taking control

Stay as actively involved with your life as you can. Try to collect up all the cancer-related bits—the hospitals, the doctors, the tests, the appointments, etc.—and put them all in one small corner of your life. Make the rest of it count—stay as actively involved in every other aspect of your life as you can. Reclaim parts of your life that you enjoy or which give you a sense of who you are, your family, your colleagues, your friends. And if you have any free time, why not use it to take up something new?

Get as much support as you feel you need. Not just practical help (fetching and carrying), but also emotional support (listening and caring). If you are worried about being a burden, think about what you would feel towards the other person if the tables were turned and they were asking you for *your* support. Practical support is important not only because it helps you physically, but because it takes stress and pressure off you at a time which is already very stressful. Emotional support is often even more important because it is often through talking to other people that we make sense of what we feel, and what is really happening in our lives. It helps us to deal with the implications of the illness and its treatment.

Take control as much as you wish. You probably know best what you need from the people offering you support, so *make it clear to other people what this is*. What you need, of course, will change over time, so on several occasions you may have to explain to those supporting you what you require. Organize your life in a way that suits you. It is you who are 'the patient' and it seems reasonable to expect people who love you to support you.

Worrying

Everyone worries. It is part of being human (and is a form of creative imagination). But worry can stop people enjoying and getting on with their lives, and it can also lead to poor sleep and unnecessary stress, so it may be helpful to know something about it.

People worry about things that are very likely to happen, and also about things that are very *un*likely to happen. This section applies to *any* kind of worry, whether realistic or not. Worry is an unpleasant side effect of our amazing ability to imagine, anticipate, and plan for the future (an ability which has allowed human beings to dominate the world).

So worrying is a very common and quite normal activity. But if you are going to worry, be sure to do it properly! There is a helpful, productive way to worry, but also a harmful, ineffective way. The two are very different.

Useless (unproductive) worrying

The way most people worry is to focus on a particular moment taken from their 'worst-case scenario'. You are going along in your life quite contentedly when you are reminded about the situation you are in (e.g. having cancer). Suddenly, a snapshot of the worst-case future pops into your mind. You imagine how you would feel and begin to get distressed, as if the event were happening now; you may feel physically tense and anxious, or depressed and sad. It is such a horrible, 'catastrophic thought' that you quickly distract yourself by thinking about something else. You calm yourself down and then try to resume whatever you were doing. But a few minutes later the same thought comes crashing into your mind again.

If this sounds familiar, read the next section.

Productive worrying

This solution may not be easy, and may even take a few goes, but a lot of people find it helps. Try really looking at your worst-case scenario *in detail* for a change. 'Unpack' what you are *really* worrying about and take a hard look at it. Often, if we try to imagine *realistically* what the future is most likely to hold (although, of course, we do not really know) we can begin to feel more confident that we, and other people we care about, will be able to cope with it, whatever it may be. Of course, really looking at your fears can be difficult and distressing, and you would be best advised to talk all this through with someone you know to be a caring and good listener.

When you think about your worst-case scenario (your 'catastrophic thought' in the section above), try thinking about what would happen *next*... for everyone concerned. What would be happening a week after that? A month after that? And so on. Talk or think it all out logically and try to imagine, *realistically*, what would happen if your worry, however unlikely, actually came to pass. This may sound ridiculously simple, but the odd thing is that people usually worry about only the worst possible *moment* in their imagination. They fail to remember that this snapshot moment in the imagined future quickly passes, and turns into something less unpleasant. Once you have thought through the worry realistically a few times with a trusted listener, you may find it does not pop into your mind quite so often.

Finally, if you worry about the possibility of a recurrence of your illness (and most people do worry about this) try to remember that, if this ever did occur, your doctors would reassess you medically and decide the most appropriate treatment for you.

Getting on with living

Sometimes, and quite understandably, people become preoccupied with their worst-case scenario (some imagined future) and spend their lives worrying about this possibility rather than getting on with their lives. The problem with using your imagination too much is that it becomes difficult to enjoy what is actually happening in the present—you begins to lose sight of the bigger picture.

It is easy for other people to remind you that it is more important to *live* your life than to worry about when it may end. It is easy for them to say 'We are all going to die one day; the important thing is to enjoy the time we have while we are alive'. It is much more difficult to live by these words when you imagine what it would be like to face the end of your life. But at the same time, a part of us perhaps knows that these words are true.

You may believe one hundred per cent that 'life is for living', yet feel afraid to be really involved with your life again. But would you decide never to go out to see a film, just in case it was sold out? Making goals and plans for yourself (with the help of friends) can feel like a risk, even tempting fate, but in time it will help rebuild your confidence and involvement. Read the section above on worrying so that you can learn to shelve your worries until those things actually need to be worried about, if ever. In time, you will once again come to appreciate that 'every moment counts'.

Other people

Other people in your life may have reacted to your illness in ways which have surprised you. Sometimes unexpected people turn out to be extraordinarily caring, and sometimes people you *thought* would be caring seem to be unsupportive. This can be a big disappointment and a source of strain within the relationship. If you feel someone close to you is finding it hard to support you effectively, you may wish to suggest that they also read this last section.

There may be some people you have chosen not to tell. Whether or not to tell people is a very personal decision. Often this decision is about balancing two genuine concerns:

(a) not wanting to create unnecessary distress among people whom we care and worry about (e.g. the very young, the very old, or those who are themselves ill, or under stress), but on the other hand...

(b) not wanting to withhold information from people who really would want to know (because secrecy can cause hurt and anger).

Again, in reaching your decision whether or not to tell a particular person, it often helps to talk through the pros and cons with someone who knows about your illness and whom you can talk to easily.

Changing relationships

Our relationships with other people often have a long history, so changes within relationships can be particularly difficult and stressful. In fact, we get so used to the people we are closest to that we often do not think about our relationship with them and may even take them for granted. We also assume lots of things about our relationships that simply may not be true. For example, children grow up and mature, but we often think of them as being younger than they are. We may think of our partners as being competent and strong, while forgetting that they can also feel scared and lost at times too. Over the years we become more dependent on our partners (and they become more dependent on us), but often we do not think about this either.

When someone becomes ill, many of their relationships change. Friends and family often do more for the patient, and although the patient may welcome this, they may also feel uncomfortable or even guilty that they are not doing as much as normal for other people. Everyone connected to the patient also has their own worries and concerns although these do not always get expressed, and this can lead to tension within relationships.

Husbands and wives (and other partnerships) sometimes find that the demands of cancer treatment put considerable strain on their relationship. There seem to be a number of reasons for this.

- Partners are usually very distressed but most of the support tends to be focused on 'the patient'; this *can* lead to resentment.

- Some people find it difficult to express their feelings (or choose not to because they fear they are being a burden) and this 'bottling up' of emotion can lead to irritation and anger within the relationship.

- Cancer can lead people to realize how much they need someone else and how dependent they have become on them. Men, in particular, often find it uncomfortable to recognize how much they may need their partners.

- Some partners believe that their role should be to be positive and cheerful *all* the time. While, of course, it is helpful to focus on the positive aspects of the situation, 'positive thinking' can be overdone if it discourages someone from talking about the things that they want, or need to talk about.

- Being either the patient *or* the partner is exhausting. Tiredness within relationships always leads to more friction.

Cancer can provoke changes which sometimes reveal the true nature of long-standing relationships. These discoveries can be positive and even lead to healthy changes within relationships, but they can *also* lead to considerable disappointment and long-term resentment.

Advice for couples facing cancer

1. Anxiety and depression are less likely to develop if the couple are able to face the stress of cancer together. Patients can support partners, as well as the other way round.

2. Try to be clear with each other about what *you* are feeling and thinking, but do not assume you know what your partner is feeling or thinking.

3. Do your best not to interrupt your partner when they are speaking; try to listen more than talk.

4. Avoid being critical of your partner; remember that it is a stressful time for *both* of you and that both of you need support.

5. Words may not always be as important as giving or receiving a hug from your partner.

6. Being overly positive, giving advice, or finding a solution is not always what is needed; try to find out instead whatever your partner would find it helpful to talk about.

7. Do not worry about saying the wrong thing—the important thing is to try to stay involved.

8. If possible, find someone in addition to your partner whom you can talk to, and get support from, on a regular basis. Depending only on your partner for support can sometimes be stressful for both of you.

Finally, every relationship is something of a journey into the unknown. The measure of any relationship is the support and companionship we give one another when the going gets tough. Couples who face the crisis of cancer together, and who are open with one another about their feelings and uncertainties, are much better able to overcome any difficulties along the way.

Index

accountability 35
activities of daily living 264
adjustment 12–13, 23, 41
  and assumptions 25–35
  individual differences 21–25
adjustment and denial 21
advocates, ethnicity 191–3
Africa, sub-Saharan, perceptions of illness 51
aged people, family support 111–13
alternative medicine *see* complementary therapy
anxiety 213, 216, 348–349
  defined 24
  see also stress; worry
Asian people
  racist attitudes 185–9
  UK vs US terminology 179
assumptions 13, 22, 25–35
  body 32–3
  clarifying and challenging 329–30
  existential–spiritual beliefs 33–5
  life trajectory 27–9
  self-worth and personal control 30–2
  social relationships 29–30
asylum seekers and refugees 194–8
  definition 194
  discrimination 197
  health/mental health 194–6
  psychological problems, treatment 197–8
  registration and information 196–7
  support 197
Australia, aboriginal perceptions of illness 50
avoidance and denial 16–17, 20–1, 53–6, 346–8
  colluding with denial 392–3

bad news 330–5
Beck Depression Inventory (BDI) 400
bereavement care 277–82
  alarm and grief 279
  anger, guilt and sadness 279–80
  chronic grief 281
  complicated grief 280–2
  delayed grief 281
  masked grief 281
  mitigation 279
  recovery from bereavement 281–2
  reviewing bereavement 280
body identity 32–3, 73–7
  gender 169–72
bone marrow transplantation (BMT) 236–8
  graft-vs-host-disease (GVHD) 236–7
breast cancer 218–20

breast reconstruction 219–20
  mastectomy vs breast conservation 219
Brief Fatigue Inventory (BFI) 403
Brief Pain Inventory 403
Brief Symptom Inventory (BSI) 400
burnout 367–8, 371–2
  Maslach Burnout Inventory 404
  prevention in healthcare professionals 380

cancer
  as catastrophe 16–35
  classification 49
  decatastrophizing 259–60
  images of 49–50
  recurrence 82–3, 266–7
Cancer Diaries Project *xxiv*
Cancer Rehabilitation Evaluation System
    (CARES) 403
carers/caring 134–9
  assessing distress among carers 137
  ethnicity 187
  supporting carers 137–9
central nervous system (CNS) tumours 223–6
  cognitive assessment 224–6
  rehabilitation 225–6
change and development 14–16
  negative aspects 15
chemotherapy and hormone therapy 231–5
  depression 254–5
  nausea and vomiting 245–7
  preparation for chemotherapy 232–4
  side-effects 234–5
children, telling about illness 106–10
choice, and consent, ethical issues 299–302
clinical context 207–93
  bereavement care 277–82
  bone marrow transplantation (BMT) 236–8
  chemotherapy and hormone therapy 231–5
  depression 253–5
  dying people 268–77
  fatigue 242–5
  general practice 208–11
  insomnia 260–2
  intense fear 255–8
  lung cancer 238–9
  nausea and vomiting 245–7
  pain 247–53
  palliative care 267–77
  prostate cancer 240–2
  radiotherapy 226–31
  recurrence 266–7

clinical context (*Continued*)
  rehabilitation 262–6
  surgery 214–26
  treatment 242–62
  worry 258–60
clinical interview, communication 323–8
cognitive adaptation, theory 26
cognitive impairment 350–1
cognitive therapy 349
cognitive-behavioural approaches to pain
    management 252–3
coherence, mental maps 11–14
colostomies 223
communication 295–362
  angry, difficult or disliked patients 351–3
  anxiety, worry and uncertainty 348–51
  assessing the whole person 321–3
  avoidance and denial 16–17, 20–1, 346–8
  clarifying and challenging assumptions 329–30
  clinical interviews 323–8
  clinically depressed or suicidal patients 342–6
  confusion/cognitive impairment 350–1
  cultural assumptions and differences 150–1,
      316–18
  dying people 270–1, 276–7
  eliciting concerns 320–30
  ethical issues 298–302
  and ethnicity 189–90
  hearing-impaired patients 340–1
  information 302–9
  interpreters 318–19
  language 319–20
  learning disabilities 338–40
  open/closed questions 325–6
  patient-centred communication 315–20
  people with special needs 338–42
  problem-solving 328
  professional distance 311–13
  professional issues 353–5
  psychiatrically ill patients 341–2
  resuscitation 335–6
  specific issues 330–48
  speech difficulties 222
  staff–patient relationships 309–15
  in terminal illness 270
  time to care 297–8
  training 355
  visually impaired patients 340
  vulnerability 336–8
complementary therapy and alternative medicine
    xxi–xxii, 389–93
  colluding with denial 392–3
  informed consent 391–2
  'spiritual abuse' 392
completion tendency 16
confidentiality 354–5
confidentiality issues 354–5
confused patients 350–1
consent
  ethical issues 299–302
  informed consent 391–2

control
  and self-worth 30–2
  stress management 409–10
  taking 413
control *see* personal responsibility/control
coping
  by 'positive thinking' 97, 115, 148–9
  defined 23
  with treatment 60–1
counselling 191–3
  need 191–2
  patronization 162
culture
  assumptions, communication 150–1, 316–18
  and ethnicity 179

delirium, differential diagnosis 225
dementia 225
denial *see* avoidance and denial
depression 213, 253–5
  chemotherapy 254–5
  clinically depressed or suicidal patients 342–6
  communication 342–6
  differential diagnosis 225
  key symptoms 343
  life trajectory 28–29
  medications associated 254
  see also suicide
diagnosis 211–14
  delays to diagnosis 56–7
  disclosure 298–9
  key concerns 212–13
  shock of diagnosis 19–20, 51–3, 68–71
  speed 211–12
diet, and ethnicity 184–5
disability
  communication 338–40
  and gender 170
  mobility 263
discharge planning 105
discrimination 197
distancing tactics 311–13
doctors 372–5
  general practice 208–11
  stress and burnout 369–75
  see also communication; healthcare
      professionals
dying 268–77
  communicating needs 270–1
  communication with doctors 276–7
  ethnicity and funerary practices 182–4
  existential/spiritual 275
  family support 272–3
  hospices 182
  life review 275–6
  life trajectory 271–2
  physical decline concerns 274–5
  practical concerns 272
  psychosocial issues 268–77
  relationship with family and friends 272–3

self-concept and control 274
see also bereavement care

Eastern perceptions of ethnicity 180–1
Edmonton Symptom Assessment Scale (ESAS) 403
emotional support 93–5
  continuity of care 217
  and integration 36–7
emotional withdrawal 100–2
emotions 4–6
  disclosure 37
  fear 5
  sadness 5–6
empathy 94
'empowerment' 150–1
encapsulation of disease 27, 72
end of treatment 80–2
  fear of recurrence 82–3
essentialism 179–80
  ethnicity 179–80
ethical issues
  communication 298–302
  consent, collaboration and choice 299–302, 391–2
  disclosure of diagnosis 298–9
ethnicity 178–94
  advocates 191–3
  communication 189–90
  cultural assumptions and communication 150–1, 316–18
  culture, definition 179
  death beliefs 268–9
  definitions 178–9
  diet 184–5
  essentialism 179–80
  interpreters 190–1
  race concept 178
  racism 185–9
  religion and death 182–4
  social class 180
  West vs East 180–1
European Organisation for Research on Treatment for Cancer (EORTC) 401–2
existential/spiritual beliefs 33–5, 77–80, 275
expectations
  about illness 49–51
  and illusions 13–14

family support 65–8, 91–145
  emotional support 93–5
  healthcare team role 102–3
  helpful and unhelpful reactions 96–8
  kinds of support needed 93–5
  living alone 110–11
  older 111–13
  partner relationships 113–34
  practical support 103–6
  roles, relationships and communication 100–2
  social context 95–6

telling children 106–10
turmoil of family 99–100
fatigue 242–5
  assessment 243–4
  fatigue management courses 245
  treatment 244–5
fear, intense 255–8
  claustrophobia 255
  needle phobia 255–6
  panic attacks 256
  treatment 256–8
Functional Assessment of Cancer Therapy–Fatigue (FACT-F) 403
Functional Assessment of Chronic Illness Therapy–(FACIT or FACT-G) 401

gender 158–72
  body image 169–72
  cancer information 164–5
  disability 170
  emotions 160–1
  gay and lesbian 124–6
  infertility 167–9
  older men 162–4
  pain 159–60
  partner relationships 120–4
  sexuality 165–7
  stigma 170–2
  support 161
  younger men 161–2
General Health Questionnaire (GHQ) 400
general practice 208–11
  bad news 331–2
  bereavement care 278
  burnout 371–2
  delays to diagnosis 56
  information 302–9
  information between professionals 353–4
  managing stress 372–3
  pain 247–53
graft-vs-host-disease (GVHD) 236–7
grief, bereavement care 277–82
guilt and self-blame 58–9, 392
Gunning's Fog Index 306

hair loss 234–5
  gender 171–2
head and neck cancers 220–2
  speech difficulties and communication 222
health beliefs, social class 153–5
healthcare professionals 61–3, 363–97
  burnout 367–8, 371–2, 380
  cancer professionals 368–79
  complementary/alternative medicine 389–93
  primary care 209–11
  providing safety, support and integration 35–7, 61–3
  requirements from patients 309–11

healthcare professionals (*Continued*)
  role in family support 102–3
  team functioning 384–5
  user involvement 386–7
  voluntary support 387–9
  see also communication; stress/management
hearing-impaired patients 340–1
homelessness 172–8
  defining 173
  health status 173–4
  psychosocial factors 175–6
  support 175, 176–7
hope 71–3
  ethnic significance 181
hormone therapy 231–5
  side-effects 129–30
hospices
  and ethnicity issues 182
  isolation 384
  palliative care 267–77
hospital admission 215–16
Hospital Anxiety and Depression Scale
    (HADS) 400
human context 1–45
human nature 3–16

illusory correlation 13
infertility issues 167–9
information 302–9
  asylum seekers and refugees 196–7
  audiotapes 307–8
  computer-based information 308
  gender 164–5
  Internet information 308
  procedural 216
  supply and demand 302–5
  support centres 308–9
  video 307
  written information 305–7
  Gunning's Fog Index 306
insight 79
insomnia 260–2
integration 21
interpreters 190–1

Japan, perceptions of illness 51

language
  communication 319–20
  and culture 6–9
  health beliefs and social class 153–5
learning disabilities, communication 338–40
Life Evaluation Questionnaire (LEQ) 402
life narrative and trajectory 14, 27–9, 271–2
living alone, family support 110–11
living with uncertainty 82–4
lung cancer 238–9

McGill Pain Questionnaire 403–4
Maslach Burnout Inventory 404
meaning of cancer 57–9
Memorial Symptom Assessment Scale (MSAS)
    402–3
menopause 131, 166–7
mental maps 8, 9–14
mind development 8–9
mobility 263
mortality, imminent spectre 52

narrative *see* life narrative and trajectory
nausea and vomiting 245–7
nurses, stress management 375–7

older people, family support 111–13

pain 247–53
  assessment 249–50
  and gender 159–60
  multidimensional 251
  patient education 249
  under-treating and under-reporting 248–9
pain management, psychological
    strategies 251–3
  cognitive-behavioural approaches 252–3
  distraction 251–2
  psychological support 251
  relaxation and imagery 252
palliative care 267–77
  resuscitation 335–6
  stress in 371
panic attacks 256
partner relationships 113–34
  advice 126–7
  communication 114–20
  communication difficulties 117–19
  dependency 116
  family support 113–34
  gay and lesbian couples 124–6
  gender differences 120–4
  healthcare implications 119–20
  mind reading 116
  partner distress 115
  positive changes 117
  'positive thinking' 97, 115
  security of relationship 116–17
  stress management 416–17
  support 117
  see also sexual problems
'patient-centred care' *xxiii*
personal context 47–89
  change 47–9
  coping with treatment 60–1
  delays to diagnosis 56–7
  existential beliefs 77–80
  practical concerns 63–5

shock of diagnosis 51–3, 68–71
  see also avoidance and denial
personal responsibility/control xx, 30–2, 58, 392
  societal expectations 149–50
physical decline, concerns 274–5
'positive thinking' 97, 115, 148–9
post-traumatic growth 18
post-traumatic stress disorder 16–17
practical concerns 63–5
  dying 272
  social class 156
  support by family 103–6
preparation
  for bad news 331–4
  for chemotherapy 232–4
  psycho-educational 20, 212
  for radiotherapy 227–8
  for surgery 216
primary care see general practice
problem-solving, communication 328
professional distance, and communication
  311–13
professionals see healthcare professionals
Profile of Mood States (POMS) 401
prostate cancer 240–2
  clinical context 240–2
  prostate specific antigen (PSA) test 240
psychiatric drugs 217
psychiatric illness, communication 341–2
psychological and social distress 400–1
psychosocial issues 47–89
  dying 268–77
psychosocial rehabilitation 264–5
purpose and hope 71–3

quality of life 38–40, 401–2
  components 38
questionnaires, self-report 399–405

race concept 178
racism 185–9
radiographers
  role 229–30
  stress management 377–9
radiotherapy 226–31
  information sources 228–9
  pelvic radiation 230–1
  preparation 227–8
  side-effects 229
reconstructive surgery 219–20
recurrence of cancer 82–3, 266–7
refugees, definition 194
rehabilitation 262–6
  activities of daily living 264
  mobility 263
  psychosocial rehabilitation 264–5
  teams 265–6
religious beliefs 34–5

differences within traditions 183
  ethnicity 182–4
  social context 182–4
  see also existential–spiritual beliefs
responsibility see personal responsibility/control
resuscitation, communication 335–6

safety 35
Schedule for the Evaluation of Quality of Life
  (SEIQOL) 402
self-report questionnaires 399–405
self-responsibility see personal
  responsibility/control
self-worth and personal control 30–2, 274
service providers, social class 156–7
sexual problems 127–34
  chemotherapy 129–30
  gay and lesbian couples 124–6
  help available 133–4
  hormone therapy 129–30
  menopause 131, 166–7
  physical damage 128–9
  psychological causes 131–3
  radiotherapy 129
  treatment side-effects 129–31
  see also gender; partner relationships
sexuality, gender issue 165–7
shock, stress management for patients 408–9
Short Form 36 (SF-36) 402
sleep 260–2
social class 152–8
  ethnicity 180
  language and health beliefs 153–5
  practicalities 156
  service providers and support 156–7
  unemployment 155
social context of patients 147–206
  see also asylum seekers/refugees; ethnicity;
    homeless
Social Problems Inventory (SPI) 401
social relationships, assumptions 29–30
social support
  defined 92–3
  see also family support
special needs, communication 338–42
speech difficulties 222
'spiritual abuse' 392
spiritual beliefs 33–5, 77–80, 275
staff–patient relationships 309–15
State-Trait Anxiety Inventory (STA) 401
stigma 170–2, 176
stress
  and burnout 367–8, 371–2, 380
  defined 365
  effects of stress 366–7
  reduction strategies 381–5
  sources 365–6
  symptoms 409
stress/management, carers 135–9

stress/management, healthcare professionals 365–86
  doctors 372–5
  nurses, radiographers 376–9
  secretaries, receptionists, porters 379
  team functioning 384–5
stress/management, patients 407–17
  advice for couples 416–17
  effect of long treatment 412
  information 408
  lifestyle changes 410–13
  living your life 415
  loss of control 409–10
  reactions of others 415–16
  shock 408–9
  taking control 413
  worrying 413–14
suicidal patients 213–14
  communication 344–5
  treatment 344
  vulnerability, communication issues 336–8
support 157
  family support 103–6
  gender 161
  homelessness 175, 176–7
  and integration 36–7
  see also emotional-; family support
surgery 214–26
  breast cancer 218–20
  CNS tumours 223–6
  continuity of care 217
  head and neck cancers 220–2
  hospital admission 215–16
  ostomies 223
  preparation 216
  psychiatric drugs 217

team functioning 384–5
testicular cancer
  prostheses 166
  younger men 161–2
top-down processing 13
treatment
  difficulties 242–62
  early phases 213–14
  excessive fear 213
  suicide risk 213–14

unemployment, and social class 155
United States
  perceptions of illness 51
  religious belief 34–5, 78
urostomies 223

visually impaired patients 340
voluntary self-help and support 387–9
vulnerability, communication issues 336–8

Western perceptions of ethnicity 180–1
WHO Quality of Life (WHOQOL) assessment
  instrument 402
worry 24, 258–60, 413–14
  about children 109–10
  decatastrophizing 259–60
  productive/unproductive 414–15
  see also stress/management, patients
writing 37
written information, Gunning's Fog
  Index 306